5th Edition

ONCOLOGY Nursing Review

Connie Henke Yarbro, MS, RN, FAAN
Adjunct Clinical Associate Professor, MU Sinclair School of Nursing
University of Missouri–Columbia
Columbia, Missouri
Editor, *Seminars in Oncology Nursing*
Destin, Florida

Debra Wujcik, PhD, RN, FAAN
Director, Cancer Clinical Trials at Meharry, Vanderbilt Ingram Cancer Center
Associate Professor, Vanderbilt University School of Nursing
Nashville, Tennessee

Barbara Holmes Gobel, MS, RN, AOCN
Patient Care Manager, Advanced Practice Nurse
Northwestern Memorial Hospital
Adjunct Faculty, Rush University College of Nursing
Rush University Medical Center
Chicago, Illinois

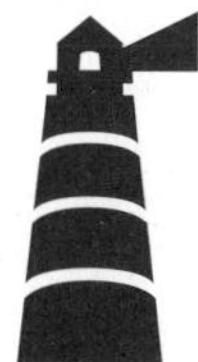

JONES & BARTLETT
LEARNING

World Headquarters
Jones & Bartlett Learning
5 Wall Street
Burlington, MA 01803
978-443-5000
info@jblearning.com
www.jblearning.com

Jones & Bartlett Learning books and products are available through most bookstores and online booksellers. To contact Jones & Bartlett Learning directly, call 800-832-0034, fax 978-443-8000, or visit our website, www.jblearning.com.

Substantial discounts on bulk quantities of Jones & Bartlett Learning publications are available to corporations, professional associations, and other qualified organizations. For details and specific discount information, contact the special sales department at Jones & Bartlett Learning via the above contact information or send an email to specialsales@jblearning.com.

Production Credits
Publisher: Kevin Sullivan
Acquisitions Editor: Amanda Harvey
Editorial Assistant: Rachel Shuster
Associate Production Editor: Cindie Bryan
Associate Marketing Manager: Katie Hennessy
V.P., Manufacturing and Inventory Control: Therese Connell
Composition: Arlene Apone
Cover Design: Kate Ternullo
Cover Image: © Ivan Mikhaylov/Dreamstime.com
Printing and Binding: Edwards Brothers Malloy
Cover Printing: Edwards Brothers Malloy

To order this product, use ISBN: 978-1-4496-3178-9

Library of Congress Cataloging-in-Publication Data
Yarbro, Connie Henke.
Oncology nursing review / Connie Henke Yarbro, Debra Wujcik, Barbara Holmes Gobel. — 5th ed.
p. ; cm.
ISBN-13: 978-1-4496-2882-6 (pbk.)
ISBN-10: 1-4496-2882-6 (pbk.)
1. Cancer—Nursing—Outlines, syllabi, etc. I. Wujcik, Debra. II. Gobel, Barbara Holmes. III. Title.
[DNLM: 1. Neoplasms—nursing—Examination Questions. 2. Neoplasms—nursing—Outlines. WY 18.2]
RC266.Y366 2012
616.99'40231—dc22

2011000678

6048

Printed in the United States of America
17 16 15 14 10 9 8 7 6 5 4

Contents

Introduction

Oncology Nursing Review is a comprehensive book and learning package to help you review content related to oncology nursing and cancer care. From the authors of the authoritative *Cancer Nursing: Principles and Practice, Seventh Edition,* this text contains nearly 1,000 multiple-choice questions with accompanying answers.

ORGANIZATION

The book is organized into 11 chapters corresponding to the areas tested on the Oncology Nursing Certification examination. The chapters include

1. Health Promotion and Disease Prevention
2. Screening, Early Detection, and Diagnosis
3. Scientific Basis for Practice
4. Cancer Treatment Modalities
5. Symptom Management
6. Psychosocial Dimensions of Care
7. Oncologic Emergencies
8. Sexuality
9. Survivorship
10. End-of-Life Care
11. Professional Performance

Each chapter represents an important content area in oncology nursing. The chapters are further divided into subsections to facilitate study of major topics within these areas.

HOW TO USE THE BOOK

There are two approaches to using *Oncology Nursing Review*. If you are just beginning to review the subject matter, you will probably want to spend more time with the book questions before you attempt the practice tests. If you are further along in your study, creating practice tests and the subsequent self-assessment can help you identify areas that need further review.

If you are just beginning to review, we recommend that you work through a small section at a time, reading the question and recording the answer. Then consult the correct answers and the explanations. Read the explanations both for the answers that you got correct and for those that you missed. A unique feature of this review book is the page number(s) provided at the end of the answer, which corresponds to additional information that you will find in *Cancer Nursing: Principles and Practice, Seventh Edition*. This feature will allow you to augment your knowledge base and clarify points that you may have overlooked or misunderstood. If you answer a question incorrectly, we encourage you to consult *Cancer Nursing: Principles and Practice, Seventh Edition*, for more information.

INSTRUCTIONS FOR USING THE ONLINE ACCESS CODE CARD

Enclosed within this review guide you will find a printed "access code card" containing an access code providing you access to the new online interactive testing program, JB TestPrep.

This program will help you prepare for the OCN® (Oncology Certified Nurse) certification exam. The online program includes the same multiple choice questions that are printed in this study guide. You can choose a "practice exam" that allows you to see feedback on your response immediately, or a "final exam," which hides your results until you have completed all the questions in the exam.

Your overall score on the questions you have answered is also compiled. Here are the instructions on how to access JB TestPrep, the online interactive testing program:

1. Find the printed access code card bound in to this book.
2. Go to http://www.jblearning.com/usecode/
3. Enter in your 10-digit access code, which you can find by scratching off the protective coating on the access code card.
4. Follow the instructions on each screen to set up your account profile and password. Please note: Only select a course coordinator if you have been instructed to do so by an institution or an instructor.
5. Contact Jones & Bartlett Learning technical support if you have any questions:
   Call: 1-800-832-0034
   Visit: www.jblearning.com and select "Tech Support"
   Email: info@jblearning.com

FINDING OUT ABOUT CERTIFICATION REQUIREMENTS

If you want to obtain the Oncology Nursing Certification, it is important for you to contact the certifying organization, the Oncology Nursing Certification Corporation (ONCC)®. The ONCC publishes a Test Bulletin, which we suggest you acquire. This bulletin provides important information about certification, including test dates, application deadlines, test center locations, eligibility criteria, and information about the test itself, as well as sample questions.

You can contact the ONCC through its website, www.oncc.org; via e-mail at oncc@ons.org; by telephone at (877) 769-ONCC or (412) 859-6104; by fax at (412) 859-6168; or by mail at 125 Enterprise Drive, Pittsburgh, PA 15275-1214.

CHAPTER 1

Health Promotion and Disease Prevention

EPIDEMIOLOGY

1.1 A research team has identified the relative risk and the frequency of a suspected etiologic factor in an entire defined population. A case-control study is conducted. What is the study *most likely* to be seeking to establish?

a. Causation
b. Attributable risk
c. A survival risk
d. Prevalence

1.2 Jana's research project is an epidemiologic study of workers in asbestos mines who are free of any cancer. Subjects are to be followed over a 10-year period, and the incidence rates of certain types of cancers are to be determined. This design is an example of a

a. Prospective study
b. Retrospective study
c. Historical prospective study
d. Historical retrospective study

1.3 Eric is a member of a research team that conducts an epidemiologic study. They determine that in a given year approximately 1 of every 12,000 American men has prostate cancer. This figure represents

a. An incidence rate
b. A mortality rate
c. A prevalence rate
d. A survival rate

1.4 The differences in incidence, mortality, and survival among various ethnic groups has been studied, and it has been determined that poverty, not race, accounts for a lower survival rate. Poverty lowers the survival rate among the many ethnic groups by

a. 5%–10%
b. 10%–15%
c. 15%–20%
d. 20%–25%

1.5 **The incidence of bladder cancer is *most common* in people with**

a. Exposure to aniline dyes and aromatic amines
b. Exposure to the parasite *Schistosoma haematobium*
c. Chronic irritation of the urothelial lining due to infections
d. A history of smoking

1.6 **Which of the following statements regarding the incidence of breast cancer is *true*?**

a. More than 50% of breast cancer occurs in women who are 61 years of age or older.
b. The incidence of breast cancer has increased, but the mortality rate—especially among African-Americans and Hispanics—has decreased.
c. A US woman's lifetime risk of developing breast cancer is approximately one out of every four women.
d. The incidence of breast cancer has increased to epidemic proportions among premenopausal women.

1.7 **The *highest* overall incidence of cancer occurs among**

a. Young adult Asian American/Pacific Islanders
b. Native Americans and Alaska Natives
c. African American men
d. Hispanics

1.8 **For cervical cancer, the average annual rate per 100,000 individuals has been *highest* among which females?**

a. Hispanic
b. Caucasian
c. Native American
d. African American

1.9 **There are two major histological types of esophageal cancer, squamous cell carcinoma (SCC) and adenocarcinoma (AC). In the United States the *highest* incidence of AC of the esophagus is found among**

a. Women aged 29–39 years
b. African American men
c. Caucasians
d. Men aged 30–40 years

1.10 **The *highest* incidence of cervical cancer occurs in women who are**

a. 30–39 years of age
b. 40–59 years of age
c. 60–69 years of age
d. 70 and older

1.11 **Which of the following has *not* been found to be associated with an increased incidence of primary brain tumors?**

a. Inhaled steroids
b. AIDS
c. Genetic disorders
d. Radiation to the head and neck area

1.12 Stomach cancer is the fourth most common cancer in the world. Which geographical locations have the *highest* incidence of stomach cancer?

a. Japan and Korea
b. East Asia
c. Central and South America
d. North America

1.13 The distribution of stomach cancer also varies according to age, sex, and ethnicity. Which of the following statements is *false*?

a. The incidence of stomach cancer rises progressively with age.
b. There is a significant male-to-female ratio in stomach cardia cancer predominance of 5:1, whereas in noncardia stomach cancer the ratio is about 2:1.
c. The prevalence of stomach cardia cancer is 2:1 in Caucasians compared with African Americans, but noncardia tumors are more prevalent (3:1) in African Americans.
d. Lower socioeconomic status and living in developing countries are associated with a decreased incidence of noncardia stomach cancer.

1.14 Which of the following statements regarding genetic predisposition to cancer is *not* correct?

a. The *BRCA1/BRCA2* gene mutations are associated with increased susceptibility to both breast and ovarian cancer.
b. The *BRCA1/BRCA2* gene mutations are more common among women with an eastern European background.
c. The *BRCA1/BRCA2* gene mutations are involved in approximately 30% of breast cancer cases.
d. Breast cancer susceptibility genes are present in less than 1% of the general population.

1.15 The overall smoking prevalence is decreasing in the United States. However, the decrease in smoking prevalence is not uniform among all groups. Which of the following statements regarding the prevalence patterns for smoking is *false*?

a. Overall smoking prevalence in women has declined more slowly than in men.
b. Approximately 3,600 adolescents, younger than age 18 begin using tobacco each day.
c. The lung cancer mortality rate for white men in the United States has peaked, but the mortality rates in women are just beginning to plateau.
d. With the predicted declines in mortality rates, the absolute number of lung cancer deaths will also decline.

1.16 Socioeconomic status (SES) is determined by income, education, occupation, or percentage below the poverty level. Racial and ethnic disparities in cancer mortality by SES has been examined by the National Cancer Institute. Which of the following statements is *false*?

a. African Americans have greater disparities in cancer mortality relative to Caucasians for each cancer site except for female lung cancer.
b. The lowest SES groups for both African Americans and Caucasians had increasing trends in cancer mortality at each cancer site except for female lung cancer.
c. The lowest SES groups of Asians and Pacific Islanders had increasing trends in female colorectal cancer and lung cancer.
d. Native Americans/Alaskan Natives had increasing trends of cancer mortality in prostate, lung, colorectal, breast, and cervical cancer.

1.17 Viruses contribute to the development of cancers. Which of the following cancer sites are associated with viruses?

a. Cervical cancer, T cell lymphoma, breast cancer
b. Burkitt's lymphoma, cervical cancer, lung cancer
c. Hepatocellular carcinoma, cervical cancer, Burkitt's lymphoma
d. Kaposi sarcoma, T cell lymphoma, pancreatic cancer

1.18 Which of the following has been associated with an increased incidence of breast cancer in women?

a. Living near high-energy electromagnetic wires
b. Radiation to chest
c. Exposure to chemicals used in hair dye
d. Cigarette smoking

1.19 Which of the following factors is *not* associated with a higher incidence of ovarian cancer?

a. Industrialized nations
b. Higher education and socioeconomic levels
c. The use of oral contraceptives
d. Family history of breast cancer

1.20 Prostate cancer is the most commonly diagnosed solid tumor in US males and the second leading cause of cancer-related deaths. Which of the following statements is *false*?

a. African American males have the highest incidence of prostate cancer.
b. African American males have the same mortality rates as Caucasian males.
c. Japanese men who emigrate to the United States have a similar incidence of prostate cancer as Caucasian men in the United States.
d. The majority of prostate cancers are diagnosed in men older than 65 years.

1.21 Mr. Allen has been exposed to asbestos in the workplace for most of his adult life (he is now 75). Mr. Eliot, 64, has smoked since he was 17. Ms. Frank, 43, calls herself "a dedicated suntanner." Ms. Smith has been a radiology technician for 20 years. Which patient is probably at *greatest risk* for cancer mortality?

a. Mr. Allen
b. Mr. Eliot
c. Ms. Frank
d. Ms. Smith

1.22 What percentage of lung cancer cases are caused by cigarette smoking?

a. 45%–50%
b. 50%–60%
c. 70%–80%
d. 85%–90%

1.23 Mr. Buck's cancer is reportedly related to his years of exposure to asbestos when he was working in construction. He is 67, worked in construction for 50 years, drinks beer occasionally, and smoked "off and on over the years." From this you can infer that Mr. Buck *most likely* has

a. Bladder cancer
b. Mesothelioma or lung cancer
c. Gastrointestinal cancer
d. Oral carcinoma

1.24 During his physical examination Mr. Pederson, a coal miner, asks you about his relative risk of developing lung cancer. The *best* response to his question would be to

a. Tell him that his risk is due to his exposure to coal.
b. Ask him about his family history of lung cancer, and explain that multiple factors cause the disease.
c. Get his demographic information, and ask him about his exposure to tobacco smoke.
d. Ask him about his diet and his smoking history.

1.25 Mr. Frank's cancer has been associated with occupational exposure to a carcinogen. He works as a chemical dye manufacturer. Of the following choices, which type of cancer is he *most likely* to have based on this small clue?

a. Bladder cancer
b. Colorectal cancer
c. Testicular cancer
d. Esophageal cancer

1.26 The leading cause of liver cancer throughout the world is

a. Chronic hepatitis B virus
b. Chronic hepatitis C virus
c. Chronic cirrhosis
d. Chronic hepatitis A virus

PREVENTION

1.27 A research study focuses on smoking cessation among a specific target population. This group's research is focusing on ____________ prevention.

a. Primary
b. Secondary
c. Tertiary
d. Integrated

1.28 You educate Miss Smith about the prevention of cervical cancer and risk-reducing behaviors. Which of the following is *not* a primary preventive strategy?

a. Limit the number of lifetime sexual partners
b. Practice safe sexual behavior
c. Have a Pap test at appropriate intervals
d. Use barrier contraceptives to reduce exposure to sexually transmitted diseases.

1.29 Mr. Holden quits smoking. He is very anxious about his risk for lung cancer and asks, "How much will my risk be affected?" You explain that the rate of decline in his risk of developing lung cancer is determined by the cumulative smoking exposure before cessation, the age when smoking began, and the

a. Degree of inhalation
b. Amount of passive smoke previously exposed to
c. Brand of cigarettes smoked
d. Amount of time that has passed since quitting

1.30 **Mr. Jantzen's wife wants him to eat more fiber because his brother had colon cancer. Which of the following sources of fiber has been shown to provide the *most* protection against colon cancer?**

a. Cereals
b. Vegetables
c. Eggs
d. Bread

1.31 **Which of the following lifestyle factors is the *most important risk* factor of oral cancer?**

a. Poor oral hygiene
b. Habitual use of alcohol and tobacco
c. Vitamin A deficiency
d. Human papillomavirus

1.32 **After her father's death from colon cancer, Ellen takes the initiative in preventing colon cancer for herself by eating less fat and more fruits and vegetables and by taking up running. She is engaged in**

a. Illness behavior
b. Sick role behavior
c. Health protective behavior
d. Information-seeking behavior

1.33 **Which of the following statements about primary prevention of skin cancers is *false*?**

a. Ultraviolet radiation is strongest during the middle part of the day.
b. For most people, sunscreen is not required on overcast days.
c. Certain medications (e.g., oral contraceptives) can make individuals photosensitive.
d. Surfaces such as sand and water can reflect more than one-half of the ultraviolet radiation onto the skin.

1.34 **Which of the following statements regarding involuntary inhalation of tobacco smoke is *not* accurate?**

a. There is an increased risk of lung cancer and heart disease among individuals who have never smoked but are living with a spouse who smokes cigarettes.
b. There is no evidence to support the idea that involuntary inhalation of tobacco smoke increases the risk of lung cancer in nonsmokers.
c. Individuals who had high levels of exposure to cigarette smoke during childhood and adolescence have a higher risk for developing lung cancer.
d. Long-term exposure to environmental tobacco smoke increases the risk of lung cancer in women who have never smoked.

1.35 **According to research, which of the following statements concerning breast health of African American women of lower socioeconomic status compared to age-adjusted Caucasian women is *not* accurate?**

a. When offered free mammograms, African American women obtained significantly fewer mammography screenings.
b. Premature deaths from breast cancer is higher in African American women (33.5% vs. 24.4% per 100,000).
c. African American women experience lower relative 5-year survival rates
d. African American women have biologically more aggressive breast cancer than Caucasian women.

1.36 Which of the following scenarios represents secondary prevention of cancer?

a. A woman at high risk for breast cancer decides to have prophylactic bilateral mastectomies.
b. A rural healthcare nurse establishes a clinic for cervical cancer education and Pap tests.
c. The Great American Smokeout is promoted to a group of individuals who want to stop smoking.
d. Celecoxib is prescribed for a patient with familial adenomatous polyposis for the reduction of colorectal adenomas.

1.37 Physical activity is one of the few known modifiable lifestyle factors, and increased exercise plays a key role in primary prevention against which of the following cancers?

a. Prostate, colon, breast
b. Colon, breast, ovarian
c. Prostate, kidney, colon
d. Pancreatic, endometrial, ovarian

1.38 Moderate to heavy alcohol intake has been linked to which of the following cancers?

a. Pancreas, stomach, proximal colon
b. Oral cavity, liver, stomach
c. Stomach, pancreas, esophagus
d. Oral cavity, larynx, bladder

1.39 Ms. Jones recently read a report from the World Cancer Research Fund and the American Institute for Cancer Research (WCRF/AICR) that made recommendations to decrease cancer risk. She has decided to modify her lifestyle and follow their recommendations. Which of the following is *not* a recommendation by the WCRF/AICR?

a. Do not use supplements to protect against cancer.
b. Increase the consumption of energy-dense foods.
c. Eat a healthy diet and be physically active for at least 30 minutes/day.
d. Avoid sugary drinks and limit alcohol to 1 drink/day.

1.40 The *most important* factors that appear to have a protective effect against the development of endometrial cancer are

a. Pregnancy, physical activity, weight management
b. Physical activity, nulliparous, weight management
c. Oral contraceptives, cigarette smoking, pregnancy
d. Nulliparous, oral contraceptives, weight management

1.41 Which of the following is *not* the most effective approach to reduce smoking in teenagers?

a. Smoking cessation interventions using nicotine patches and gum
b. Smoking cessation programs using multiple recruitment strategies
c. Smoking cessation programs offered in structured settings (e.g., schools, sports clubs)
d. Smoking cessation programs that provide psychosocial support and life management skills

1.42 Ms. Ellis tells you that her adult daughter is pressuring her to give up suntanning. "I've had a good tan for over 20 years," she says. "I like it. Is my daughter being a little hysterical?" You explain that long-term exposure to the sun has been associated with skin cancer and also with

a. Colorectal cancer
b. Breast cancer
c. Leukemia
d. Cancer of the lip

1.43 Local and national efforts to curb smoking in public places have gained support due to research findings concerning lung cancer in never-smoking lung cancer patients. Which of the following statements regarding lung cancer incidence or survival in never-smoking lung cancer patients is *false*?

a. The greater the exposure to secondhand smoke, the shorter the lung cancer patient's survival.
b. Secondhand smoke is associated with worse survival among never-smoking lung cancer patients.
c. Secondhand smoke increases risk of lung cancer for heavy smokers as well as light smokers.
d. Lifetime never-smokers with lung cancer likely represent a genetically susceptible subgroup.

1.44 Effective cancer control is influenced most by which of the following?

a. Government policy
b. Routine chest x-rays
c. Hygiene
d. A low-fat diet

1.45 The Breast Cancer Prevention Trial tested the ability of which of the following to prevent breast cancer in healthy women at high risk for the disease?

a. Sulindac
b. Retinoic acid
c. Tamoxifen
d. Beta-carotene

1.46 Nonsteroidal anti-inflammatory drugs have been purported to prevent which of the following?

a. Bladder cancer
b. Breast cancer
c. Colorectal cancer
d. Prostate cancer

ANSWER RATIONALES

Please note: All page numbers referenced in the Answer Rationales sections refer to the textbook *Cancer Nursing: Principles and Practice, Seventh Edition*, by Connie Henke Yarbro, Debra Wujcik, and Barbara Holmes Gobel (Jones & Bartlett Learning, © 2011).

Epidemiology

1.1 The answer is b.
Attributable risk is the difference in the incidence or death rates between the group exposed to some factor and unexposed groups. It estimates the number of disease cases that can be attributed to or explained by the exposure (e.g., the majority of lung cancer cases can be attributed to cigarette smoking). Page 40.

1.2 The answer is a.
In this prospective (cohort) study, subjects (miners) are being selected with varying degrees of exposure to the suspected factor (asbestos). They have not experienced the outcome thought to be associated with the factor (lung cancer or some other cancer). They are then being followed over time to see whether the outcome (e.g., a type of cancer) occurs. Page 42.

1.3 The answer is c.
The prevalence rate is the total number of cases—new and existing—in a given population during a specific time period, in this case 1 year. It is a function of both incidence and duration. In other words, the higher the survival rate (duration) for a type of cancer, the higher its prevalence rate will be. Page 39.

1.4 The answer is b.
In the late 1970s the question of the role of poverty in the differences in incidence, mortality, and survival of different ethnic groups was first raised. The disproportionate number of African Americans in the lower socioeconomic strata accounted for the increased incidence. However, a landmark report by Freeman concluded that poverty, not race, accounted for the 10%–15% lower survival rate from cancer in many ethnic groups. Page 87.

1.5 The answer is d.
All four factors play some role in the development of bladder cancer. However, a history of smoking is present in up to 50% of those diagnosed with bladder cancer. Page 1081.

1.6 The answer is a.
The incidence of breast cancer increases with age. More than 50% of breast cancer occurs in women who are 61 years of age or older. Page 1092.

1.7 The answer is c.
The highest overall cancer incidence rates occur among African American men followed by White, Hispanic, Asian American/Pacific Islander, and Native Americans and Alaska Natives. Page 57.

1.8 The answer is a.
For cervical cancer, the average annual rate per 100,000 individuals has been highest among Hispanic females. Page 57.

1.9 The answer is c.
Squamous cell carcinoma is more prevalent among Asians and African Americans, while AC is more prevalent among Caucasians. Page 1296.

1.10 The answer is b.
New cervical carcinomas remain highest in women aged 40–59. Page 55.

1.11 The answer is a.
Increased incidence of primary brain tumors is associated with all these choices except inhaled steroids. Page 1148–1149.

1.12 The answer is a.
Japan and Korea have the *highest* incidence of stomach cancer in the world. Noncardia stomach cancer has high incidence rates in East Asia and Central and South America. Low incidence rates are seen in South Asia, North America, North and South Africa, Australia, and New Zealand. Page 1684.

1.13 The answer is d.
There is an *increased* incidence of noncardia stomach cancer for those individuals of lower socioeconomic status and living in developing countries. The incidence of stomach cancer rises progressively with age, with the peak incidence occurring between 50 and 70 years. Stomach cancer is more predominant in males. The prevalence of stomach cardia cancer is higher in Caucasians as compared to African Americans, but noncardia tumors are more prevalent in African Americans. Page 1684.

1.14 The answer is c.
The genes account for only a small proportion (approximately 5%–10%) of all breast cancers. The *BRCA1* and *BRCA2* gene mutations are associated with increased susceptibility to breast and ovarian cancer, and are more common among people of eastern European (Ashkenazi Jewish) background occurring in 1 in 40 women of this descent. These breast cancer susceptibility genes are present in less than 1% of the general population. Page 148, 1094.

1.15 The answer is d.
Even with the predicted declines in mortality rates, the absolute number of lung cancer deaths will continue to rise because of the increasing size of the population. Page 98.

1.16 The answer is c.
The lowest SES groups of Asians/Pacific Islanders had *declining* trends in female colorectal and lung cancer. All the other statements are true. Page 56.

1.17 The answer is c.
Viruses contribute to approximately 15%–20% of cancers worldwide. Hepatocellular cancer is associated with hepatitis B virus, cervical cancer with human papillomavirus (types 16 and 18), and Burkitt's lymphoma with the Epstein-Barr virus. Page 50.

1.18 The answer is b.
A risk of breast cancer has been associated with exposure of the breast to ionizing radiation therapy for a broad spectrum of health problems, including chronic mastitis, and thymus disorders, especially if the exposure occurred before the age of 40. Mantle radiation for Hodgkin's disease is associated with an increased risk relative to age during treatment. Page 1096.

1.19 The answer is c.
The use of oral contraceptives provides long-term protection against ovarian cancer. With the exception of Japan, industrialized nations have the highest incidence of ovarian cancer. Women with higher educational and socioeconomic levels tend to delay childbearing, have

fewer children, and have a higher incidence of ovarian cancer. A family history of breast cancer or ovarian cancer are risk factors. Page 1548.

1.20 **The answer is b.**
The mortality rate of African American males is twice that for Caucasian males. The other statements are true. Page 1610.

1.21 **The answer is b.**
Mr. Eliot is at greatest risk. Cigarette smoking is the largest single preventable cause of premature death and disability and the major single cause of cancer mortality. Individuals such as Ms. Smith who is exposed to ionizing radiation or Mr. Allen who is exposed to high levels of asbestos and other respiratory carcinogens in the workplace also have an increased risk, but it is not the single major cause of cancer mortality. Cancers of the skin—most often caused by excessive sun exposure—are the most common cancers in humans, but they too are not the major single cause of cancer mortality. Page 51, 98.

1.22 **The answer is d.**
It is estimated that 85%–90% of lung cancer cases are caused by cigarette smoking. Page 1426.

1.23 **The answer is b.**
Asbestos, a carcinogenic fiber, is most commonly associated with mesothelioma. However, asbestos is also a major risk factor for lung cancer because of its synergism with tobacco smoke. Data do not support an association between gastrointestinal cancer and asbestos. Page 1427.

1.24 **The answer is c.**
It is misleading to suggest that coal poses the most obvious risk. By asking Mr. Pederson for demographic information, the nurse would be able to assess his exposure to air pollution and possibly his exposure to radon (certain areas have been identified as higher in radon activity than others). Because tobacco has an interactive and synergistic effect on the development of lung cancer when combined with other carcinogens, this would also be a good factor to explore. Genetics and diet have a less significant effect on the development of lung cancer. Page 1426–1428.

1.25 **The answer is a.**
One of the strongest risk factors for bladder cancer involves occupational exposure to naphthylamine, benzidine, and aniline dyes. Smoking is also an important exogenous risk factor. Page 1081.

1.26 **The answer is a.**
Chronic hepatitis B virus infection is the leading cause of hepatocellular carcinoma throughout the world. Page 1401.

Prevention

1.27 **The answer is b.**
Primary prevention is the avoidance of exposure to carcinogens; secondary prevention is the prevention of promotion by smoking cessation, changes in diet, and administration of chemopreventive agents presumed to act on promotion. Tertiary prevention consists of arresting, removing, or reversing a premalignant lesion to prevent recurrence or progression to cancer. Page 116.

1.28 **The answer is c.**
Obtaining a Pap test at appropriate intervals is secondary prevention and a screening method. The other measures are primary strategies, which include measures to avoid carcinogen exposure and improve health practices. Page 116, 1190.

1.29 The answer is a.
There is a gradual decrease in the former smoker's risk of dying from lung cancer; eventually the risk is almost equivalent to that of a nonsmoker. The rate of decline of risk after cessation of smoking is determined by the cumulative smoking exposure before cessation, the age when smoking began, and the degree of inhalation. Filtered cigarettes allowed smokers to inhale more deeply. Page 1426.

1.30 The answer is b.
Some studies of differing epidemiologic designs support the hypothesis that high fiber intake is protective against colon cancer. However, other studies report no benefit from dietary fiber. In studies in which the source of fiber has been examined, fiber from vegetables appears protective against colon cancer, whereas the data for cereal fibers are less supportive of a protective effect. Page 47, 97.

1.31 The answer is b.
The synergistic use of both alcohol and tobacco has long been implicated in the etiology of oral cavity malignancies. Approximately 75% of patients with oral cancer drink alcohol, and 90% of patients have a history of tobacco use. Poor oral hygiene and deficiencies in vitamin A have also been connected to the development of oral cavity tumors. Human papillomavirus has been implicated as a causative agent in a subset of oral squamous cancers. Page 1340.

1.32 The answer is c.
Health-protective lifestyle behaviors (primary prevention) consists of actions taken by people to protect, promote, or maintain their health. Page 96.

1.33 The answer is b.
Sunscreen should always be applied on overcast days because 70%–80% of ultraviolet radiation can penetrate cloud cover. Page 1660.

1.34 The answer is b.
A meta-analysis found a 29% increased risk of lung cancer in women whose husbands were smokers. Inhalation of secondhand smoke poses an elevated risk of lung cancer for both smokers and never-smokers. Page 1427.

1.35 The answer is d.
Whether African American women have biologically more aggressive breast cancer than Caucasian women has not been determined by any large-scale clinical trial. African American women of lower socioeconomic status obtain fewer mammograms, experience premature deaths, and have a lower survival rate. Page 1134.

1.36 The answer is b.
Although education regarding cervical cancer is a primary prevention strategy, the use of Pap test screening is a secondary method of cancer prevention. A, C, and D are measures of primary cancer prevention. Page 96, 100, 116.

1.37 The answer is a.
Exercise plays a role in primary prevention for prostate, colon, and breast cancer. Emerging evidence suggests increased exercise may be protective against kidney and ovarian cancer. There are inconsistent findings on the association between pancreatic and endometrial cancer. Page 48.

1.38 The answer is d.

Moderate to heavy alcohol use has been linked to cancers of the oral cavity, larynx, bladder, esophagus, rectum, and distal colon. The association of alcohol consumption with cancers of the stomach, proximal colon, and pancreas are less well established. Page 48.

1.39 The answer is b.

Ms. Jones should limit, not increase, the consumption of energy-dense foods, which are processed foods with sugar and fat. High-dose supplements can affect the risk of different cancers. A healthy balanced diet is the best source of nourishment. Page 97.

1.40 The answer is c.

The two most important factors that appear to have a protective effect against the development of endometrial cancer are oral contraceptives and cigarette smoking because they reduce the estrogenic stimulation on the endometrium. However, risks of developing lung cancer far outweigh protection against endometrial cancer. Pregnancy and weight management also reduces the risk of endometrial cancer. Page 1283–1284.

1.41 The answer is a.

Approximately 3,600 adolescents begin using tobacco each day. Interventions utilizing the administration of nicotine patches or gum along with bupropion were not found to be as effective for adolescents as the other approaches. Page 98–99.

1.42 The answer is d.

Long-term exposure to the sun has been associated with cancer of the lip. Lip malignancies occur most frequently on the lower lip. Page 1340.

1.43 The answer is c.

Secondhand smoke poses an elevated risk of lung cancer for heavy smokers as compared to light smokers suggesting that heavier smokers could have already acquired more tobacco-related mutations. Secondhand smoke exposure is associated with worse survival in early-stage non-small cell lung cancer patients, especially for secondhand smoke exposure at the workplace. These individuals also had the shortest survival. Page 1427.

1.44 The answer is a.

National, state, and local governments have an impact on cancer control through legislation. Cancer control efforts are affected by the monies specifically appropriated to cancer control in the National Institutes of Health budget. The government can influence advancement in this area by setting national goals for cancer control, such as those in the *Healthy People 2010* document. Page 108.

1.45 The answer is c.

The Breast Cancer Prevention Trial tested tamoxifen as a chemopreventive agent in a randomized double-blind trial. Page 104–105.

1.46 The answer is c.

An example of how chemoprevention may potentially be applied to high-risk populations is the use of nonsteroidal anti-inflammatory drugs for the prevention of colorectal cancer. Page 1212.

CHAPTER 2

Screening, Early Detection, and Diagnosis

RISK FACTORS FOR CANCER

2.1 A primary risk factor for breast cancer is

a. Age in the 30- to 45-year group
b. Family history of breast cancer
c. Two or more heterosexual relationships
d. Lower socioeconomic status

2.2 Which of the following statements regarding the *BRCA2* gene mutation is *true*?

a. The *BRCA2* gene mutation is associated with postmenopausal breast cancer.
b. The *BRCA2* gene mutation is only associated with breast cancer.
c. The *BRCA2* gene mutation is genetically related to the *BRCA1* gene.
d. The *BRCA2* gene mutation is related to breast cancer in men.

2.3 Hepatocellular carcinoma is often associated with

a. A long history of smoking
b. Obesity
c. Cirrhosis
d. A bacterial infection

2.4 Individuals with esophageal cancer typically have a history of

a. Occupational exposure to radiation
b. Obesity
c. *Helicobacter pylori* infection
d. Heavy alcohol intake

2.5 Which of the following risk factors is *not* associated with the development of cervical carcinoma?

a. Nulliparous
b. Human papillomavirus
c. Women exposed to diethylstilbestrol (DES) in utero
d. Immunosuppression

2.6 **Although the exact etiology of multiple myeloma is not known, certain factors increase the risk. Which of the following is the most recognized and *most common* risk factor for multiple myeloma?**

a. Obesity
b. High doses of ionizing radiation
c. Positive family history of lymphatohematopoietic cancer
d. Monoclonal gammopathy of undetermined significance (MGUS)

2.7 **Which of the following risk factors is associated with an increased incidence of papillary thyroid cancer?**

a. Exposure to ionizing radiation
b. Diet low in iodine
c. History of goiter
d. Inherited gene mutation

2.8 **Gastric cancer is associated with numerous risk factors. Which of the following is the *strongest* risk factor for the development of stomach cancer?**

a. Tobacco use
b. *Helicobacter pylori* infection
c. High intake of smoked or salted meats and fish
d. Alcohol consumption

2.9 **Which of the following are risk factors for vaginal carcinoma?**

a. Human papillomavirus, genital warts, and cervical carcinoma in situ
b. Human papillomavirus, HIV, and maternal use of diethylstilbestrol (DES)
c. Cervical carcinoma in situ, HIV, and human papillomavirus
d. HIV, genital warts, and number of sex partners

2.10 **Although the cause has not been established, certain occupations increase an individual's risk of developing a glioma or a meningioma, including**

a. Exposure to wood dust
b. Exposure to rubber
c. Exposure to chemicals in pesticides, herbicides, and fertilizers
d. Exposure to nickel

2.11 **Of the factors listed, the one that places a woman at *highest* risk for the development of ovarian cancer is**

a. Occupational exposure
b. Many sexual partners
c. Diethylstilbestrol (DES) use by the mother
d. A history of breast cancer

2.12 **Which of the following statements regarding ovarian cancer risk in families is *not* correct?**

a. Women who have two or more first-degree relatives with a history of ovarian cancer have a significantly increased risk for ovarian cancer.
b. Ovarian cancer is an autosomal dominant mode of inheritance with variable penetrance.
c. A woman who has one first-degree relative with ovarian cancer has an overall risk that is two to four times the average risk of having ovarian cancer.
d. Ovarian cancer tends to be common among lower-income groups, especially African American, Hispanic, and Native American women.

2.13 **Which of the following statements regarding breast cancer risk is *not* accurate?**

a. Only 5%–10% of all breast cancers are due to tumor-suppressor genes *BRCA1* and *BRCA2*.

b. Female carriers of a *BRCA1* mutation are at much greater risk of developing breast and ovarian cancer.

c. A woman with a strong family history of breast cancer has a 10% chance that her cancer is caused by an inherited mutation in the *BRCA1/BRCA2* gene.

d. Most women (70%) who develop breast cancer have no known risk factors.

2.14 **High-risk factors for cutaneous melanoma (CM) include all of the following *except***

a. Skin pigmentation

b. A persistently changed or changing mole

c. The presence of a precursor lesion such as dysplastic nevi

d. Oral contraceptives

2.15 **Kidney cancer has been consistently linked to which of the following risk factors?**

a. Cigarette smoking

b. Caffeine ingestion

c. Heredity

d. Asbestos

SCREENING

2.16 **Alexis, 27, brings her mother Margie, 48, in for a clinical breast exam. Both women have avoided regular medical care because they fear the discovery of problems. During the course of the interview, you discover that neither is familiar with the rationale behind regular breast self-examinations (BSEs) or mammography. As part of your patient education plan, you tell them which of the following?**

a. Alexis should have a clinical breast exam every year but should perform BSE monthly; her mother should do both every 6 months.

b. Margie should begin getting mammograms annually. Her daughter should get one every 2 years.

c. Margie is the only one who should be getting clinical breast exams at this time; Alexis will, too, at 30 years of age.

d. Alexis should have a clinical breast exam every 3 years; Margie, every year.

2.17 **A patient arrives at a clinic for cancer risk assessment. The most significant risk factors for the patient are listed below. Based on this information, you determine that one risk factor is specific to the individual yet outside the individual's control. This patient's risk factor is**

a. Cigarette smoking

b. Exposure to asbestos

c. Air pollution

d. Familial polyposis

2.18 **Which of the following statements is *not* true regarding prostate-specific antigen (PSA)?**

a. PSA is elevated only in men who have prostate cancer.

b. When tumor destroys the natural tissue barrier, PSA enters the bloodstream.

c. PSA levels are used as a screening test for prostate cancer.

d. Procedures such as biopsies can cause false PSA levels.

2.19 In your community seminar, when you explain the proper technique for breast self-examination, you should *not* include which of the following instructions?

a. For the visual inspection note symmetry, size, and shape of the breasts.
b. Examine yourself in front of the mirror with your arms relaxed at your sides.
c. Examine yourself in front of the mirror with your hands pressed on your hips.
d. Examine yourself in front of the mirror with your arms folded behind your back.

2.20 A student nurse under your supervision is about to perform her first breast examination on a patient with known pathology. You know she is using proper technique when she tells you

a. "I should palpate the normal breast first."
b. "It is important to press firmly to detect subtle differences beneath the cutaneous layers."
c. "After the patient is supine, I will start at the armpit and palpate in increasingly small circles, slowly moving in toward the center and finishing at the nipple area."
d. "The patient can have the examination in an upright position if she is more comfortable."

2.21 The *most widely* used screening programs have been for the early detection of

a. Breast and cervical cancer
b. Breast and colon cancer
c. Colon and cervical cancer
d. Breast and prostate cancer

2.22 Nurses must communicate to patients about the accuracy of screening tests. All of the following are attributes of an effective screening test *except*

a. The *sensitivity* of a screening test is its ability to detect those individuals with cancer.
b. The *specificity* of a screening test is its ability to identify those individuals with cancer.
c. A *true-positive test* is a normal test for cancer in an individual who has cancer.
d. A *true-negative test* is a normal test in an individual who does not have cancer.

2.23 Which of the following tests is recommended by the American Cancer Society to screen for polyps and colorectal cancer in asymptomatic individuals ages 50 and above?

a. Flexible sigmoidoscopy every 2 years
b. Digital rectal examination
c. Colonoscopy every 10 years
d. Double-contrast barium enema every 10 years

2.24 The American Association for the Study of Liver Diseases recommends surveillance of patients at high risk for developing hepatocellular carcinoma (HCC). Which of the following groups of patients do *not* require surveillance?

a. Patients with autoimmune hepatitis
b. Africans over the age of 20
c. Hepatitis B (HBV) carriers who are Asian
d. Individuals with a family history of HCC

2.25 You are providing a community education program on cancer prevention when a participant asks what is cancer screening and is it important if you are healthy and have no problems. Your *most appropriate* response is

a. Screening for genetic abnormalities that put individuals at high-risk for developing cancer is a form of cancer screening.
b. Cancer must be measurable and detectable to be detected on a screening examination.
c. Cancer screening is aimed at individuals with no symptoms with the goal of finding disease when it is more easily treated.
d. Screening tests seek to decrease both the morbidity and mortality associated with cancer.

2.26 **The single *most important* factor in whether an individual has ever had a screening test is**
- a. Recommendation by a nurse
- b. Recommendation by a family member
- c. Recommendation by a friend who has cancer
- d. Recommendation by a physician

EARLY DETECTION

2.27 **One of the early signs of ovarian cancer is**
- a. Frequent urinary tract infections
- b. Thin bloody vaginal discharge
- c. Heavy and painful menstruation
- d. Bloating

2.28 **Physical recognition of cutaneous melanoma by practitioners and those at risk can be initiated by using the ABCDE rule. In this rule *C* stands for**
- a. Change in symmetry
- b. Crusting or bleeding
- c. Color irregularity
- d. Cause

2.29 **Which of the following statements about dysplastic nevi (DN) is *not* correct?**
- a. DN is nonfamilial.
- b. Most persons affected by DN have a large number of abnormal nevi.
- c. The total number of DNs is an indicator of risk for developing malignant melanoma.
- d. DNs may develop throughout life and show clinical features similar to normal moles.

2.30 **One way that basal cell carcinoma (BCC) is distinguished from squamous cell carcinoma (SCC) is by its**
- a. Common occurrence on the head and hands
- b. Lower incidence
- c. Slower growth rate
- d. Less well-demarcated margins

2.31 **Which of the following is the *most likely* presenting symptom in a patient with Hodgkin's lymphoma?**
- a. Edema in the upper part of the body
- b. Enlarged cervical lymph nodes
- c. A palpable mass in the axillary or inguinal lymph nodes
- d. An upper respiratory infection

2.32 **Ms. Allison notices a "funny discoloration" on her arm and comes in for an examination. She tells you that her brother died at age 38 from a common skin cancer. Ms. Allison's brother *most likely* had and you should be suspicious for**
- a. Squamous cell carcinoma
- b. Basal cell carcinoma
- c. Melanoma
- d. Leukoplakia

2.33 Mr. Eliot, 64 and a smoker for 17 years, has an undifferentiated neoplasm arising in the proximal right bronchus. Which symptom *most typically* reflects this?

a. Barrel chest
b. Bulges on the thorax
c. Breathlessness
d. Superior vena cava obstruction

2.34 Mrs. Johns is pregnant and discovers a mass in the upper-outer quadrant of her left breast. Following her physical exam the physician is *most likely* to order which of the following tests?

a. Ultrasound
b. Fine-needle aspiration
c. Mammogram (diagnostic)
d. PET scan

2.35 Mrs. Blase presents with a continuous sore throat, referred pain in her jaw, and increased difficulty chewing and swallowing. These symptoms are an indication of which type of cancer?

a. Cancer of the larynx
b. Esophageal cancer
c. Cancer of the oral cavity
d. Cancer of the salivary gland

2.36 The *most common* presenting symptom of testicular cancer is

a. A small hard mass in the scrotum
b. A dragging sensation
c. Swelling
d. Dull aching or pain in the scrotal area

2.37 Early detection of gastric cancer is *unlikely* because

a. The cancer metastasizes readily.
b. People tend to self-medicate themselves for gastrointestinal distress.
c. Risk factors for the disease have not yet been identified.
d. None of the diagnostic tests or procedures currently available accurately detect gastric cancer in its early stages.

RISK-REDUCTION GUIDELINES

2.38 Once the elements of a cancer risk assessment are collected (e.g., personal medical history, history of exposures to carcinogens, family history) the risk must be interpreted to the individual in understandable terms. This is often accomplished by using various risk terms. Which of the following terms is *not* accurate?

a. Absolute risk measures the occurrence of cancer (incidence or mortality) in the general population.
b. Relative risk compares the incidence or deaths among those with a particular risk factor compared to those without the risk factor.
c. Attributable risk is the amount of disease within the population that could be prevented by alteration of a risk factor.
d. Proportional risk factor implicates which disease an individual will eventually develop.

2.39 Chemoprevention focuses on individuals or subpopulations known to be at increased risk for developing a malignancy. All of the following statements about chemoprevention are true *except*

a. Chemoprevention refers to the use of natural or synthetic agents to interrupt the carcinogenic process.
b. Chemoprevention refers to compounds manufactured into pill, capsule, ointment, or liquid form.
c. Chemopreventive agents include food components ingested as part of a regular diet.
d. Chemopreventive agents are often derived from food compounds or supplements.

2.40 Most chemopreventive agents are administered through a clinical trial. Which of the following individuals most likely would *not* be considered for a chemoprevention trial?

a. An individual who has smoked for 20 years
b. A 40-year-old female with dense breasts
c. A 55-year-old black male with a PSA of 0.5 ng/mL
d. A 63-year-old woman who has a history of benign breast disease

2.41 Your patient, Mrs. Smith, who has ovarian cancer and a *BRCA1* gene mutation, asks you if her 35-year-old daughter should have risk-reduction surgery to prevent her from developing ovarian cancer. Your *best* advice to her is which of the following?

a. For your daughter to fully understand her risk she should go through a formal risk assessment and see a genetic health professional before she makes any decision.
b. She is at risk for ovarian cancer, and it would be worthwhile for her to consider a prophylactic oophorectomy.
c. Your daughter should be followed closely, and she may want to talk to her physician about oral contraceptives to suppress ovulation.
d. Since she is asymptomatic, she should have a yearly physical examination that includes a bimanual rectovaginal examination and discuss tubal ligation with her physician.

2.42 Which statement is the *best* reason to recommend risk-reduction bilateral mastectomy for a woman with high genetic risk of breast cancer?

a. Removal of the breasts before cancer detection lowers risk by 90%.
b. Removal of the breasts before cancer detection lowers risk by 95%.
c. Removal of the breasts will decrease the risk of ovarian cancer.
d. Removal of the breasts will decrease the risk of both ovarian and breast cancer.

2.43 The American Cancer Society recommends that all women who are sexually active or who are 21 years of age or older have a Pap smear performed

a. Every 3 years with new liquid-based Pap test
b. Every 2 years with a regular Pap test
c. Biannually
d. Annually with regular Pap test

2.44 Surveillance recommendations for carriers of hereditary nonpolyposis colon cancer-associated mutations (Lynch syndrome) include which of the following?

a. Colonoscopy beginning at age 40; repeat every 2 years
b. Transvaginal ultrasound and endometrial aspirate annually, starting at age 40
c. Colonoscopy beginning at ages 20–25; repeat every 1–2 years
d. Transvaginal ultrasound and endometrial aspirate every 2 years starting at age 30

2.45 The most important risk-reduction strategies for the prevention of colon cancer include all of the following *except*
a. Weight reduction to appropriate weight for height
b. Regular exercise
c. Eating 5 or more fruits and vegetables per day
d. Reducing intake of concentrated carbohydrates

2.46 The *most significant* reduction in prostate cancer risk is
a. Men who take nutritional supplements of selenium and vitamin E
b. Men who take finasteride
c. Men who have an annual digital rectal examination
d. Men who have a high dietary intake of antioxidants

2.47 The most important risk-reduction behaviors for the prevention of cervical cancer include all of the following *except*
a. Limit the number of lifetime sexual partners.
b. Maintain a lifetime monogamous relationship.
c. Take oral contraceptives.
d. Use barrier contraceptives.

DIAGNOSTIC TESTING

2.48 Ms. Edwards, a patient with cancer, is being assessed for abnormal bleeding. She is to receive a prothrombin time test. This test is a measure of
a. Coagulation deficiencies in the intrinsic pathways
b. The concentration of functional factors in plasma
c. Platelet plug formation
d. Diminished or absent coagulation factors

2.49 The individual who has recently had an ultrasound-guided percutaneous needle biopsy of the liver must be monitored closely for symptoms of
a. Spinal cord compression
b. Hematemesis
c. Hemorrhage
d. Headache

2.50 A patient with a brain tumor is suspected of having possible hemorrhage. The test *most likely* needed to determine this is
a. Noncontrast computed tomography (CT)
b. CT with contrast
c. Magnetic resonance imaging
d. Cerebral angiography

2.51 During the physical exam of a new patient you notice that he has small red eruptions on his upper and lower extremities. He appears pale and states that he is exhausted most of the time. A diagnostic test will be suspicious for which of the following?
a. Severe anemia and bleeding
b. Disseminated intravascular coagulopathy
c. Thrombocytopenia
d. Leukemia

2.52 **Tumor markers are most often used as adjuncts to diagnosis for several cancers or used to monitor disease progression and response to treatment. Of the following markers and associated malignancy, which is *not* true?**

a. Elevated CA-125 may increase the level of suspicion of ovarian cancer.
b. Elevated CA 27-29 may indicate recurrent breast cancer.
c. Elevated carcinoembryonic antigen may indicate poor prognosis of colon cancer.
d. Elevated alpha-fetoprotein (AFP) may indicate prostate cancer.

2.53 **Mr. Jones reports frequent episodes of hematuria. His doctor assesses him for possible bladder cancer. Of the following tests, which is the *most* definitive to diagnose bladder cancer?**

a. Urine cytology
b. Cystoscopy with biopsy
c. Intravenous pyelogram
d. CT scan

2.54 **Magnetic resonance imaging (MRI) is useful in detecting cancers but does have some limitations, which includes all of the following *except***

a. It exposes the patient to ionizing radiation.
b. Patients with tattooed eyeliner may experience irritation and edema around the eye.
c. Sedation may be required for claustrophobic patients.
d. Injury may occur in patients with any ferrous metal in the body.

2.55 **When providing instructions for patients undergoing positron emission tomography (PET) you will emphasize all of the following *except***

a. Patients must fast for at least 8 hours prior to the procedure.
b. Fasting glucose must be within a normal range.
c. Patients are to avoid chewing gum and exercise before the exam.
d. The radiotracer is given to the patient the night before the exam.

2.56 **Ms. Anderson presents to her physician with the complaints of recurrent infections and chest pain. Her physician orders numerous laboratory tests and does a bone marrow biopsy aspirate that shows more than 30% plasma cells. This is indicative of what disease?**

a. Chronic myelogenous leukemia
b. Acute myelogenous leukemia
c. Multiple myeloma
d. Metastatic lung cancer

2.57 **The presence of the following molecular markers help diagnose specific types of leukemia in all of the following *except***

a. BCR-ABL fusion gene in CML
b. PML-RARα oncogene in APL
c. Flt protein in AML and APL
d. IgV gene in ALL

2.58 **Of the tests that are available to help determine the presence of disseminated intravascular coagulation (DIC), which of the following tests are specific and sensitive for DIC?**

a. International normalized ratio
b. Fibrinogen level and platelet level
c. Plasminogen level and plasmin α-2-antiplasmin level
d. D-dimer assay and the fibrin degradation product (FDP) titer

2.59 A patient is found to have a large tumor mass associated with high levels of parathyroid hormone-related protein but normal levels of 1,25-dihydroxyvitamin D and normal intestinal absorption rates. Bone absorption is found to exceed bone formation. The *most likely* diagnosis is

a. Primary hyperparathyroidism
b. Multiple myeloma
c. Humoral hypercalcemia of malignancy (HHM)
d. Hodgkin's disease

ANSWER RATIONALES

Please note: All page numbers referenced in the Answer Rationales sections refer to the textbook *Cancer Nursing: Principles and Practice, Seventh Edition,* by Connie Henke Yarbro, Debra Wujcik, and Barbara Holmes Gobel (Jones & Bartlett Learning, © 2011).

Risk Factors for Cancer

2.1 The answer is b.
The primary risk factors for breast cancer are increasing age, family history of breast cancer, history of benign breast disease, late age at first live birth, nulliparity, early age at menarche, late age at menopause, higher socioeconomic status, being Jewish, estrogen replacement therapy, exposure of the female breast to ionizing radiation in infancy, mammographic parenchymal patterns that are dense, having complex fibroadenomas, and being single. Page 1093.

2.2 The answer is d.
BRCA2 gene mutation has been identified on the long arm of chromosome 13 (13q12-13). This mutation seems to be associated with male breast cancer and early-onset female breast cancer. It is not genetically related to *BRCA1*, and the *BRCA2* gene mutation has been associated with prostate cancer, pancreatic cancer, malignant melanoma, and carcinoma of the fallopian tube and peritoneum. Page 147.

2.3 The answer is c.
The majority of hepatocellular carcinomas (HCC) cases occur in people with chronic liver disease or cirrhosis. Other risk factors for HCC include environmental and chemical toxins, alcohol and smoking, hereditary factors, and hepatitis B and hepatitis C viruses. Page 1400–1401.

2.4 The answer is d.
The major risk factors for esophageal cancer are heavy alcohol intake and heavy tobacco use. Poor nutrition, obesity, vitamin deficiency, anemia, and poor oral hygiene may be contributing factors. *Helicobacter pylori* infection may provide protection against the development of esophageal cancer. Page 1296–1297.

2.5 The answer is a.
Cervical cancer is rare in women who are nulliparous or in lifetime monogamous relationships. Females exposed to diethylstilbestrol in utero have a higher incidence of clear cell adenocarcinoma of the cervix and vagina. Human papillomaviruses (HPV) are members of the family of DNA tumor viruses that can cause cellular hyperproliferation and a variety of warty infections. HPV 18 is the most common papillomavirus found in women with adenocarcinoma of the cervix, and HPV 16 is more commonly associated with squamous carcinoma. Immunosuppression and HIV infection are higher risk for cervical cancer. Page 1189–1191.

2.6 The answer is d.
The most recognized and common risk factor for multiple myeloma is monoclonal gammopathy of undetermined significance (MGUS). In addition to the other risk factors listed, male gender, increasing age and African American ethnicity are additional factors. Page 1515.

2.7 The answer is a.
Ionizing radiation is the only known environmental cause for papillary thyroid cancer. This is especially true in children exposed to high levels of radioactive fallout from nuclear accidents. Follicular thyroid cancer is more common in parts of the world in which people's diet is low in iodine. Anaplastic thyroid cancer is associated with a history of goiter, and about 1 out of 5 medullary thyroid cancers result from an inherited gene mutation. Page 1259–1261.

2.8 The answer is b.
Helicobacter pylori is the strongest risk factor for the development of stomach cancer. Approximately 59% of stomach cancer in developing countries and 63% in developed countries can be attributed to *H. pylori*. High intake of excessive salt such as smoked or salted meats and fish are associated with increased risk, and smoking continues to be considered a risk factor. Alcohol does not appear to contribute to the etiology of stomach cancer. Page 1685.

2.9 The answer is a.
Human papillomavirus (types 16 and 18), cervical cancer, and genital warts are risk factors for vaginal cancer. Maternal use of DES and numerous sexual partners are also associated with vaginal cancer. HIV has not been implicated in the development of vaginal cancer. Page 1730.

2.10 The answer is c.
Although many chemicals are carcinogenic in animals and produce brain tumors the substances that have been tested include chemicals in pesticides, herbicides, and fertilizers. Page 1149.

2.11 The answer is d.
Hormonal factors such as nulliparity, infertility, and estrogen therapy have been connected to the development of ovarian cancer. A family history of breast cancer or colon cancer doubles the risk of ovarian cancer. Page 1550.

2.12 The answer is d.
Ovarian cancer tends to be more common among white upper-income groups in highly industrialized countries. Jewish women experience a 40% higher incidence rate than do African American, Hispanic, and Native American women. Page 1547–1550.

2.13 The answer is c.
A woman with a strong family history of breast cancer is generally defined as having four or more genetically related women affected with the disease; women who have inherited a mutation on *BRCA1* and *BRCA2* have up to an 85% risk of developing breast cancer by age 70. Page 147, 1094.

2.14 The answer is d.
Multiple etiologic and risk factors are associated with skin cancers. High-risk factors for cutaneous melanoma (CM) include a persistent changed or changing mole and the presence of irregular pigmented precursor lesions, including dysplastic nevi, congenital nevi, and lentigo maligna. Other possible risk factors for CM include ultraviolet (UV) radiation, age, hormonal factors, immunosuppression, and a previous history of melanoma. There is no conclusive evidence regarding the use of oral contraceptives and the increased risk of CM. Page 1653–1656.

2.15 The answer is a.
Cigarette smoking has been linked persistently to kidney cancer by both cohort studies and epidemiologic. Obesity and hypertension are additional risk factors. The links to occupational exposures (lead, asbestos) and genetics are less frequent. Page 1635.

Screening

2.16 The answer is d.
Women in Alexis' age category (20–30 years of age) should have a clinical breast physical exam every 3 years, and women older than 40 years should have a breast physical examination every year. Breast self-exam (BSE) is an option for women starting in their 20s. Yearly mammograms are recommended starting at age 40. Page 126.

2.17 The answer is d.
Choice *a* is individual but under the person's control; choice *b* is typically a group risk factor shared by persons from the same occupation; choice *c* is typically a group risk factor shared by persons from the same geographic residence. Only choice *d*, an inherited condition, is both specific to the individual and, at the same time, outside the person's control. Page 117–119.

2.18 The answer is a.
Conditions other than prostate cancer can give rise to elevated PSA levels. Page 1612.

2.19 The answer is d.
During a proper breast self-examination, the woman should stand in front of the mirror, noting the size, shape, and symmetry of her breasts. She should examine herself with her arms relaxed at her side, with her hands pressed on her hips, and with her arms overhead, but not with her arms folded behind her. Page 1099–1100.

2.20 The answer is a.
The examiner should palpate the normal breast first. It is important to press very lightly (not firmly) and gently to detect subtle differences. When the patient is supine, the examiner starts at the areolar area and palpates in increasingly wider concentric circles. Finally, the patient is to be in a supine position. Page 1099–1100.

2.21 The answer is a.
The most widely used screening programs have been for the early detection of cancers of the cervix and breast. Prior to screening, cervical cancer was the leading cause of death among women. Page 107.

2.22 The answer is b.
The *specificity* of a test is its ability to identify those individuals who do not have cancer. Page 106, 124.

2.23 The answer is c.
Colonoscopy is recommended every 10 years; flexible sigmoidoscopy every 5 years; double contrast barium enema every 5 years. Page 126.

2.24 The answer is a.
Lack of data precludes an assessment of whether surveillance would be beneficial for patients with autoimmune hepatitis. Page 1400–1403.

2.25 The answer is c.
All the statements are true, but choice *c* is the most appropriate response in this situation. Page 116.

2.26 The answer is a.
There is a far greater chance that the individual will actually go on to have appropriate screening when a nurse recommends screening to an individual. Page 130–131.

Early Detection

2.27 The answer is d.
Ovarian cancer is typically asymptomatic in its early stages. As the disease progresses women may experience bloating, vague abdominal discomfort, leading to loss of appetite, flatulence, or urinary frequency. More often than not, these symptoms are no more than annoying and are not taken seriously by the patient and her physician. By the time a diagnosis of ovarian cancer is made, approximately 70% have advanced stage ovarian cancer. Page 1554.

2.28 The answer is c.
Physical recognition of cutaneous melanoma by practitioners and those at risk can be initiated by using the ABCDE rule. In this rule, A = asymmetry, B = border irregularity, C = color irregularity, D = diameter greater than 0.6 cm, and E = elevation or evolving. Page 1665.

2.29 The answer is a.
DN are familial or nonfamilial. People who have a family history of DN and/or malignant melanoma have a 100-fold increase of developing malignant melanoma over their lifetime. Page 1652–1654.

2.30 The answer is c.
BCC is the least aggressive type of skin cancer and has its origins in either the basal layer of the epidermis or in the surrounding dermal structures. It is most commonly found on the nose, eyelids, cheeks, neck, trunk, and extremities. It grows slowly by direct extension and has the capacity to cause major local destruction. Metastasis is rare and most often occurs in the regional lymph nodes. SCC, on the other hand, may arise in any epithelium. It is most commonly found on the head and hands. It is more aggressive than BCC, has a faster growth rate, less well-demarcated margins, and a greater metastatic potential. Metastatic disease is usually first noted in the regional lymph nodes. Page 1666–1667.

2.31 The answer is b.
Three-fourths of lymphoma patients present with enlargement of cervical or supraclavicular lymph nodes, but enlarged axillary or inguinal nodes may be the presenting symptoms. Such nodes are characteristically painless, firm, rubbery in consistency, freely movable, and of variable size. Weakness, fatigue, and general malaise may be a part of the presenting picture. Page 1462.

2.32 The answer is c.
There are three types of skin cancer: basal cell carcinoma, squamous cell carcinoma, and melanoma. However, melanoma is the most common skin cancer to result in death. Page 1651.

2.33 The answer is d.
Superior vena cava obstruction is a common complication of lung cancer; approximately 65% of these cases are caused by undifferentiated neoplasms arising in proximal right bronchi. Barrel chest is associated with pulmonary emphysema or normal aging. Bulges on the thorax are often a manifestation of a neoplasm on the ribs. Breathlessness is a more generalized indication of obstruction of the lungs. Page 996, 1434.

2.34 The answer is a.
Ultrasound is the imaging modality of choice in a young woman, a pregnant woman, or a lactating woman who has not discovered any lumps or other signs of cancer. Fine-needle aspiration is also appropriate. Page 1107.

2.35 The answer is c.
Persistent sore throat and difficulty chewing and swallowing, are indications of cancer of the oral cavity. Referred pain is an important sign that can indicate induration, ulceration, or pressure affecting adjacent nerves. As the lesion increases in size, the individual may experience difficulty chewing foods and swallowing. Page 1341–1343.

2.36 The answer is a.
The most common sign of testicular cancer is a painless, small hard mass in the scrotum. However, a dragging sensation, swelling, dull aching, or pain in the scrotal area also may be a presenting symptom. Page 1700.

2.37 The answer is b.
The earliest symptoms of gastric cancer, such as a sense of fullness or heaviness and moderate distention after meals, are usually vague. Home remedies and self-medications are often used successfully for a while until other symptoms appear. Because of the elusive nature of gastric disorders, this type of cancer is usually quite advanced by the time medical attention is sought. Page 1687.

Risk-Reduction Guidelines

2.38 The answer is d.
Proportional risk does not implicate which disease an individual will develop. Page 117.

2.39 The answer is c.
Food components ingested as part of a regular diet are not considered chemopreventive agents. Page 100.

2.40 The answer is b.
Chemoprevention trials target high-risk individuals with a personal or family history of the disease, known exposure to a carcinogen or history of a prior malignancy. Although the female has dense breasts and is at moderate risk for breast cancer, she should discuss with her doctor the benefits of adding MRI screening to her yearly mammogram. Page 104, 126.

2.41 The answer is a.
She should have a thorough cancer risk assessment and genetic counseling so she will have the necessary facts about her risk, the alternatives for dealing with her risk, and consideration of the options available to her. Women at high risk may elect to take medicine to suppress ovulation or consider prophylactic oophorectomy at the completion of childbearing. Page 145, 1552.

2.42 The answer is a.
For women at high risk of hereditary breast and cancer (HBOC), risk-reducing bilateral mastectomy (RRBM)—the removal of both breasts before a breast cancer is detected—lowers breast cancer risk by 90%. RRBM does not decrease the risk of ovarian cancer. Page 147–150.

2.43 The answer is d.
The American Cancer Society currently recommends that all women who are or have been sexually active for 3 years or who are 21 years of age or older should have annual Pap tests or every 2 years using the newer liquid-based Pap test. Page 126.

2.44 The answer is c.

Colonoscopy with removal of polyps is recommended beginning at ages 20–25, repeating every 1–2 years. Transvaginal ultrasound and/or endometrial biopsy and CA-125 are recommended annually, starting at ages 25–35. Page 151–154.

2.45 The answer is d.

Most important risk-reduction strategies are weight control, exercise, diet, and taking a baby aspirin or NSAID daily, if at risk and appropriate. Page 1212.

2.46 The answer is b.

Research has shown that men who took finasteride as part of the Prostate Cancer Prevention Trial (PCPT) had a lower incidence of prostate cancer. The selenium and vitamin E cancer prevention trial (SELECT) was stopped because there was a higher incidence of prostate cancer in men taking vitamin E and increased incidence of diabetes in men taking selenium. Page 105–106.

2.47 The answer is c.

Modifying sexual behavior, thereby limiting a woman's exposure to oncogenic human papillomavirus, will prevent cervical cancer. This includes barrier contraceptives and limiting sexual partners. Oral contraceptives are not a risk-reducing behavior for prevention of cervical cancer. Page 1190.

Diagnostic Testing

2.48 The answer is d.

This screening test is called prothrombin time. Choice *a* is the activated partial prothromboplastin test, choice *b* is the specific factor assays test, and choice *c* is the bleeding time test. Page 755, 758.

2.49 The answer is c.

Because most liver tumors are highly vascular, the person having an ultrasound-guided percutaneous needle biopsy of the liver must be monitored closely for intra-abdominal hemorrhage. In general, this procedure is rapid, safe, and commonly used; however, some clinicians strongly believe that needle biopsies should be avoided at all costs if there is any potential for curative resection, because of the potential for seeding and spreading the cancer during the procedure. Page 186, 1406.

2.50 The answer is a.

Noncontrast CT can be performed rapidly and is the technique of choice for evaluating acute hemorrhage. Contrast is then administered to delineate the margins and extent of blood–brain barrier disruption. Magnetic resonance imaging is the more definitive and preferred imaging study for the individual with a central nervous system tumor. Cerebral angiography may be used to confirm that the lesion in question is a vascular malformation or an aneurysm rather than a neoplasm. Page 175, 1159.

2.51 The answer is c.

Manifestations of thrombocytopenia are easy bruising; bleeding from gums, nose, or other orifices; and petechiae on the upper and lower extremities. Page 750.

2.52 The answer is d.

Alpha-fetoprotein (AFP) is elevated in 80% of hepatocellular cancer and 60% of nonseminomatous germ cell cancer, but not prostate cancer. Page 171.

2.53 The answer is b.

Cystoscopy with biopsy is the test of choice for a definitive diagnosis. CT scan is used for staging and follow-up. Sensitivity is low with urine cytology, and a pyelogram evaluates the entire genitourinary system. Page 174, 1083.

2.54 The answer is a.

An advantage of MRI is that it does not expose the patient to ionizing radiation like a CT scan does. Page 181–184.

2.55 The answer is d.

The radiotracer is injected, inhaled, or swallowed at the time of the test and will take 30–60 minutes for absorption. Vigorous exercise before the test, chewing gum, and talking can give a false-positive appearance. Page 177–178.

2.56 The answer is c.

Bone marrow plasmacytosis with 30% plasma cells and bone pain in back or chest are indications for multiple myeloma. Page 1517–1524.

2.57 The answer is d.

The immunoglobulin variable gene (IgV) is found in chronic lymphocytic leukemia (CLL), not ALL. Page 1371–1373.

2.58 The answer is d.

Of the tests that are available to help diagnose DIC, only the D-dimer assay and the FDP assay are sensitive and specific for DIC. Page 933–934.

2.59 The answer is c.

In humoral hypercalcemia of malignancy (HHM), patients secrete high levels of parathyroid hormone-related protein but have normal levels of 1,25-dihydroxyvitamin D and normal intestinal absorption rates. Osteoblastic and osteoclastic activities are "uncoupled" so that bone resorption exceeds bone formation. Hypercalcemia and hypercalciuria thus occur. Page 945, 950.

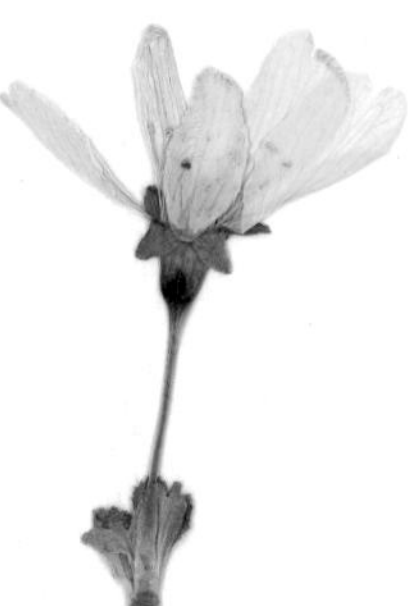

CHAPTER 3

Scientific Basis for Practice

CARCINOGENESIS

3.1 In clonal selection

a. Mutation in the genome of a cell may confer a survival advantage on that cell.
b. A cell becomes weaker with each mutation.
c. Oncogenes are destroyed.
d. Telomeres develop, which are completely duplicated during cell division.

3.2 A patient asks you to describe the "types of things that cause cancer." Because of her interest in "types" of causes, you might begin by explaining that cancer is ordinarily classified as being caused by a combination of factors that include

a. Biological, physical, or chemical
b. Viral, dietary, or familial
c. Genetic, dietary, and environmental
d. Genetic, familial, and environmental

3.3 One encouraging aspect of research into tumor-associated viruses is the discovery of

a. Their direct tumor causation
b. Their promise for prevention through development of vaccines from animal forms of the viruses
c. Their promise for prevention through inactivation
d. Similar viruses in animals that have been eliminated by vaccines made from attenuated viruses

3.4 Which of the following is *not* true of carcinogenesis and chemoprevention?

a. Chemoprevention is the most promising form of host modification, using nutrients or pharmacological agents to inhibit or reverse carcinogenesis.
b. Proto-oncogenes are most likely involved in initiation and promotion of cancer.
c. Chemoprevention has the potential for both secondary and tertiary prevention, but by definition it cannot be useful in primary prevention.
d. Agents that inhibit carcinogenesis generally are classified by the point in the process at which they are effective.

3.5 **Asbestos, the major carcinogenic fiber, is related to which of the following diseases?**
a. Gastrointestinal cancer
b. Bladder cancer
c. Mesothelioma
d. Renal cancer

3.6 **Fat and fiber are two dietary factors that appear to be correlated with the occurrence of colorectal cancer. It is thought that they operate by affecting, in opposite ways, the**
a. Conversion of ionized bile salts into insoluble compounds
b. Rate of uptake of calcium by the gastrointestinal tract
c. Breakdown of carcinogenic compounds by digestive enzymes
d. Exposure of the gastrointestinal tract to promoters of carcinogenesis

3.7 **Mrs. Harris has hepatocellular carcinoma and states she never drank alcohol in her life and cannot understand how she could have liver cancer. You explain that although the cause is not really known, hepatocellular carcinoma is associated with all of the following *except***
a. Chronic hepatitis B virus infection
b. Chronic hepatitis C virus infection
c. Human papillomavirus
d. Macronodular cirrhosis

3.8 **One of the most exciting developments in the mechanism of carcinogenesis is the discovery of a relationship between the mucosa-associated lymphoid tissue (MALT) lymphoma and which bacteria?**
a. *Helicobacter pylori*
b. *Escherichia coli*
c. *Staphylococcus aureus*
d. *Pseudomonas aeruginosa*

IMMUNOLOGY

3.9 **The macrophage**
a. Manufactures interleukin-3, -4, and -6 and alpha- and gamma-interferon to aid in its ultimate function of target cell wall damage
b. Is a glycoprotein product that initiates effector defense functions
c. Is a primary initiator to an inflammatory immune response
d. Is a short-lived white blood cell that responds to bacterial invasion

3.10 **Diseases such as Kaposi sarcoma that are common in AIDS are referred to as opportunistic. This is because they**
a. Affect any or all organs and tissues in the body
b. Normally occur in a benign state in most individuals
c. Occur in patients with preexisting immunodeficiency
d. Affect only HIV-infected individuals who have other diseases

3.11 **Which of the following *best* describes what cytokines do?**
a. They bind to surface receptors of target cells and act as regulators of cell growth or as mediators of defense functions.
b. They are capable of nonspecific tumor cell killing.
c. They are sedentary cells located in the spleen.
d. They facilitate the attachment of a natural killer cell and other cytotoxic cells.

3.12 Each of the following is an important function of the body's immune system *except*
a. Protecting the body against injury from foreign substances
b. Preserving the body's internal environment
c. Preventing the growth of aberrant cells that might develop into neoplasms
d. Providing support and nourishment to the body's genetic machinery

3.13 The body can generally respond to a nonself invader cell more quickly and powerfully the second time it encounters such a cell than it did the first time, even if months have passed between invasions. Which of the following cells is *most closely* related to this ability?
a. Polymorphonuclear granulocytes
b. Memory B lymphocytes
c. Natural killer cells
d. Mononuclear phagocytes

3.14 Antibody is the final product in the differentiation of
a. B lymphocytes
b. Helper T lymphocytes
c. Mononuclear phagocytes
d. Suppressor T lymphocytes

GENETICS

3.15 A patient asks, "What are tumor-suppressor genes?" As part of your answer, you explain that tumor-suppressor genes code for proteins that _________ growth-promoting factors.
a. Enhance
b. Fuel
c. Inactivate
d. Duplicate

3.16 The *p53* gene is
a. A potent oncogene
b. The most frequently mutated gene in human cancer
c. The "guardian of the oncogene"
d. Protected from DNA viruses

3.17 Mr. Henderson's cancer is said to have been induced by familial carcinogenesis. From this, you can assume that in his case certain genes
a. Caused cancer by functioning to excess
b. Caused cancer by their absence
c. Acted as growth promoters
d. Lost their ability to prevent malignant growth by their loss of homozygosity

3.18 The ras oncogenes
a. Have a screening usefulness of about 45%
b. Function early in the process of carcinogenesis as signal transducers
c. Function late in the process of carcinogenesis
d. Are not effective as targets for early detection

3.19 Genes that predispose for the development of cancer are generally transmitted in an autosomal dominant fashion. Which is *not* true?
a. Individuals who harbor a mutated gene have a 50% chance of passing the mutated gene on to their children.
b. Every affected person in a pedigree has an affected parent.
c. The pattern of transmission is usually vertical, meaning successive generations are affected.
d. Half of affected persons in a pedigree have an affected parent.

3.20 Which of the following statements *best* describes the significance of the *BRCA1* gene?

a. It is an inherited gene that identifies women who are ensured of having breast cancer during their premenopausal years.
b. It is an inherited gene mutation that identifies families at significant risk for breast cancer and ovarian cancer.
c. It is an inherited gene mutation that identifies women likely to have breast cancer in their postmenopausal years.
d. It is an inherited gene that is present in over 90% of women with breast cancer.

3.21 Approximately what percentage of people with cancer have an increased risk for cancer due to a hereditary predisposition?

a. 5%–10%
b. 20%–25%
c. < 5%
d. > 25%

3.22 Which of the following statements regarding our understanding of the genetic susceptibility in breast cancer and ovarian cancer is *not* correct?

a. The *BRCA1* gene mutation is associated with increased susceptibility to both breast and ovarian cancer.
b. The *BRCA2* gene mutation is associated only with an increased susceptibility to ovarian cancer.
c. One of the gene mutations is estimated to be present in approximately 15% of breast cancer cases.
d. The genes are associated with breast cancer diagnosed at an early age.

3.23 Which of the following statements regarding genetic susceptibility to colon cancer is *not* correct?

a. Individuals who have a first-degree relative with colorectal cancer have double the risk for developing colon cancer.
b. Adenomatous polyps are considered to be precursors of colorectal carcinoma.
c. An inheritable autosomal dominant trait is found in families with a high incidence of colon cancer.
d. Individuals who have familial adenomatous polyposis (FAP) syndrome are at a 50% risk for developing cancer of the colon.

3.24 Which of the following variables appears to be the *best* descriptive determinant of cancer risk?

a. The mortality rates for Japanese Americans with stomach cancer are significantly higher than for the white American population.
b. As more women smoke, more women are developing lung cancer.
c. A study of Johns Hopkins medical students found that 55 students who later developed cancer perceived themselves as less close to their parents than did their healthy counterparts.
d. Familial aggregates of cancer have been found to occur.

3.25 Which of the following cancer-causing mutations is transmitted to the next generation at birth?

a. Oncogene mutations
b. Germ cell mutations
c. Somatic mutations
d. Antioncogene mutations

3.26 A genetic variant on chromosome 8 was recently discovered and is thought to be useful in accomplishing which of the following?

a. Identify individuals at risk for lung cancer
b. Identify men at risk for prostate cancer
c. Determine susceptibility to chemotherapy
d. Determine susceptibility to hormonal therapy

3.27 During follow-up counseling for your 47-year-old patient with hereditary breast cancer, you mention that she should consider genetic counseling even though her cancer is *not* due to *BRCA1* or *BRCA2*. To clear up her confusion, you explain which of the following?

a. Women younger than age 50 with hereditary breast cancer have a significant risk of developing contralateral breast cancer in the next 20 years.
b. It is just precautionary to ensure she does not develop cancer that is due to *BRCA1* or *BRCA2*.
c. Counseling would help her decide whether or not she is a candidate for adjuvant chemotherapy.
d. Counseling would help her decide whether or not she is a candidate for prophylactic oopherectomy.

SPECIFIC CANCERS

3.28 Ms. Jantzen will soon begin induction therapy for acute myelogenous leukemia. As her oncology nurse you explain that the goal of therapy is to cause severe bone marrow hypoplasia, using

a. Busulfan and hydroxyurea
b. Cytosine arabinoside and daunorubicin
c. Vincristine, prednisone, L-asparaginase, and daunorubicin
d. Chlorambucil and cyclophosphamide

3.29 Which of the following statements about lymphomas is correct?

a. Non-Hodgkin's lymphoma (NHL) is distinguished from Hodgkin's disease (HD) primarily on the basis of its different clinical manifestations.
b. Lymphomas are predominantly a malignancy of the lymphocyte.
c. There seems to be a single malignancy for all stages in the developmental sequence from primitive to mature lymphocyte.
d. In general, B-lymphocyte malignancies are more aggressive than T-lymphocyte malignancies.

3.30 The *most common* form of skin cancer is

a. Basal cell carcinoma
b. Squamous cell carcinoma
c. Malignant melanoma
d. Superficial spreading melanoma

3.31 Ms. Smith, who has acute myelogenous leukemia (AML), is in complete remission after two courses of induction therapy. She is beginning postremission therapy, in which she will receive very high doses of the same drugs used for induction therapy. She asks, "What's the point of this? I'm so sick of treatment. I'm in remission, aren't I?" You explain that this type of postremission therapy is

a. Consolidation therapy to prevent leukemic recurrence related to minimal residual disease
b. Intensification therapy to treat substantial toxicities, including extended myelosuppression and cerebellar dysfunction
c. Maintenance therapy, which is used to help prevent a recurrence in some specific cases
d. Central nervous system prophylaxis to prevent leukemic recurrence related to minimal residual disease

3.32 You are the new oncology nurse in a large hospital. On your first day you meet Mr. Jackson. His physician neglects to tell you what type of leukemia Mr. Jackson has, but he says to you, "He still has the Philadelphia chromosome, so we don't exactly have a cure yet." From this you are able to discern that Mr. Jackson has

a. Acute lymphocytic leukemia
b. Acute myelogenous leukemia
c. Chronic lymphocytic leukemia
d. Chronic myelogenous leukemia

3.33 The glioblastoma multiforme

a. Is most common in individuals who are between 30 and 50 years of age
b. Has less necrosis than anaplastic astrocytoma
c. Is the most common adult primary brain tumor
d. Is the least aggressive brain tumor

3.34 Which of the following conditions is *commonly* associated with colorectal carcinoma?

a. Appendicitis or gallbladder disease
b. Hemorrhoids
c. Anal condylomata acuminata
d. Chronic ulcerative colitis

3.35 Multiple myeloma is a cancer of which of the following cell types?

a. T lymphocyte
b. Granulocytes
c. Monoclonal lymphocyte
d. Plasma cells

3.36 In determining the progression of bladder cancer, the *most important* feature is the

a. Degree of hematuria present
b. Presence of bladder neck obstruction
c. Depth of penetration into the bladder wall
d. Presence of pain in the suprapubic region

3.37 Mrs. Carry asks you to explain the relationship among tumor size, node involvement, and prognosis. Which of the following statements is *most accurate*?

a. Smaller tumors with positive node involvement have the best prognosis.
b. Larger tumors with negative node involvement have the best prognosis.
c. Smaller tumors with negative node involvement have the worst prognosis.
d. Larger tumors with positive node involvement have the worst prognosis.

3.38 The prognosis for a patient with Hodgkin's disease is *most closely* related to

a. Elevated lactic dehydrogenase level
b. Histologic type
c. Abdominal lymph node involvement
d. Stage at presentation

3.39 Which of the following patients with prostate cancer is *most likely* to be given "watchful waiting" as a treatment choice?

a. Frank, who is 37, recently married, and still hopes to have children
b. Harold, who is 76 and enjoying an active retirement with his wife
c. Byron, who is 56 and has poorly differentiated localized disease
d. Phil, who is 40 and has a high-grade tumor

3.40 Of the following factors related to cutaneous melanoma prognosis, the one *most closely* correlated with decreased survival rates in patients with stage I cutaneous melanoma (CM) is

a. Anatomic level of tumor invasion
b. Tumor location
c. Clark level
d. Tumor thickness

3.41 A poor prognosis for survival in a patient with AIDS-related Kaposi sarcoma includes all of the following *except*

a. History of fever, night sweats, and weight loss
b. CD4 cell count > $200/mm^3$
c. Karnofsky performance status of < 70%
d. History of opportunistic infection or thrush

3.42 Mr. James has been told by his physician that he has a high-grade seminoma of the testis. His doctor seemed encouraged by this, but your patient is concerned that a high-grade tumor might be associated with a poor prognosis. Which of the following statements might help to clarify the issue for Mr. James?

a. High-grade seminomas respond poorly to radiation and surgery but are curable with chemotherapy.
b. High-grade tumors have a brief tumor cell doubling time, which means they are more susceptible to the cell kill effects of chemotherapy.
c. High-grade seminomas tend to be more like the cell of origin and therefore metastasize infrequently.
d. A high-grade seminoma is curable by surgery, whereas chemotherapy is used for palliation only.

3.43 The *most favorable* prognostic factor for a patient with small cell lung cancer (SCLC) is

a. Female gender
b. Normal serum lactic dehydrogenase
c. Limited-stage disease
d. Good performance status

3.44 Alicia is diagnosed with breast cancer and is confused about prognostic indicators and how tests on her tumor will determine the type of treatment she should receive. Which of the following would be appropriate points to clarify for this patient regarding what the test results mean for her treatment and prognosis?

a. The hormone receptor analysis is used to determine the likelihood of metastases.
b. The hormone receptor analysis and assessment for the presence or absence of the human growth factor receptor (HER2) gene are used to decide what type of treatment is needed for metastatic disease.
c. The hormone receptor analysis and assessment for the presence or absence of the human growth factor receptor (HER2) gene are used to determine treatment strategies and prognosis for both local and advanced disease.
d. Women who have tumors that are positive for the hormone receptor do not require further treatment beyond surgery.

3.45 The prognosis for a patient with colorectal cancer is probably poorest if which of the following exists?

a. Venous and lymph node invasion
b. High blood pressure
c. Location of the tumor above the peritoneal reflection
d. Squamous cell involvement

3.46 Mr. Black presents to the physician's office with complaints of fatigue, loss of appetite, and generalized itching. Which of the following diagnoses is *least likely* to be associated with these presenting symptoms?

a. Prostate cancer
b. Multiple myeloma
c. Small cell lung cancer
d. Leukemia

3.47 During the initial history and physical the patient states that the most annoying symptom he has is constant itching and a burning sensation on the lower legs. These symptoms often intensify after consuming alcoholic beverages. Which of the following cancer diagnoses is *most often* associated with these symptoms?

a. Small cell lung cancer
b. Hodgkin's disease
c. Kaposi sarcoma
d. Acute myelogenous leukemia

3.48 Ten-year-old Liza is to be assessed for possible acute myelogenous leukemia (AML) and acute lymphocytic leukemia (ALL). This proves to be quite a challenge because the two have similar symptoms. Liza has ALL and begins treatment with a combination of vincristine, prednisone, and L-asparaginase. The physician begins to express strong hopes for a remission, but Liza's mother takes you aside and says, "My husband's aunt died of AML at age 40—and she was very robust and athletic! What hope does a mere 10-year-old have? Liza's not exactly robust to begin with, and she's so young." Which of the following answers is correct?

a. The physician is aware that the prognosis is grimmer when ALL affects children but that psychosocial support for Liza can make a world of difference in survival rate.
b. Age and athletic ability have been shown to make no difference in the demographics of remission and survival rates in ALL.
c. Complete remission is achieved in 93% of children with ALL, as opposed to 70%–75% in adults.
d. Remission rates in patients with ALL depend on etiology and stage of disease and are not reflected by age or activity levels.

3.49 Corticosteroids and nonsteroidal anti-inflammatory drugs (NSAIDs) are commonly used in the treatment of patients with brain tumors. Which of the following are considered anticipated side effects of this therapy?

a. Hypertension and hypoglycemia
b. Hypotension and hypoglycemia
c. Hyperglycemia and peptic ulceration
d. Hypertension and hyperglycemia

3.50 The *most common* sites of occurrence for chondrosarcoma are the

a. Femur, tibia, patella, and metatarsal
b. Vertebrae and shoulder girdle
c. Shoulder girdle, hip girdle, and trunk
d. Mandible and maxilla

3.51 The anemia associated with multiple myeloma is believed to be caused by

a. The effects of radiation
b. A normochromic iron deficiency
c. The replacement of erythrocyte precursors with plasma cells
d. Erythrocyte destruction by white blood cells

3.52 Ms. Drake has myelodysplastic syndrome (MDS). She reports being asymptomatic for a prolonged time and asks you why she still has to endure ongoing monitoring. The *best* explanation you can offer is that

a. T-cell abnormalities increase the risk of opportunistic infections.
b. Compliance with the prescribed treatment delays or prevents the onset of symptoms.
c. All patients with MDS eventually develop anemia, thrombocytopenia, and/or neutropenia.
d. All patients with MDS eventually develop acute leukemia.

3.53 A 60-year-old woman reports a flesh-colored, raised, firm papule on the top of her nose. It is examined and found to be a squamous cell carcinoma (SCC). How do SCCs differ from most basal cell carcinomas (BCCs)?

a. They tend to be less aggressive than BCCs, even though they have faster growth rates.
b. Their margins are well demarcated, as compared with those of the BCCs.
c. They tend to have greater metastatic potential.
d. They tend to bleed easily.

3.54 Which of the following statements about dysplastic nevi (DN) is *not* correct?

a. DN may be familial or nonfamilial.
b. Most persons affected by DN have about 25–75 abnormal nevi.
c. DN develop from precursor lesions of cutaneous melanoma.
d. A distinctive feature of DN is a "fried egg" appearance with a deeply pigmented papular area surrounded by an area of lighter pigmentation.

3.55 The phase of cutaneous melanoma tumor growth that is characterized by invasion into and through the dermis is the

a. Radial phase
b. Vertical growth phase
c. Nodular phase
d. Acral lentiginous phase

3.56 All of the following statements regarding primary central nervous system lymphoma (PCNSL) are correct *except*

a. PCNSL is often associated with acquired or congenital immunosuppression.
b. PCNSL is generally disseminated within the central nervous system at diagnosis.
c. Patients with PCNSL show no evidence of a systemic lymphoma.
d. Patients with PCNSL often present with enlarged cervical lymph nodes.

3.57 A common manifestation of central nervous system lymphoma is

a. A change in personality
b. Syndrome of inappropriate antidiuretic hormone (SIADH)
c. Frontal headache
d. Spinal cord compression

3.58 The occurrence of non-Hodgkin's lymphoma (NHL) in persons infected with HIV appears to be related to

a. The destruction of helper T cells as a result of infection by cytomegalovirus
b. Decreased levels of serum protein/albumin as a result of internal coalesced lesions
c. Opportunistic infections of the central nervous system related to toxoplasmosis
d. The proliferation of B lymphocytes as a result of Epstein-Barr virus (EBV) and HIV infection

3.59 Common symptoms of carcinoma of the nasal cavity and paranasal sinuses include all of the following *except*

a. Diplopia
b. Hyperesthesia of the cheek
c. Taste changes
d. Headache pain

3.60 The three classic signs of a pancreatic tumor located in the head of the pancreas are progressive jaundice, pain, and

a. Profound weight loss
b. Projectile vomiting
c. Confusion
d. Hyperkalemia

3.61 The cancer *most often* associated with malignant ascites is

a. Ovarian cancer
b. Pancreatic cancer
c. Breast cancer
d. Esophageal cancer

3.62 Approximately what percentage of women with ovarian carcinoma eventually develop ascites?

a. 90%
b. 80%
c. 60%
d. 30%

3.63 Which of the following clinical manifestations typically occur in patients with a cancer of the sigmoid colon?

a. Anemia and a vague, dull, persistent pain in the upper-right quadrant
b. Abdominal pain and melena
c. Sensations of incomplete evacuation and tenesmus
d. Bright red bleeding through the rectum

3.64 Assessments completed on a patient with cancer of the right colon usually find which of the following?

a. A palpable mass
b. Polyps in the rectum
c. Anemia
d. High levels of carcinoembryonic antigen

3.65 The *most common* clinical symptom associated with esophageal cancer is

a. Other gastrointestinal cancers
b. Superior vena cava syndrome
c. Dysphagia and weight loss
d. Xerostomia

3.66 Stan has a well-differentiated tumor on his true vocal folds that seems to be growing slowly. Stan's tumor is *most likely* to be which kind of tumor?

a. Subglottic
b. Supraglottic
c. Glottic
d. Periglottic

3.67 Most small cell lung cancer (SCLC) tumors

a. Are not associated with necrosis
b. Are responsible for 55% of all lung cancers
c. Are centrally located, developing around a main bronchus, and eventually compressing the bronchi externally
d. Have a longer doubling time than that of any other lung cancer type

3.68 The *best* method to establish a histopathological diagnosis of chemotherapy-induced pulmonary toxicity is

a. A sputum specimen
b. Fiber-optic bronchoscopy
c. Thoracotomy
d. Needle biopsy

3.69 Mrs. Mura has chronic myeloma and has recently begun to complain of blurred vision, headache, drowsiness, and occasional confusion. These symptoms may be caused by all of the following *except*?

a. A high concentration of proteins that increases serum viscosity
b. Vascular sludging
c. Hyperviscosity syndrome
d. Chronic effects of steroid use

3.70 In determining the survival rate for persons with cancer of the renal pelvis, the *most important* factor seems to be

a. The stage of the tumor
b. Whether or not radiotherapy was used in treatment
c. Whether or not the tumor is hormone sensitive
d. The age and physical condition of the patient at diagnosis

3.71 The phase of cutaneous melanoma tumor growth that is characterized by focal deep penetration of atypical melanocytes into the dermis and subcutaneous tissue is the
a. Radial phase
b. Vertical growth phase
c. Nodular phase
d. Acral lentiginous phase

3.72 A liver tumor may be suspected if laboratory tests reveal elevated levels of
a. Gastrin
b. Cholesterol
c. Alpha-fetoprotein
d. Amylase

3.73 Mr. Elliot presented to the outpatient ambulatory care center with a complaint of recent-onset generalized itching. This itching, or pruritus, could be related to all of the following *except*
a. Central nervous system malignancies
b. Hodgkin's disease
c. Occult metastases
d. Non-Hodgkin's lymphoma

CLASSIFICATION

3.74 Important features of tumor classification systems include all *except*
a. Allows for tumors to be classified by their biological behavior
b. Allows for tumors to be classified by their tissue of origin
c. Provides clinical and prognostic information
d. Provides information about who will benefit from chemotherapy

3.75 A benign tumor
a. Is well circumscribed or encapsulated and appears to be orderly
b. Is not made up of cells similar to those of its parent tissue
c. Invades the organs from which it originated and is made up of cells that are similar in size and shape
d. Has its own blood supply

3.76 Cervical intraepithelial neoplasia (CIN) stage III is characterized by neoplastic changes involving up to full thickness of the epithelium with no areas of stromal invasion or metastases. CIN III is also known as
a. Preclinical invasive carcinoma
b. Carcinoma in situ
c. Adenocarcinoma
d. Verrucous carcinoma

3.77 Two patients have been diagnosed with bronchogenic cancer. You know this does not mean that both patients will necessarily have a similar symptomatology or course of treatment because bronchogenic cancers are grouped into two broad categories:
a. Small cell lung cancer and non-small cell lung cancers
b. Adenocarcinoma and large cell carcinoma
c. Heterogeneous and histologic
d. Hyperplasia and carcinoma in situ

3.78 The *primary* objective of classification and staging of malignant tumors is to do which of the following?

a. To provide the information necessary for treatment planning
b. To identify individuals who might be candidates for research studies
c. To recommend the best cancer center for treatment
d. To determine what insurance will cover

3.79 In the TNM staging system

a. cTNM indicates that assessment has been obtained clinically.
b. cTNM indicates whether carcinogenesis has occurred.
c. rTNM indicates that remission of the cancer is occurring.
d. aTNM indicates that the cancer has been detected on first assessment.

3.80 Stage groupings involve

a. Combining the various classification elements of tumor site, regional lymph node involvement, and the presence or absence of metastasis
b. Two main staging periods: pretreatment and posttreatment
c. Two main staging periods: clinical diagnostic staging and pretreatment staging
d. Combining the various classification elements of tumor site, regional lymph node involvement, and the presence or absence of metastasis posttreatment

3.81 After a course of treatment Ms. Trent's treatment response is evaluated. This reevaluation or restaging

a. Makes possible the redesignation of a more appropriate stage to be referenced throughout the remaining course of the illness, replacing the stage ascribed at the time of diagnosis
b. Focuses attention on the disease parameters that were positive at diagnosis
c. Determines whether the patient is eligible to participate in a clinical trial
d. Helps the physician plan for maintenance therapy

3.82 Tumors of unknown origin occur in 2%–5% of patients diagnosed with cancer each year. All of the following factors are true *except*

a. Most tumors of unknown origin are adenocarcinomas
b. The prognosis is generally poor, from 9–12 months
c. Prognosis is predicted by serum albumin levels, and performance status
d. Patients with adenocarcinoma of unknown origin have a higher median survival than those with neuroendocrine carcinoma of unknown origin

3.83 The American Joint Committee on Cancer (AJCC) staging system for lung cancer uses

a. Eight stages, each of which is distinct relative to treatment and 5-year survival statistics
b. The TNM letters
c. The simple two-stage system
d. Two defining terms—limited-stage disease and extensive-stage disease—to stage lung cancers

3.84 Which of the following statements about the staging of Hodgkin's disease (HD) is correct?

a. Stage II malignancy is determined by a positive bone marrow biopsy.
b. Stage determination is important because it influences what treatment option will be used.
c. Stage II presentation is usually indicative of a more aggressive HD type.
d. HD rarely presents as stage II.

3.85 Accurate staging of a patient with Hodgkin's disease is *least likely* to include which of the following procedures?

a. A chest radiograph
b. An exploratory laparotomy
c. Blood chemistries, including liver and kidney function tests
d. A complete blood count

3.86 The *most important* objective of solid tumor staging is which of the following?

a. Provide information regarding risk factors.
b. Provide the necessary information for individual treatment planning.
c. Identify individuals at high risk for disease recurrence.
d. Determine performance status and eligibility for research protocols.

3.87 Treatment of advanced intermediate/high-grade non-Hodgkin's lymphoma is *most likely* to involve

a. Invasive surgery
b. High doses of topical radiation
c. Combination chemotherapy
d. Cyclophosphamide combined with radiation

3.88 A primary tumor is one that is histologically confirmed to arise from a specific site of tumorigenesis, whereas a secondary tumor refers to

a. A tumor that arises in another site after the primary tumor has been discovered
b. A tumor of unknown origin
c. A metastatic tumor resembling the primary tumor histologically
d. A second primary cancer that is histologically different from the primary tumor

3.89 Grading a malignant neoplasm is a method of classification based on histopathologic characteristics of the tissue. Which is *not* considered to be a primary objective of grading?

a. Establishing the aggressiveness or degree of malignancy of tumor cells
b. Providing prognostic information for all cancers
c. Quantifying information to assist in treatment planning
d. Determining the stage of disease of selected cancers

3.90 Mr. Fleischman's cancer is given an American Joint Committee on Cancer (AJCC) classification of G2. This means his cancer is

a. Undifferentiated
b. Well differentiated
c. Poorly differentiated
d. Moderately well differentiated

3.91 Histopathologic type refers to

a. A qualitative assignment given to a lesion at a site other than the original site that is of the same cell type as the original; this is used to determine metastatic tumors
b. A quantitative assessment of the extent to which the tumor resembles the tissue of origin
c. A qualitative assessment whereby a neoplasm is categorized in terms of the tissue or cell type from which it has originated
d. A qualitative assignment that indicates that a lesion at a site other than the original site is of a different cell type than the original tumor; this is used to indicate a second primary cancer

3.92 The least threatening prostate cancers are those that

a. Feature large tumor volume
b. Have a Gleason grade of 3–5
c. Originate in the peripheral zone
d. Are indolent

3.93 The primary application of flow cytometry analysis in solid tumors is to do all *except* which of the following?

a. Determine DNA content (ploidy)
b. Determine the percentage of cells synthesizing DNA (the S-phase fraction)
c. Determine tumor behavior to predict prognosis
d. Is more useful in solid tumors than blood tumors

COMMON METASTATIC SITES

3.94 The *most common* site of metastasis for tumors of the bone is the

a. Gastrointestinal tract
b. Central nervous system
c. Liver
d. Lungs

3.95 All of the following are common metastatic sites for breast cancer *except* the

a. Brain
b. Liver
c. Bone
d. Gastrointestinal tract

3.96 During the initial workup Mr. Smith, who has testicular cancer, complains of low back pain that has been present for about 1 month. This may indicate

a. Metastatic disease to the lumbar spine
b. That the cancer has spread to the prostate
c. That the cancer has spread into the retroperitoneal lymph nodes
d. That the pain is unrelated to testicular cancer and other causes should be explored

3.97 Patients with metastatic disease to the bone who have little benefit from nonsteroidal anti-inflammatory drugs (NSAIDs) and steroids are *most likely* to benefit from which of the following systemic therapies?

a. Mithramycin
b. Zoledronic acid
c. Saline hydration
d. Calcitonin

3.98 Tumor spreads from the primary site to bone by all of the following mechanisms *except*

a. Direct extension to adjacent bone
b. Arterial embolization
c. Direct venous spread
d. Surgical seeding

3.99 Treatment of metastases to the bone may include surgery, chemotherapy, and/or radiotherapy. When radiation therapy is used, the primary goal often is to

a. Eliminate the need for surgical intervention
b. Palliate pain
c. Decrease the likelihood of further metastases
d. Treat the primary cancer

3.100 **Beth has slowly progressing ascites due to liver failure associated with metastatic ovarian carcinoma. She is uncomfortable from the pressure and asks what can be done. All of the following supportive measures are appropriate to manage her discomfort *except***

a. Fluid and sodium restriction
b. Diuretic therapy
c. Paracentesis
d. Sclerosing chemotherapy

3.101 **Andrea has ovarian cancer and complains of abdominal fullness. In this patient the presence of shifting dullness during percussion would be indicative of which of the following?**

a. Abdominal carcinomatosis
b. Liver enlargement
c. Ascites
d. Recurrent cancer

3.102 **Malignant peritoneal effusion (ascites) is caused by all of the following *except***

a. Obstruction of diaphragmatic lymphatics
b. Tumor seeding of the peritoneum
c. Humoral factors that cause increased capillary leakage of proteins
d. Perforation of the bowel

3.103 **Your patient with ascites has had a paracentesis and removal of 1–2 liters repeatedly in the past and is calling now with a request for another tap because the fluid has come back and she is uncomfortable. Your response is based on knowledge of which of the following?**

a. Sclerosis with instillation of chemotherapy is the most effective treatment.
b. Draining the peritoneum only makes fluid accumulate faster.
c. Repeated paracentesis can lead to severe protein depletion.
d. Paracentesis can lead to tumor seeding.

3.104 **In the presence of a known bone tumor, symptoms such as hemoptysis, cough, fever, weight loss, and malaise may indicate**

a. Pulmonary metastases
b. Pernicious anemia
c. Radiotherapy toxicity
d. Infection

3.105 **Mr. Svensen has had treatment for a primary kidney tumor, which was completely eradicated. Now, however, the surgeon discovers a biopsy-proven metastatic lesion in the lung. The metastatic site seems to be solitary, and Mr. Svensen is very healthy otherwise. Given these limited clues, what method of treatment will be used for his metastatic lesion?**

a. Chemotherapy to provide systemic control of metastasis
b. Cytoreductive surgery to reduce the mass so combination therapy will be effective
c. Combination radiation and chemotherapy
d. Surgical resection

RESEARCH PROTOCOLS AND CLINICAL TRIALS

3.106 **A phase IV clinical trial is designed for all *except***

a. To address the use of drugs, usually in combination, with cure as the goal of therapy
b. To answer questions regarding various doses and schedules
c. To offer new information regarding risks and toxicities
d. Comparison to standard therapy

3.107 A major barrier for both patients and institutions to participation in national studies is which of the following?

a. Trials sponsored by drug companies pose a financial burden for most oncology programs.
b. The National Cancer Institute rarely is committed to research to prevent cancer because success is fairly limited; thus, it only consistently supports research to improve the quality of life for those who develop cancer.
c. Third-party payers often do not cover experimental treatment, which includes all research trials.
d. Standard-of-care treatments are covered by the research sponsor.

3.108 The reliability of a measure can be said to depend on all *except*

a. The homogeneity or consistency of the items on the measurement scale
b. The extent to which the measure produces the same score when applied at two different times or in two different ways
c. Test–retest or alternative form and interrater repeatability
d. Publication in a peer-reviewed journal

3.109 Content validity

a. Need not depend on the degree to which the scale superficially appears to measure the construct
b. Includes the degree to which the items represent the range of significant attributes
c. Includes statistical evidence to support inferences
d. Must include the physical and psychological domains but not the social one (which is covered under construct validity)

3.110 The Quality of Life Index (QLI)

a. Was originally a patient-rated scale of five areas of functioning (activity, daily living, health, support, and outlook)
b. Can distinguish cancer patients with terminal illness from those with recent disease or active treatment
c. Is probably the best example of a "cancer-specific" scale that in reality measures generic health concepts
d. Is used in NCI-sponsored clinical trials.

3.111 Evelyn uses the Functional Living Index—Cancer (FLIC) scale to assess a group of patients to determine the impact of cancer on daily issues. The degree to which this scale superficially appears to measure the construct in question is referred to as

a. Face validity
b. True content validity
c. Construct validity
d. Criterion validity

3.112 In a research study four basic elements are required to be included in the informed consent document. Which of the following is *not* one of these essential elements?

a. Compensation
b. Understanding
c. Comprehension
d. Competence

3.113 The *primary* ethical struggle in clinical research is which of the following?

a. Accurate documentation
b. Patient participation
c. Construct and execution of the study
d. Institutional review boards

ANSWER RATIONALES

Please note: All page numbers referenced in the Answer Rationales sections refer to the textbook *Cancer Nursing: Principles and Practice, Seventh Edition,* by Connie Henke Yarbro, Debra Wujcik, and Barbara Holmes Gobel (Jones & Bartlett Learning, © 2011).

Carcinogenesis

3.1 The answer is a.
In clonal selection, mutation in the genome of a cell may confer a survival advantage on that cell. The cell grows stronger, not weaker, with each mutation. The cancer cell is immortal because it seems to lack the "biologic clocks" like telomeres, which are not completely duplicated during cell division and thus grow progressively shorter until the chromosome can no longer replicate. In cancer the final common path of action is through oncogenes, the growth-promoting genes: Oncogenes must be mutated or relocated to be activated. Page 4.

3.2 The answer is c.
Carcinogenesis is influenced by genetic, dietary, and environmental factors, even though it is likely that human carcinogenesis involves a combination of factors. Page 96.

3.3 The answer is c.
Tumor-associated viruses probably are necessary but not sufficient for tumor causation. The discovery of cancer-causing viruses in humans shows some promise for cancer prevention in that similar viruses in animals have been eliminated by vaccines made from the attenuated (inactivated) viruses. Page 50.

3.4 The answer is c.
Chemoprevention is the most promising form of host modification, using nutrients or pharmacological agents to inhibit or reverse carcinogenesis. Proto-oncogenes are most likely involved in initiation and promotion of cancer. The theoretical disruption of carcinogenesis at several points provides the rationale for use of chemopreventive agents. Agents that inhibit carcinogenesis generally are classified by the point in the process at which they are effective. Chemoprevention has the potential for primary, secondary, and tertiary prevention. Page 100.

3.5 The answer is c.
Asbestos is related to about 2000 cases of mesothelioma annually in the United States. Asbestos causes more bronchogenic cancers than mesotheliomas because of its synergism with tobacco smoke. Lung cancer is rare in asbestos workers who do not smoke. There is a long latent period between exposure and the onset of mesothelioma. Data do not support an association between asbestos and gastrointestinal, bladder, or renal cancer. Page 49.

3.6 The answer is d.
It is believed that dietary factors affect the exposure of the gastrointestinal tract to promoters of carcinogenesis. Fats increase the production, and change the composition, of bile salts. These altered bile salts are converted into potential carcinogens. Fiber decreases the effects of fatty acids and may actually protect against the disease, even in the presence of a high-fat diet. Fiber may limit the time the colon is exposed to cancer promoters by speeding intestinal transit time. Page 46, 1208–1209.

3.7 The answer is c.
Hepatocellular carcinoma is associated with chronic hepatitis B and C, viral infection, macronodular cirrhosis, schistosomias and other parasitic infections, environmental carcinogens, and organic materials. Smoking has also been associated with the development of hepatocellular carcinoma. Page 1400.

3.8 The answer is a.
The relationship between *H. pylori* and MALT lymphoma has been determined, and after treatment with antibiotics to eradicate the bacteria the lymphoma was resolved. Page 1477.

Immunology

3.9 The answer is c.
The macrophage is a primary initiator to an inflammatory immune response. It originates in the bone marrow, circulates as a monocyte, and becomes a macrophage when it enters a tissue at a site of infection. The macrophage is also a secretory cell manufacturing key pyrogenic cytokines such as interleukin-1, tumor necrosis factor, and interleukin-6. Page 719.

3.10 The answer is c.
AIDS-related diseases such as Kaposi sarcoma, non-Hodgkin's lymphoma, and primary central nervous system lymphoma are referred to as opportunistic because they occur in patients with preexisting immunodeficiency. This immunodeficiency can be the result of HIV infection (which destroys the immune system), therapeutic immunosuppression (e.g., chemotherapeutic agents used in organ transplantation), or primary immunodeficiency (e.g., as the result of a genetic defect). These malignancies normally occur at a low incidence and in a more benign form. An AIDS-related opportunistic disease that is not a malignancy is *Pneumocystis carinii* pneumonia. Page 1041.

3.11 The answer is a.
Cytokines are glycoprotein products of immune cells. They bind to surface receptors of target cells and act as regulators of cell growth or as mediators of defense functions. Natural killer cells are capable of killing transformed cells. Lymphokine-activated killer cells are a special population of cytotoxic cells used in cancer therapy that comprise primarily natural killer cells, which are capable of nonspecific tumor cell killing. B lymphocytes are sedentary cells located in lymph nodes and spleen. Page 28–30.

3.12 The answer is d.
The classic function of the immune system is that cited in choice *a*, distinguishing self from nonself and destroying foreign substances. Homeostasis and surveillance are other important functions. Page 24.

3.13 The answer is b.
B memory cells (memory B lymphocytes), along with T memory cells (memory T lymphocytes), make up the recall component of the immune system. They have memory of antigens previously recognized by the body and deal with a particular antigen each time it is encountered. Page 30–31.

3.14 The answer is a.
B lymphocytes form plasma cells that produce specific immunoglobulins when stimulated by helper T lymphocytes and an encounter with a foreign antigen. Antibody is an antigen-specific immunoglobulin that is synthesized and secreted by a mature plasma cell, the final cell of B-lymphocyte differentiation. Each plasma cell produces only one type of antibody, and each antibody is specific for only one type of antigen. Page 30–31.

Genetics

3.15 The answer is c.
Suppressor proteins "turn off" cell growth. Because the genes coding for these proteins have an opposite function to that of oncogenes, they are called antioncogenes. Because they suppress malignant growth, they are also called tumor-suppressor genes. Page 12.

3.16 The answer is b.
The *p53* gene is one of the most important of the tumor-suppressor genes. Not only is it the most frequently mutated, but when it is not mutated another abnormal gene blocks the *p53* protein. The protein product of *p53* is the "guardian of the genome." DNA viruses produce proteins that inactivate the *p53* protein. Page 12, 591. (Associated with glioblastoma, page 1148; endocrine malignancies, page 1272; and esophageal cancer, page 1297.)

3.17 The answer is b.
Familial carcinogenesis is based in large part on a group of genes that, when mutated, cause cancer by their absence; that is, they seem to prevent cancer when they are functioning normally. These protective genes are the cancer-suppressor genes. The loss of the normal copy of a gene by the process of mitotic recombination is referred to as loss of heterogeneity or reduction to homozygosity because the cell becomes homozygous for the abnormal gene, thus losing its ability to prevent malignant growth. Page 12.

3.18 The answer is b.
The ras oncogenes appear to function early in the process of carcinogenesis and may be a good target for early detection. Page 11–12.

3.19 The answer is d.
Genes that predispose for cancer development are generally transmitted in an autosomal dominant fashion, meaning that individuals who harbor a mutated gene have a 50% chance of passing the mutated gene on to their children. Inheritance of the altered gene confers an increased risk for developing cancer. The pattern of transmission seen with cancer susceptibility genes is usually vertical, meaning successive generations are affected; depending on the disease, males and females are generally equally affected. Page 137–139.

3.20 The answer is b.
Inheritance of the *BRCA1* susceptibility gene is associated with a strong likelihood that the effect of the mutation will result in the disease for families with multiple breast and ovarian cancers (90%) as well as for those with breast cancers diagnosed before the age of 45 (70%). Page 145–148, 1097–1098.

3.21 The answer is b.
Most people believe cancer risk is increased simply because someone in the family has cancer, which is not true. For example, breast cancer is estimated to have a familial component in only about 10%–20% of cases. Page 137.

3.22 The answer is b.
The *BRCA2* gene is associated with an increased susceptibility to both breast and ovarian cancer. Page 145–148, 1097–1098.

3.23 The answer is d.
Individuals who have a first-degree relative with colorectal cancer have double the risk for developing adenomatous polyps, which are considered to be precursors of colorectal carcinoma. Persons who have a FAP have 100% risk of developing colorectal cancer. Page 1206–1208.

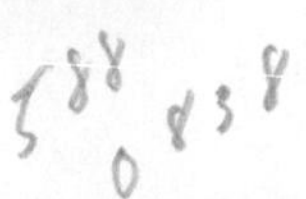

3.24 The answer is d.
Data regarding the genetic basis of cancer have been derived from a number of sources, including familial patterns, which have been studied in an attempt to elicit features of the transmission of neoplastic tendencies. Page 119–120.

3.25 The answer is b.
Germ cell mutations are transmitted to the next generation at birth and are responsible for hereditary (familial) cancer. Most human cancers result from a combination of acquired and inherited mutations with alterations of both oncogenes and antioncogenes. Page 137.

3.26 The answer is b.
The genetic variant on chromosome 8 may account for 8% of prostate cancers in men of European descent and 16% of prostate cancers in African American men. Tests for this genetic variant could help identify men who would benefit from earlier or more frequent prostate cancer screening. Page 1611.

3.27 The answer is d.
After 20 years the probability of developing contralateral breast cancer is approximately 27% among women with hereditary breast cancer compared to 5% among women with breast cancer in the general population. The risk of contralateral breast cancer is highest among women with hereditary breast cancer that is diagnosed before the age of 50. More than 40% of women in this group develop contralateral breast cancer during the 20 years after their initial breast cancer diagnosis. Adjuvant hormone therapy reduces the risk of contralateral breast cancer. Page 1124–1125.

Specific Cancers

3.28 The answer is b.
The cornerstone of induction therapy in acute myelogenous leukemia is the cell cycle-specific antimetabolite cytosine arabinoside, plus an anthracycline such as daunorubicin. Page 1381–1383.

3.29 The answer is b.
Lymphomas are preeminently a malignancy of the lymphocyte. However, there seems to be a separate malignancy for each sequential stage in the developmental sequence from primitive to mature lymphocyte. At each stage of development, the potential exists for the normal maturing lymphocyte to be transformed into a cancer cell. Once transformed, the new clone of malignant cells follows the behavioral pattern of the stage of the lymphocyte at which the transformation occurred. For example, if the function of the maturing cell at the time it is transformed is secretion of an antibody, the tumor cells continue to secrete that normal protein in abnormal quantities. HD and NHL are distinguished on the basis of the Reed-Sternberg giant cells in NHL. The information in choice *d* is reversed. Page 1459–1462.

3.30 The answer is a.
Basal cell carcinoma is the most common form of skin cancer in whites and outnumbers squamous cell carcinoma by a ratio of 3:1. Nonmelanoma skin cancers, including basal cell carcinoma, have a higher incidence but a lower metastatic potential and mortality rate than malignant melanoma. Malignant melanoma has a much lower incidence but a mortality rate that is triple that of the nonmelanoma cancers. Increased mortality is directly related to its high potential for metastasis. Page 1666–1667.

3.31 **The answer is a.**
The purpose of postremission therapies is to prevent leukemic recurrence related to minimal residual disease. The four types of postremission therapies are consolidation therapy, intensification therapy, maintenance therapy, and bone marrow transplant. Consolidation therapy consists of one or two courses of very high doses of the same drugs used for induction (up to 30 times the induction doses of cytosine arabinoside for AML). Intensification regimens use different drugs in the hope that they will not be cross-resistant. Maintenance therapies use lower doses for a prolonged period of time. Maintenance therapy is not currently recommended for the treatment of AML. Page 1383.

3.32 **The answer is d.**
Approximately 90% of patients with chronic myelogenous leukemia have the diagnostic marker Philadelphia chromosome Ph^1. Page 593.

3.33 **The answer is c.**
The glioblastoma multiforme is the most common adult primary brain tumor. It is most common in individuals who are 50 or older. It shares all the characteristics of anaplastic astrocytoma plus necrosis. Page 1148, 1161–1162.

3.34 **The answer is d.**
A number of predisposing conditions have been associated with an increased risk of colorectal cancer. These include chronic ulcerative colitis, Crohn's disease, familial polyposis, and a strong family history of predisposition to colon cancer and familial adenomatous polyposis. Page 1221–1222.

3.35 **The answer is d.**
In multiple myeloma the malignant cell is the plasma cell, the functional mature cell that differentiates and develops from the B lymphocytes. Page 1515.

3.36 **The answer is c.**
Although gross hematuria, bladder neck obstruction, and pain in the suprapubic region can all be clinical manifestations of bladder cancer, the most important indicator of disease progression is the depth of tumor penetration into the bladder wall. Page 1083.

3.37 **The answer is d.**
The larger the tumor and the more positive nodes involved, the worse the prognosis is. Page 189–190.

3.38 **The answer is d.**
For Hodgkin's disease, prognosis is most closely related to stage of disease. Age and the total number of lymph node groups involved (independent of stage) are other prognostic factors, whereas for non-Hodgkin's lymphoma prognosis is most closely related to histologic type. Page 1471.

3.39 **The answer is b.**
For patients over 70, watchful waiting may be an appropriate option. Research has yet to demonstrate that for those with stage A or B cancer treatment is more beneficial than watchful waiting. For men under 70, a physician may often be reluctant to offer watchful waiting, and there is evidence that for younger men with moderately or poorly differentiated localized prostate cancer, treatment may offer a survival advantage. Page 1616, 1765.

3.40 **The answer is d.**
Microstaging describes the level of invasion of the CM and maximum tumor thickness. The two parameters that are used in assessing the depth of invasion are the anatomic level of

invasion, or the Clark level, and the thickness of tumor tissue, or the Breslow level. The prognosis for patients with metastatic disease at the time of diagnosis is poor, with most dying within 5 years. As CM thickness increases, survival rates decrease. Thus the Breslow level has consistently proved to be a significant prognostic variable in stage I CM. Page 1673.

3.41 The answer is b.

Factors associated with a poor prognosis in AIDS-related Kaposi sarcoma (KS) include CD4 cell count < 200/mm^3; history of systemic "B" symptoms such as fever, weight loss, and night sweats; history of opportunistic infections; Karnofsky performance status < 70%; tumor-associated edema or ulceration; gastrointestinal KS; or KS in visceral organs. Page 1041.

3.42 The answer is b.

Ninety percent of patients with seminoma are curable by radiation and chemotherapy. Because they are extremely sensitive to radiation and chemotherapy, the stage of the disease at diagnosis is insignificant. High-grade tumors are known to undergo rapid cell division; they double their tumor volume quickly. Because most drugs are active against cells that are undergoing cell division, seminomas are more susceptible to the cell kill effects of chemotherapy. Page 1706–1707.

3.43 The answer is c.

Limited-stage disease is the most favorable prognostic factor in SCLC. A good ambulatory performance status, female gender, and normal lactate dehydrogenase are also favorable prognostic factors for SCLC. Poor prognostic factors include weight loss, impaired immunocompetence as measured by delayed hypersensitivity skin testing, and Cushing's syndrome. Page 1441.

3.44 The answer is c.

Hormone receptor analysis reveals whether a tumor is positive for the estrogen and progesterone receptor. If the tumor is positive for hormone receptors, then hormonal manipulation can be used for treatment. Patients with hormone receptor-negative tumors tend to have a poorer prognosis. Women whose tumors are positive for the *HER2* receptor gene are candidates for trastuzumab (Herceptin) therapy whether they have local or metastatic disease. Presence of the gene indicates a poorer prognosis. Page 1111–1112.

3.45 The answer is a.

Poor prognosis has been associated with obstructing or perforating carcinomas, occurrence in young people, location of the tumor below the peritoneal reflection, lymph node involvement, venous invasion, hepatic metastasis, and invasion of the bowel wall. Page 1222–1223.

3.46 The answer is a.

Presenting symptoms for prostate cancer rarely include generalized itching. The other diagnoses are commonly associated with generalized itching, as are vulvar cancer, gastric adenocarcinoma, central nervous system tumors, and Hodgkin's disease and non-Hodgkin's lymphoma. Page 1615.

3.47 The answer is b.

In patients with Hodgkin's disease, itching is often constant and manifests as a burning sensation in the lower legs. These patients also report pruritus and painful lymph nodes after alcohol consumption. Page 1463.

3.48 The answer is c.

Although it is possible to achieve complete remission in 93% of children with ALl drug treatment—even with the addition of an anthracycline—produces remissi only 70%–75% in adults with ALL. Page 1384–1386.

3.49 The answer is d.

Adverse effects of corticosteroids and NSAIDs together include hypertension, hyperglycemia, immunosuppression, and psychiatric reactions. Although corticosteroids were previously believed to cause peptic ulcers, this effect probably occurs more with the concomitant use of NSAIDs. Page 1180–1182.

3.50 The answer is c.

Chondrosarcoma is a tumor arising from either the interior medullary cavity of the cartilage (central chondrosarcoma) or from the bone through malignant changes in benign cartilage tumors (peripheral chondrosarcoma). The most frequent sites for this cancer are the shoulder girdle, hip girdle, and trunk. Less common sites include the bones of the hands and feet. Page 1074.

3.51 The answer is c.

A multifactorial model for multiple myeloma-associated anemia has been postulated, including the replacement of erythrocyte precursors with plasma cells. Page 1518–1519.

3.52 The answer is c.

All patients with MDS eventually develop life-threatening anemia, thrombocytopenia, and/or neutropenia. Regular evaluation of patients with MDS is important to monitor the need for supportive therapy with red blood cells, platelets, or antibiotics. MDS can transform to acute leukemia; however, this does not occur in all patients with MDS. Page 1391.

3.53 The answer is c.

SCC is more aggressive than BCC because it has a faster growth rate, less well-demarcated margins, and a greater metastatic potential. SCC appears as a flesh-colored or erythematous raised firm papule. It is usually confined to areas exposed to ultraviolet radiation. Page 1666–1667.

3.54 The answer is c.

DN may develop throughout life. They may be familial or nonfamilial. The age-adjusted incidence of melanoma is approximately 15 times higher among persons with DN as compared to the general population. DN are often larger than 5 mm and can number from 1 to 100. They appear typically on sun-exposed areas, especially on the back, but also may be seen on the scalp, breasts, and buttocks. Pigmentation is irregular, with mixtures of tan, brown, and black or red and pink. A distinctive feature is a "fried egg" appearance. Page 1653.

3.55 The answer is b.

Melanoma has two growth phases. In the radial phase tumor growth is parallel to the skin surface, risk of metastasis is slight, and surgical excision is usually curative. The vertical growth phase is marked by deep penetration into the dermis and subcutaneous tissue. Penetration occurs rapidly, increasing the risk of metastasis. Page 1667.

3.56 The answer is d.

The incidence of PCNSL has increased dramatically in recent years, primarily due to the AIDS epidemic. Of patients diagnosed with PCNSL, about 95% have a brain lesion, and 50% of these lesions are multifocal. These lymphomas are primarily of B-cell origin confined to a single extranodal site. Page 1038–1039.

3.57 The answer is a.

Central nervous system lymphoma commonly causes neurologic dysfunction, apathy, confusion, and/or personality changes. It does not typically cause the headaches that are common to brain tumors, spinal cord compression, or SIADH. Page 1039.

3.58 The answer is d.

AIDS-associated NHLs are typically intermediate- to high-grade B-cell malignancies. They appear to be associated with a rise in polygonal B-cell lymphoproliferation that results from EBV and HIV infection. AIDS-NHL has been associated with persistent generalized lymphadenopathy, suggesting polyclonal B-cell activation. One possibility is that once HIV infection occurs, EBV may trigger lymphocyte proliferation that remains unchecked as a result of HIV-induced immune dysfunction. This proliferation, in turn, may allow the expression of two oncogenes, resulting in a polygonal or monoclonal NHL. Page 1036, 1481.

3.59 The answer is c.

Choices *a*, *b*, and *d*, along with excessive lacrimation and swelling of the cheeks or orbit, are all clinical manifestations of carcinoma of the nasal cavity and paranasal sinus. Page 1341.

3.60 The answer is a.

A classic triad is apparent with cancer of the head of the pancreas: progressive jaundice, profound weight loss, and pain. Jaundice, which is precipitated by common bile duct obstruction, is the presenting symptom in 80% of all cases of cancer of the head of the pancreas and is the symptom that inevitably leads individuals to seek medical attention. Page 1587.

3.61 The answer is a.

Malignant peritoneal effusion (ascites) is most common in patients with ovarian cancer. Page 1566–1567.

3.62 The answer is c.

Over 60% of women with ovarian cancer develop ascites at some time before death. The appearance of ascites in patients with advanced disease is prognostically grim, and palliation is usually all that can be offered. Life expectancy is a few months. Page 1566.

3.63 The answer is b.

Cancers of the sigmoid colon are most often manifested by abdominal pain and melena. The manifestations in choice *a* are those of a tumor of the right colon; manifestations in choices *c* and *d* are those of rectal cancer. Page 1221.

3.64 The answer is a.

Because the transverse colon is the most anterior and movable part of the colon, tumors here are more accessible to detection by palpation. Other possible symptoms that might have been determined by inspection, auscultation, palpation, and percussion of the abdomen include distention of the abdomen, enlarged and visible abdominal veins, occult blood in the stool, and enlarged lymph nodes or organs (especially the liver). Diagnostic examination by fiber-optic colonoscopy confirms the presence of the tumor. Anemia is more likely to occur with cancer of the right colon. Polyps in the rectum may be present and may indicate the patient was at high risk for colorectal cancer. Carcinoembryonic antigen, although useful in evaluating the efficacy of treatment, is of limited value in the detection of colon cancer. Page 1220–1221.

3.65 The answer is c.

An esophageal tumor gets so large that it can interfere with the ability to swallow saliva, food, and liquids. Weight loss occurs along with a potential for aspiration pneumonia. Nutrition support, pulmonary hygiene, and aspiration precautions should be a focus of nursing care for the person with esophageal cancer. Page 1313.

3.66 The answer is c.

The glottic area includes the true vocal folds and the anterior and posterior glottic commissures. Tumors in this area tend to be well differentiated, grow slowly, and metastasize late.

Lesions that lie superior to a horizontal plane passing through the floor of the ventricles and including the epiglottis, aryepiglottic folds, arytenoids, and ventricular bands (false cords) are classified as supraglottic. Page 1354.

3.67 **The answer is c.**
Most SCLC tumors are centrally located, developing around a main bronchus as a whitish-gray growth that invades surrounding structures, eventually compressing the bronchi externally. Necrosis is frequently seen, and SCLC is responsible for 25% of all lung cancers, not 55%. Its doubling time is shorter, not longer, than that of any other lung cancer type. Page 1433.

3.68 **The answer is b.**
The best method to establish a histopathologic diagnosis is to obtain involved tissues by means of an open-lung biopsy or a fiber-optic bronchoscopy. Page 493.

3.69 **The answer is d.**
The patient's symptoms could be caused by hyperviscosity syndrome, a rare occurrence in myeloma patients caused by a high concentration of proteins that increases the serum viscosity and vascular sludging. Page 1520.

3.70 **The answer is a.**
Five-year survival rates have slowly improved to approximately 62% for all stages of disease, 87% for patients with localized disease, and 9% for stage IV disease. Page 1638–1639.

3.71 **The answer is b.**
Melanoma has been classified into several types, including lentigo maligna, superficial spreading, nodular, and acral lentiginous. Each type is characterized by a radial and/or vertical growth phase. In the radial phase, tumor growth is parallel to the skin surface, risk of metastasis is slight, and surgical excision is usually curative. The vertical growth phase is marked by focal deep penetration of atypical melanocytes into the dermis and subcutaneous tissue. Penetration occurs rapidly, increasing the risk of metastasis. Page 1667.

3.72 **The answer is c.**
Alpha-fetoprotein is a tumor marker that is elevated in the serum of 70%–90% of individuals with primary hepatocellular carcinoma, but because levels of alpha-fetoprotein are not specific for liver cancer, histologic diagnosis is required. Page 1405.

3.73 **The answer is c.**
Generalized pruritus may be an early sign of systemic disease as with Hodgkin's disease and T-cell lymphomas. In central nervous system malignancy, pruritus can present as a paraneoplastic syndrome. Page 1384–1386.

Classification

3.74 **The answer is d.**
The most relevant classification systems will communicate clinical and prognostic information. The tumors may be classified not only by their biological behavior (benign versus malignant) but also by their tissue of origin. Page 185–187.

3.75 **The answer is a.**
A benign tumor is well circumscribed or encapsulated; microscopically, it appears orderly and comprises cells similar to those of its parent tissue. A malignant tumor invades both the organs from which it originated and eventually the surrounding tissues, and it is made up of cells that vary greatly in size and shape. Page 188.

3.76 The answer is b.
The term *carcinoma in situ* describes a lesion characterized by full-thickness neoplastic change with no evidence of stromal invasion or metastases. Page 1044.

3.77 The answer is a.
Bronchogenic cancers are grouped into small cell lung cancer and non-small cell lung cancers, which include squamous cell carcinoma, adenocarcinoma, and large cell carcinoma. Many tumors are heterogeneous, containing cells from more than one histologic type. In both types of cancer, both hyperplasia and carcinoma in situ occur. Page 1432–1433.

3.78 The answer is a.
There are multiple objectives of solid tumor staging, but the most important is to provide the necessary information for individual treatment planning. Other reasons for using a uniform staging system are to give prognostic information, to assist in treatment evaluation, to facilitate the exchange of information and comparative statistics among the treatment centers, and to stratify individuals who may be eligible for clinical trials. Page 189–192.

3.79 The answer is a.
In the TNM system the extent of the primary tumor (T) is evaluated on the basis of depth of invasion, surface spread, and tumor size. The absence or presence and extent of regional lymph node (N) metastasis are considered, and the presence of distant metastasis (M) is assessed. The system is further classified by whether the assessment is obtained clinically (cTNM or TNM), after pathologic review (pTNM), at the time of retreatment (rTNM), or on autopsy (aTNM). Page 190.

3.80 The answer is a.
Stage groupings involve combining the various classification elements of tumor site, regional lymph node involvement, and the presence or absence of metastasis. It involves two main staging periods: pretreatment and retreatment. The two aspects of pretreatment staging of a previously undiagnosed cancer are clinical diagnostic staging, for patients who have had a biopsy, and postsurgical resection-pathologic staging, which includes a complete evaluation of the surgical specimen by a pathologist. Page 189–191.

3.81 The answer is b.
Restaging focuses particular attention on the disease parameters that were positive at diagnosis, to signal a search for any remaining evidence that treatment should continue. Restaging does not imply that if a remission is obtained the patient reverts to a lesser disease stage. The stage ascribed at the time of diagnosis is the one referenced throughout the illness. Page 189–191.

3.82 The answer is d.
Most tumors of unknown origin are adenocarcinomas and have a poor prognosis. Patients with neuroendocrine carcinomas of unknown origin have a higher median survival time (33 months) than those with adenocarcinomas (9 months). Page 189.

3.83 The answer is b.
The AJCC staging system for lung cancer uses the letters T, N, and M. T designates primary tumor and is divided into categories relative to size, location, and invasion. N, with three categories, represents regional lymph node status. M designates the absence or presence of distant metastases. Lung cancer is also divided into eight stages, each of which is distinctive relative to treatment and 5-year survival statistics. Small cell lung cancer is usually staged using a simple two-stage system. Because most small cell lung cancer patients have metastatic disease at the time of diagnosis, this system describes the extent of disease as either "limited" or "extensive." Page 1440–1442.

3.84 The answer is b.

Determination of the stage of disease in HD is important because it influences which treatment option (radiation therapy or combination therapy) is used. Radiation is very effective for localized HD and is therefore used in early-stage disease. Chemotherapy is more effective than radiation for late-stage disease, when the number of lymph node groups involved is greater, but it also is as effective as radiation in early-stage disease. Non-Hodgkin's lymphoma, on the other hand, is almost always treated with chemotherapy because it usually presents at an advanced stage. A positive bone marrow biopsy indicates a stage IV tumor. A stage II presentation for HD is more likely to indicate a slow-growing malignancy; it is not at all uncommon. Page 1463–1464.

3.85 The answer is b.

All the other choices, along with a history and physical examination, are standard procedures used in the staging of lymphoma. Other procedures, including a computed tomography of the chest and abdomen, a bone marrow biopsy, a percutaneous liver biopsy, a lower limb lymphangiogram, and an exploratory laparotomy, may be done if there is evidence of lymph node involvement below the diaphragm, hepatomegaly or abnormal liver function, extension of the lymphoma to mediastinal lymph nodes, or splenomegaly. Positive results on these tests often indicate a stage IV disease. Page 1465–1468.

3.86 The answer is b.

There are multiple objectives of solid tumor staging, but the most important is to provide the necessary information for individual treatment planning. Page 189–192.

3.87 The answer is c.

Whereas intermediate-grade tumors can be treated with either chemotherapy or radiation therapy, depending on the stage at presentation, advanced intermediate/high-grade lymphoma is treated with combination chemotherapy. Cyclophosphamide, the most active and effective agent, is commonly used in combination with other agents. Initial responses are usually dramatic but are not long-lived; relapse typically occurs in 4–6 weeks following discontinuation of chemotherapy. In addition, treatment-related neutropenia is severe and sometimes precipitates an opportunistic infection. Page 1468–1470.

3.88 The answer is c.

A secondary or metastatic tumor resembles the primary tumor histologically. A second primary lesion refers to an additional histologically separate malignant neoplasm in the same patient. Page 187.

3.89 The answer is b.

For selected tumors the grade is considered more significant than anatomic staging in terms of prognostic value and treatment. In soft tissue sarcomas, the grade is the primary determinant of stage of disease and of prognosis. In other tumors, such as melanoma, testicular cancer, and thyroid cancer, histologic grading has no useful application. Page 191–192.

3.90 The answer is d.

A G2 rating means the tumor is moderately well differentiated. The AJCC recommends the following grading classification:

GX = grade cannot be assessed
G1 = well differentiated
G2 = moderately well differentiated
G3 = poorly differentiated
G4 = undifferentiated Page 191.

3.91 **The answer is c.**

Histopathologic type is a qualitative assessment whereby a neoplasm is categorized in terms of the tissue or cell type from which it has originated. Histopathologic grade is a quantitative assessment of the extent to which the tumor resembles the tissue of origin. A lesion with the same cell type but at a site other than the original site indicates a metastatic tumor; a different cell type originating from another lesion anywhere in the body indicates a second primary cancer. Page 188–189.

3.92 **The answer is d.**

Clinically important cancers include features such as large tumor volume, Gleason grades 3–5, an invasive proliferative pattern of growth, elevated PSA, and origination in the peripheral zone. These cancers threaten the patient's life because they progress to fatal metastatic cancers. The vast majority of prostate cancers do not threaten the patient's life and are termed indolent. Page 1616.

3.93 **The answer is d.**

The primary application of flow cytometry analysis in solid tumors has been to determine DNA content and the percentage of cells synthesizing DNA. Normal DNA is characterized as diploid and contrasts with abnormal disorganized DNA that is aneuploid. The value of the information in solid tumors is not well established. Page 171–172.

Common Metastatic Sites

3.94 **The answer is d.**

Although some bone tumors metastasize to the lymph nodes (e.g., Ewing's sarcoma), few, if any, seem to metastasize to the central nervous system or liver. Most of the more common bone tumors metastasize to the lungs. Whether or not these metastases develop and when depends on the stage and aggressiveness of the disease process. Page 1055.

3.95 **The answer is d.**

Breast cancer primarily metastasizes to the bone, liver, lungs, nodes, and brain—but not the gastrointestinal tract. Page 1127.

3.96 **The answer is c.**

A complaint of low back pain frequently indicates that the cancer has spread into the retroperitoneal lymph nodes. Page 1703–1705.

3.97 **The answer is b.**

Bisphosphonates such as pamidronate and zoledronic acid effectively palliate pain in patients who have metastatic disease, especially in situations where NSAIDs and steroids are no longer effective. Zoledronic acid has been found to be more effective than pamidronate. Page 1131, 1628.

3.98 **The answer is d.**

The three mechanisms by which a tumor spreads from the primary site to bone are (1) direct extension to adjacent bones, (2) arterial embolization, and (3) direct venous spread through the pelvic and vertebral veins. Page 15–18.

3.99 **The answer is b.**

Radiation to the involved sites is used primarily to relieve pain, improve bone strength, and improve neurological deficits. Page 251.

3.100 The answer is d.
Ascites can become severe in advanced disease. Palliative measures to control ascites include fluid and sodium restriction, diuretic therapy, paracentesis, and albumin administration. Page 1666–1668.

3.101 The answer is c.
The physical examination to test for ascites includes percussion to assess for shifting dullness to ascertain the presence of fluid and shifting of fluid as the patient changes positions. Page 1666–1668.

3.102 The answer is d.
The most common cause of ascitic fluid buildup is tumor seeding of the peritoneum, resulting in obstruction of the diaphragmatic and abdominal lymphatics. The tumor itself may secrete humoral factors that cause increased capillary leakage of proteins and fluids into the peritoneum. Page 1666–1668.

3.103 The answer is c.
Removal of 2–3 liters of fluid and repeated paracentesis can lead to severe protein depletion, postural hypotension, and electrolyte abnormalities. Although sclerosing therapy is effective in treating pleural effusions, it is less successful with ascites. Page 1666–1668.

3.104 The answer is a.
Metastatic spread in bone cancer occurs primarily to the lungs by the hematogenous route. Symptoms of pulmonary metastases include weight loss, malaise, hemoptysis, cough, chest pain, and fever. Page 1055.

3.105 The answer is d.
Surgery may be used to resect a metastatic lesion if the primary tumor is believed to be eradicated, if the metastatic site is solitary, and if the patient can undergo surgery without significant morbidity. Page 237.

Research Protocols

3.106 The answer is d.
Postmarketing or phase IV studies are usually designed to answer questions regarding other uses, doses, and schedules as well as new information regarding risks and toxicity of a new treatment. Page 221–223.

3.107 The answer is c.
A major barrier for both patients and institutions to participation in national studies is that third-party payers often do not cover experimental treatment, which includes all research trials. Trials sponsored by drug companies generally do not pose a financial concern for oncology programs. The National Cancer Institute clearly is committed to research to prevent cancer as well as to improve the quality of life for those who develop cancer. Page 228–229.

3.108 The answer is d.
Two synonyms for *reliability* are *repeatability* and *consistency*. Repeatability is the extent to which a measure, applied two different times (test–retest) or in two different ways (alternative form and interrater), produces the same score. Consistency is the homogeneity of the items of a scale. Reliability is not a fixed property of measure, and it cannot be assumed to be generalizable. Page 40.

3.109 The answer is b.

Content validity includes both face validity (the degree to which the scale superficially appears to measure the construct in question) and true content validity (the degree to which the items accurately represent the range of attributes covered by the construct). Content validity does not include statistical evidence to support inferences made from tests, but it should cut across at least three broad domains (e.g., the physical, psychological, and social) to be considered valid from the perspective of item content. Page 40.

3.110 The answer is c.

The QLI is probably the best example of a "cancer-specific" scale that in reality measures generic health concepts. It was originally a physician-rated scale of five areas of functioning (activity, daily living, health, support, and outlook). It has been shown to distinguish cancer patients with terminal illness from those with recent disease or active treatment, as was once popularly assumed. Page 1826.

3.111 The answer is a.

The degree to which a scale superficially appears to measure the construct in question is referred to as face validity. The degree to which the items accurately represent the range of attributes covered by the construct is called true content validity. Criterion validity includes both concurrent and predictive validity. Data collected simultaneously with the scale data provide evidence of concurrent validity; data collected after the scale data provide evidence for predictive validity. Construct validity extends criterion validity to test the scale in question against a theoretical model and adjusts it according to results to help refine theory. Page 40.

3.112 The answer is a.

Legal, regulatory, medical, and ethical groups have described the process of informed consent to contain four essential elements: understanding, comprehension, voluntariness, and competence. Page 225–226.

3.113 The answer is b.

The primary ethical struggle in clinical research is that comparatively few individuals accept the risk of being research subjects in order to benefit others and society. Ethicists raise the point that asking subjects to bear the risk of harm for the good of others creates the potential for maltreatment or misuse. Page 225–226.

CHAPTER 4

Cancer Treatment Modalities

MAJOR TREATMENT MODALITIES

Vascular Access Devices

4.1 Following administration of cyclophosphamide and fluids via an implanted port, your patient complains of chills, which she states she has had in the past after her chemotherapy. You take her temperature and note a slight elevation. The *best* subsequent nursing action would be

a. Let her go home, and instruct her to call with any temperature elevation.
b. Notify the doctor, and prepare to draw blood cultures.
c. Keep her for two more hours, and then recheck her temperature.
d. Vigorously flush the catheter to avoid thrombus formation.

4.2 Which of the following skin disinfection solutions has been found to provide the *best* protection against central venous catheter colonization in hospitalized patients?

a. 2% aqueous chlorhexidine
b. 70% isopropyl alcohol
c. 10% povidone-iodine
d. Sterile water

4.3 Which of the following is a *major* advantage of the peripherally inserted central catheter?

a. It does not require frequent flushing because of the one-way valve.
b. Dressing changes are simpler and more cost-effective.
c. It can be inserted at home by a certified nurse.
d. It has a separate designated port for blood withdrawal.

4.4 The cause of extravasation in implanted ports is generally which of the following?

a. The caustic nature of the drugs
b. Misplaced or displaced needle
c. Use of a coring needle
d. Inserting the needle firmly against the needle stop

4.5 **Your patient has had an implanted port for 4 months. He is currently due for routine cisplatin and 5-fluorouracil. Following access with a Huber point needle, the port flushes easily with no evidence of swelling or pain. However, there is no blood return despite repositioning. The *most appropriate* nursing action would include which of the following?**

a. Avoid using the port if there is no blood return.
b. Infuse fluids for 1 hour then check again for blood return.
c. Send patient for a dye study to assess for sheath formation.
d. Follow institutional protocol for tissue plasminogen activator.

4.6 **An Ommaya reservoir is generally placed underneath the skin of the scalp overlying the cranium with the catheter extending to the ventricle of the brain. The purpose of this catheter placement is which of the following?**

a. Measurement of intracerebral pressure
b. Treat brain metastases
c. Injection of chemotherapeutic agents
d. Injection of chemotherapeutic agents through the intrathecal route

4.7 **Which of the following statements describes the *best* reason to use peripherally inserted central catheters (PICCs)?**

a. PICCs are excellent for long-term intermittent infusional therapy.
b. PICCs can be inserted at the bedside by certified nurses.
c. PICCs do not require sterile external site care and routine flushing.
d. PICC lines are used for short term intermittent infusional therapy.

4.8 **Which of the following is the *best* statement regarding use of the epidural implanted port?**

a. Epidural ports are used to administer intrathecal or epidural medications, including chemotherapy and analgesics.
b. To prevent infection, only medication with preservative is instilled or infused into the port.
c. The port is flushed with preservative-free heparin after each use.
d. A standard 24-gauge needle and meticulous sterile technique are used to access epidural ports.

4.9 **Mr. Archer has had an implanted port for 4 weeks and recently complained of pain in his right neck and shoulder, just above the catheter insertion site. On examination you notice slight swelling over the neck, face, shoulder, and arm. He also complains that his arm is cold at times and there is some tingling in his arm and shoulder. What is the *most appropriate* action to take?**

a. These symptoms are normal following port placement and should resolve in 2–3 weeks. Have him return to the clinic in a week if he is not better.
b. Flush the line with heparin to make sure it is not clotted.
c. Notify the physician to examine the patient. A venogram will probably demonstrate a venous thrombosis.
d. Notify the physician to obtain an order for a tissue plasminogen activator. The patient probably has a fibrin sheath formation around the tip of the catheter.

4.10 **Ms. Charles needs a peripheral intravenous injection of doxorubicin, a known vesicant. When giving a vesicant through a peripheral vein, the *most important* step is**

a. To maintain a blood return throughout the injection
b. To use a smaller-gauge, steel needle
c. To use a vein below the vein used for venipuncture
d. To administer the vesicant as quickly as possible to decrease the risk of extravasation

4.11 Which of the following factors should influence the choice of catheter used in the blood cell transplant (BCT) process for a patient?

a. The patient undergoing BCT requires a catheter that is stiffer than the traditional central venous catheter used for autologous bone marrow transplant (ABMT).
b. The stiff catheters used in ABMT are not necessary in BCT pheresis because there is a less rapid withdrawal of blood in BCT.
c. Low volume and pressure are needed during pheresis.
d. The patient undergoing BCT needs a catheter similar to the ones used for ABMT.

4.12 Alfred is a patient with colon cancer who is scheduled to have a vascular access port placed before beginning continuous infusion of 5-fluorouracil. He has recently experienced diarrhea and fever of unknown origin. His hemogram reveals a hemoglobin of 11.0 g/100 mL, a white blood cell count of 2000/mm^3 with an absolute neutrophil count of 750/mm^3, and platelets of 92,000/mm^3. His surgeon has delayed his port placement for another week. The *likely* cause of this delay is which of the following?

a. Diarrhea is a common cause of fever of unknown origin.
b. Platelets less than 100,000/mm^3 are associated with bleeding during surgery.
c. Neutropenia is the primary risk factor for infection with vascular access catheters.
d. Anemia is associated with postoperative complications.

Surgery

4.13 Mr. Vance just had gastric surgery and needs both radiation and chemotherapy. Why would these both be given after surgery?

a. Sometimes it is difficult for the surgeon to assess before surgery whether invasion has occurred and excision is the best choice.
b. Most likely, the tumor was found to be invading nearby tissues that could not be surgically resected, and micrometastases is a potential problem.
c. Both radiation and chemotherapy are needed to remove any systemic disease.
d. Mr. Vance was known to have metastases prior to surgery.

4.14 You have recently become part of a new interdisciplinary oncology team. You are aware that situations lending themselves best to surgical treatment include all factors *except*

a. Slow-growing tumors that consist of cells with prolonged cell cycles
b. An ability to achieve resection of the entire tumor mass as well as a margin of safety of normal healthy tissue surrounding the tumor
c. Embedded tumors
d. Malignancies diagnosed at an early or localized stage

4.15 Stereotactic biopsy is used to accomplish which of the following?

a. Several biopsies are obtained from samples of tissue from different locations.
b. Radiographic images are used to create three-dimensional views of a tumor.
c. "Sound" waves are recorded in stereo to outline a tumor.
d. Biopsies are used to diagnose metastatic disease.

4.16 Which of the following lung tumor types is thought to be nonresectable because it is of neuroendocrine origin?

a. Small cell lung cancer
b. Large cell lung cancer
c. Squamous cell lung cancer
d. Adenocarcinoma of the lung

4.17 Within a week of surgery for esophageal cancer, contrast studies are likely to be done to check for

a. Local edema
b. Any signs of residual tumor
c. Anastomotic leaks
d. Swallowing ability

4.18 All of the following are possible contraindications to hepatic resection for liver cancer *except*

a. Jaundice
b. Severe cirrhosis
c. Chemotherapy failure
d. Ascites

4.19 In women, radical cystectomy includes removal of the

a. Bladder, urethra, uterus, ovaries, fallopian tubes, and the anterior wall of the vagina
b. Bladder, urethra, and anterior wall of the vagina only
c. Bladder and urethra only
d. Bladder only

4.20 A new patient, Charles, undergoes transurethral resection of the prostate (TURP). He asks if this will cure the disease. The *best* response is

a. TURP is sometimes found to cure prostate cancer, but the chances diminish with increasing tumor involvement.
b. TURP is used to treat symptoms of bladder outlet obstruction.
c. TURP is required to prove cancer is present.
d. TURP is used to cure prostate cancer.

4.21 Postoperative care of an individual who has undergone palliative surgery for pancreatic cancer includes all of the following *except*

a. Administration of pancreatic enzyme supplements
b. Providing a diet that is low in fat, is high in protein, and includes a glass of red wine with lunch and dinner
c. Observing for hemorrhage, hypovolemia, and hypotension
d. Examining stools for steatorrhea

4.22 Your patient is newly diagnosed with lung cancer and is scheduled to undergo a pneumonectomy. You schedule a preoperative teaching session to instruct the patient and family on smoking cessation. The rationale for this action is based on which of the following?

a. Patients who quit smoking before surgery have less immunosuppression and less infection postoperatively.
b. Smoking cessation strategies are for the family, because the patient should not be around smoke postoperatively.
c. Risk of death is significantly higher in patients who continue to smoke within 4 weeks of surgery.
d. There is no benefit at this point to encourage smoking cessation.

4.23 Which of the following conditions is benign and iatrogenic in origin and is usually secondary to radical cancer surgery?

a. Pericardial effusion
b. Lymphedema
c. Pleural effusion
d. Anasarca

4.24 A woman who is about to have a modified radical mastectomy for diffuse multicentric breast cancer states, "Having a lymph node dissection is all right with me. I want all the cancer cells taken out if they are there." The *most appropriate* nursing response is which of the following?

a. The axillary dissection could cause lymphedema depending on the number of nodes removed.
b. The purpose of the lymph node dissection is staging; it is not a therapeutic procedure.
c. Because her disease is all over the breast, it is a good idea that she is having a more extensive dissection under her arm.
d. If any nodes are left behind, radiation can always be used.

4.25 A woman with a history of modified radical mastectomy with axillary dissection and radiation therapy completed chemotherapy 6 months ago and calls concerned about slight swelling and redness in her affected arm. On questioning her you learn that she has recently been to Europe. What is the *appropriate* nursing action and why?

a. She should keep the arm elevated. Slight swelling is common following exposure to compression changes in an airplane.
b. The swelling is probably due to the flight and the fact that she probably carried a suitcase. She should wear a sleeve. The redness is a problem. She should be on antibiotics, so she should see her doctor as soon as possible.
c. Keep the arm elevated. If it is not better in a week, call back.
d. She needs a diuretic and an antibiotic, so she should see her doctor.

Radiation

4.26 The biological effects on tissue from fractionated radiation therapy depend on the four *R*s of radiobiology, which are

a. Redistribution, reevaluation, reoxygenation, repair
b. Repair, resimulation, redistribution, reoxygenation
c. Repair, redistribution, repopulation, reoxygenation
d. Reoxygenation, redistribution, radiosensitivity, repair

4.27 Breast-conserving radiotherapy after conservative breast surgery is to prevent local recurrence. The treatment techniques used include all of the following *except*

a. Whole breast radiotherapy
b. MammoSite Radiation Therapy
c. High-dose-rate brachytherapy
d. Proton therapy

4.28 An important advantage of megavoltage equipment over conventional or orthovoltage equipment used in radiotherapy is that it

a. Is more effective in treating surface lesions
b. Is more tissue and skin sparing
c. Delivers radioisotopes to the site of the tumor
d. Limits release of dangerous heavy ions and negative pi-mesons

4.29 The possibility of contamination of equipment, dressings, and linens is greatest when radioactive isotopes are delivered as

a. Implants
b. Colloids or solutions
c. Molds
d. Ovoids separated by a spacer

4.30 Compounds that assist in maximizing the tumor cell kill achieved with radiation while minimizing injury to normal tissues are called

a. Radioantagonists
b. Radiosensitizers
c. Oxygen-enhancement ratios
d. Linear energy transfer

4.31 Nurses are often involved with managing the side effects that result from radiotherapy. To minimize the degree of the symptoms experienced, the nurse should schedule to see most patients

a. Immediately after the first fractionated dose
b. On completion of the scheduled 5-week course
c. At the end of the first week
d. 10–14 days after treatment has begun

4.32 Simulators are used in treatment planning for radiotherapy to localize a tumor and to

a. Define the volume to be treated with radiotherapy
b. Remove a section of a tumor for a laboratory evaluation
c. Reduce the size of a tumor before surgical resection
d. Prepare a histopathologic profile of a tumor

4.33 Radiation effects take place primarily at the level of

a. Cells
b. Tissues
c. Organs
d. The whole body

4.34 One of the primary goals of dose fractionation is to

a. Redistribute cell age within the cell cycle, making normal cells less radiosensitive.
b. Allow tumor cells to repopulate, making them more vulnerable to the late consequences that occur if new growth was inhibited.
c. Deliver a dose sufficient to prevent tumor cells from being repaired while allowing normal cells to recover before the next dose is given.
d. Provide time between treatments for normal cells to reoxygenate, thus making them less radiosensitive.

4.35 The late effects of radiation that are often seen 6 months or more after radiotherapy are the result of

a. Cell damage in which mitotic activity is temporarily altered in some way
b. Acute damage that occurs to tissues and organs outside the treatment field
c. The organism's attempt to repair the damage inflicted by ionizing radiation
d. Acute site-specific reactions to treatment

4.36 Hank received prostatic brachytherapy with implantation of seeds of iodine-125. Which of the following is *not* included as part of your patient education plan for Hank and his family?

a. Implants may be permanent or temporary.
b. The urine may be strained to retrieve any dislodged seeds.
c. A condom should be worn during sexual intercourse for the first 2 months following implantation.
d. Hank must remain hospitalized until the source that emits gamma radiation has completely decayed so he is not a source of radiation to those around him.

4.37 Your patient is scheduled to have intensity-modulated radiation therapy with low-energy nonthermal light-emitting diode (LED) photomodulation following lumpectomy for stage II breast cancer. Which of the following teaching points is *most appropriate* to describe the purpose of LED photomodulation?

a. Photomodulation promotes skin repair and collagen buildup.
b. Photomodulation promotes radiation effect on the possible tumor cells.
c. Photomodulation enhances the skin-saving effects of modern radiation therapy.
d. Photomodulation enhances oxygen exposure to neighboring tissues.

4.38 Fatigue associated with radiation therapy is most often associated with all of the following *except*

a. An accumulation of cell-destruction end products
b. Increased energy requirements to repair damaged epithelial tissue
c. Age, diagnosis, or stage of disease at diagnosis
d. Pain, depression, and weight loss

4.39 Which of the following side effects is *least likely* to occur as a result of radiation therapy?

a. Alterations in organ function (e.g., decreased vaginal lubrication)
b. Enhanced hormonal activity (e.g., overstimulation of the hypothalamus or pituitary)
c. General or psychologic side effects of therapy that can alter sexual function (e.g., diarrhea, loss of sexual desire)
d. Primary organ failure (e.g., ovarian failure)

4.40 Rosa is about to receive radiation therapy for the first time. She says, "I have such sensitive skin. I'm worried about the effect radiation could have on my skin." The *best* advice you can give Rosa is

a. Gently wash the skin with lukewarm water and mild soap.
b. She can still use a safety razor in the treatment field.
c. Wear sunblock products with at least 15 SPF.
d. Use mild lotions on all treatment areas to reduce dry skin.

4.41 Which of the following is *not* true regarding radiation-induced skin reactions?

a. Higher doses given over shorter periods of time to larger volumes result in more severe acute skin reactions.
b. Electrons produce greater skin reactions than photons.
c. Placing tissue-equivalent material on the skin creates a skin-sparing effect during radiation therapy, minimizing dose at the level of the skin.
d. When treatment is targeted at areas of skin apposition, increased reaction secondary to warmth and moisture can be expected.

4.42 Following radiation therapy to the chest, your patient plans a trip to Bermuda. You instruct her to use a sunscreen with an SPF of 30 or more because radiation has undoubtedly affected her skin via

a. Skin-sparing effect during radiation therapy
b. Slower rate of melanin production in new epidermal cells in the radiation field
c. Faster rate of melanin production in new epidermal cells in the radiation field
d. Destruction of lymphocytes in the irradiated epidermis

4.43 Three months after sentinel lymph node biopsy (SLNB) your patient complains of tenderness and soreness at the site. The *most appropriate* response to her complaint would include which of the following?

a. She should call her doctor to report these symptoms because they are unusual.
b. She probably bumped herself and should not be concerned.
c. These sensations are common for up to 6 months after SLNB, and she should not worry.
d. Tenderness this long after the procedure could mean hematoma formation, and hot packs could help.

4.44 About 1 month after whole brain radiation your patient's wife calls, stating that her husband is more sleepy, lethargic, and complaining of fatigue and lack of appetite. The physician states that the patient's tumor has decreased in size as expected. Therefore your response would include which of the following nursing interventions?

Somnolence Syndrome

a. Reassure the family that these symptoms are expected and will gradually improve.
b. Reassure the family that the symptoms are not related to radiation and are more likely the flu.
c. Explain that these symptoms could mean the cancer has returned, and they should make an appointment to see the doctor.
d. Explain that this side effect can last up to a year.

4.45 Complications and side effects of radiotherapy for esophageal cancer include all of the following *except*

a. Esophageal stricture
b. Radiation pneumonitis
c. Skin reaction
d. Nausea and vomiting

4.46 A patient's prostate cancer has recurred, and he is receiving radiation to a portal including the prostate, periprostatic tissue, and pelvic lymph nodes. Possible complications of radiation to this area include all of the following *except*

a. Constipation and bowel narrowing
b. Urinary incontinence
c. Lower extremity edema
d. Cystitis

4.47 Your patient with prostate cancer is scheduled to undergo brachytherapy. Part of his preprocedural preparation includes instructions on a low-residue diet and antidiarrheal agents. The *primary* purpose of these instructions is which of the following?

a. Prevent gastrointestinal irritation to the gastrointestinal mucosa
b. Prevent diarrhea from the radiation
c. Prevent bowel movements while implants are in place
d. Prevent contamination of the operative field

4.48 The *most common* injury to the large bowel that occurs following radiotherapy is

a. Increased bowel motility
b. Proctosigmoiditis
c. Abdominal cramping
d. Loose watery stools

4.49 Larson is receiving radiation to his posterior hypopharynx. Your teaching would include all of the following points regarding the effects of radiation on taste *except*

a. He can expect to experience alterations of taste about 2–3 weeks into treatment.
b. The most severely affected taste qualities are salt and bitter.
c. Sweet taste is generally least affected.
d. Taste returns within 2 weeks of completion of therapy

4.50 Approximately what percentage of persons who receive mediastinal irradiation for Hodgkin's disease experience pericardial toxicity?

a. 20%
b. 30%
c. 50%
d. 70%

4.51 Delayed radiation injury to the heart can manifest as all of the following *except*

a. Pericarditis
b. Cardiomyopathy
c. Congestive heart disease
d. Cardiac tamponade

Targeted Therapy

4.52 Allen has non-small cell lung cancer and has begun treatment with gefitinib (Iressa), an epidermal growth factor receptor–tyrosine kinase inhibitor. Which of the following is considered to be a common side effect of this treatment?

a. Anaphylaxis
b. Hypotension
c. Skin rash
d. Pancytopenia

4.53 Which of the following side effects are *most often* associated with cetuximab therapy?

a. Hair loss, fatigue, constipation
b. Fatigue, hair loss, nausea, and vomiting
c. Acnelike rash, swelling and redness of the nails, malaise
d. Blood clots, disorientation, fever

4.54 The *primary* mechanism of action of an epidermal growth factor receptor monoclonal antibody (e.g., cetuximab) is which of the following?

a. It disrupts mitosis by spindle binding
b. By attaching to the receptor, it blocks the signaling agents
c. By attaching to the signaling agent, it prevents attachment to the receptor
d. It disrupts the cell dividing process

4.55 While teaching your patient about cetuximab the *most important* point you would be certain to include is

a. Infusion reactions such as tightening in the throat, hoarseness, and rash can occur with the first infusion or with subsequent infusions.
b. If a mild infusion reaction occurs, the cetuximab would be discontinued permanently.
c. If a reaction does not occur with the first infusion of cetuximab, it will not occur with subsequent infusions.
d. Infusion reactions are preventable with medications.

4.56 The primary action of bevacizumab (Avastin) is to accomplish all of the following *except*?

a. Increase nitric oxide production, thus regulating vascular tone
b. Inhibit blood vessel formation
c. Block blood flow at the tumor site, thereby increasing efficacy of chemotherapy
d. Inhibit vasodilation

4.57 Patients who receive bevacizumab can complain of headache and experience severe (grade 3) hypertension. The occurrence of these two relatively serious side effects is due to which of the following?

a. Bevacizumab was infused too rapidly.
b. Bevacizumab decreases vascular endothelial growth factor, which decreases nitric oxide production.
c. Bevacizumab reduces nitric oxide production, which results in vasodilation.
d. Bevacizumab increases vascular endothelial growth factor, which decreases nitric oxide production.

4.58 Your patient has been on bevacizumab (Avastin) for 3 months and complains that testing his urine for protein results in delay of his treatment, and he believes it can be stopped after all this time. To increase his compliance with therapy and to help him understand his treatment, you would most likely respond with which of the following?

a. These are doctor's orders and must be followed.
b. Vascular endothelial growth factor impairs glomerular endothelial cells.
c. The bevacizumab can impair the ability of the kidneys to filter proteins.
d. Agree to test his urine for proteins with every other treatment.

4.59 Recombinant humanized monoclonal antibodies directed against vascular endothelial growth factor are effective in impeding tumor growth based on which of the following basic facts regarding how tumors grow?

a. Tumors grow exponentially rather than at the same rate over time.
b. Tumors cannot grow beyond 1–2 mm without establishing a new blood vessel system.
c. Tumors require certain proteins to supply the tumor with nutrients.
d. Tumors invade regional blood vessels to gain blood and nutrients for tumor growth.

4.60 Rituximab is a monoclonal antibody used to treat patients with non-Hodgkin's lymphoma. During the initial infusion a patient begins to shake and complains of feeling very cold. The first nursing intervention is

a. Stop the infusion, and administer diphenhydramine and acetaminophen as well as bronchodilators and epinephrine, as needed.
b. Slow the infusion to 50% of the previous rate until symptoms have resolved, because the reactions are related to the infusion rate.
c. Monitor the patient for cardiac arrhythmias because arrhythmias and angina have been reported with rituximab infusion.
d. Stop the infusion, start oxygen therapy and notify the physician.

4.61 Mrs. Andrews has just begun her first dose of cetuximab. One-third of the way through the infusion she complains of feeling cold. She is experiencing a shaking chill and has a temperature of 101.4°F. Your interventions include all of the following *except*

a. Stop the infusion, and notify the physician that the patient is having a reaction to the cetuximab therapy.
b. Monitor vital signs, and administer diphenhydramine and acetaminophen as directed.
c. Inform the patient that people who react to the cetuximab the first time are more likely to react more intensely with each subsequent treatment.
d. Resume the infusion at a slower rate when vital signs are stable.

4.62 Shortly after beginning therapy with an epidermal growth factor receptor inhibitor your patient experiences a macular papular rash over 25% of his body. The *best* intervention at this time is

a. This is a mild rash, and only water-based skin products should be used to minimize dryness.
b. This is a moderate rash that requires antibiotics for treatment.
c. This is a mild rash, and the patient may use cortisone cream.
d. This is a moderate rash that requires clindamycingel for treatment.

4.63 Overexpression of epidermal growth factor receptors has been found to correlate with a poor prognosis in which of the following?

a. Breast cancer, bladder cancer, glioblastoma
b. Breast, ovary, endometrial
c. Bladder, kidney, glioblastoma
d. Glioblastoma, astrocytoma, breast cancer

4.64 Epidermal growth factor receptors have recently been found to be an important prognostic indicator in breast cancer. Which of the following statements regarding the relationship between epidermal growth factor receptors and breast cancer is *false*?

a. The presence of the epidermal growth factor receptor means that a woman is most likely to be estrogen receptor (ER) and progesterone receptor positive.
b. The presence of the epidermal growth factor receptor means the patient has a poor prognosis.
c. Inhibiting growth factor receptors is therapeutic in women with breast cancer.
d. The presence of the epidermal growth factor has implications for selection of chemotherapy protocols.

4.65 Vascular endothelial growth factor (VEGF) stimulates endothelial cell growth. Which of the following is considered to be the primary trigger for activation of VEGF?

a. Apoptosis
b. Anemia
c. Thrombocytopenia
d. Tumor hypoxia

4.66 Which of the following *best* describes tumor angiogenesis?

a. A process whereby tumor cells are able to divide despite low hemoglobin
b. A response to tumor hypoxia
c. A process whereby tumors create their own vascular network
d. A process whereby tumors are deprived of a vascular network

Biotherapy

4.67 Which of the following substances is *not* a cytokine?

a. Alpha-interferon
b. Interleukin-2
c. Levamisole
d. Tumor necrosis factor

4.68 Flulike syndrome, specifically fever, is common when biological agents are administered. This fever is believed to be due to which of the following physiological mechanisms?

a. Infection causes the fever, and vasoconstriction causes the shivering.
b. Pyrogenic pathogens stimulate the release of endogenous cytokines that act on the thermal brain centers to create an increase in the body's temperature set point.
c. The hypothalamic temperature set point is lowered as the level of endogenous pyrogens increases.
d. Tachyphylaxis is common with biological agents and is a normal physiological response to the antigen-antibody response.

4.69 The following statements about Bacillus Calmette-Guérin (BCG) are true *except*:

a. BCG is approved for intravesical instillation as treatment of invasive cancer of the bladder.
b. BCG instillation sets off a cytokine cascade that produces both inflammatory and infectious processes.
c. BCG is contraindicated when the patient has an infection, recent surgery, or hypersensitivity to BCG product.
d. Common side effects of BCG instillation include painful urination and fever.

4.70 Biologic response modifiers are

a. Agents that restore, augment, or modulate host antitumor immune mechanisms
b. Agents that bind with cell surface receptors
c. Cells or cellular products that have direct antitumor effects
d. Biologic agents that have other biologic antitumor effects

4.71 Among the therapeutic cellular activities of interferons are all of the following *except*

a. Antiviral activity—protecting a virally infected cell attack by another virus
b. Immunomodulatory activity—interacting with T lymphocytes that stimulate the cellular immune response
c. Antiproliferative activity—directly inhibiting DNA and protein synthesis in tumor cells
d. Immunoregulatory activity—mediating the proliferation and activation of hematopoietic factors

4.72 Cytokines are glycoprotein products of immune cells that share all of the following properties *except*

a. They bind to surface receptors and regulate cell growth.
b. They mediate and regulate immune defense functions of the body.
c. They produce synergistic effects in the cytokine network.
d. They direct lymphocyte migration.

4.73 Mr. Ely has recently been told he will be starting interleukin-2 therapy as part of a research protocol. Which of the following is *not* considered a side effect of interleukin-2 therapy?

a. Moderate hair loss
b. Moderate to severe itching
c. Rapid weight gain
d. Nausea, vomiting, and diarrhea

4.74 Shortly after beginning treatment with a biologic response modifier your patient complains of intense chills and a headache. She informs you that she has been septic in the past and fears this may be happening again. The *best* nursing action in this situation would include which of the following?

a. Monitor her temperature and treat her symptoms with opiates/acetaminophen or benzodiazepines depending on the severity.
b. Stop the infusion, and notify the doctor because this could be a serious allergic reaction.
c. Consider administering the dose in the evening so the patient can sleep through the worst of the symptoms.
d. Stop the infusion, and notify the doctor to see if blood cultures should be obtained.

4.75 When patients are receiving biotherapy as their primary treatment for cancer, corticosteroids are generally avoided for which of the following reason(s)?

a. Corticosteroids mask a fever that is therapeutic.
b. Corticosteroids may block the effects of biotherapy on the immune system.
c. Corticosteroids promote prostaglandin synthesis.
d. Corticosteroids enhance the mechanism of action of biotherapy.

4.76 Hematopoietic growth factors act on the stem cells to specifically mediate all of the following steps in hematopoiesis *except*

a. Cellular proliferation
b. Cellular differentiation
c. Stem cell maturation
d. Programmed cell death

4.77 Granulocyte and granulocyte-macrophage colony-stimulating factors

a. Increase febrile episodes
b. Decrease myelosuppression
c. Increase mucositis
d. Decrease anorexia

4.78 Hematopoietic growth factors (HGFs) are given to prevent infection in potentially neutropenic patients. These injections achieve which of the following?

a. Decrease the time from the administration of the drug to the onset of the nadir
b. Decrease the activity of mature cell lineages, thereby preserving them for the period of neutropenia and infection
c. Enhance phagocytosis, antibody-dependent cytotoxicity, and chemotaxis
d. Enhance neutrophil regeneration

4.79 Which of the following is *not* considered a primary reason to administer colony-stimulating factors to patients receiving chemotherapy?

a. To permit administration of full doses of the chemotherapy agents
b. To decrease infectious complications
c. To shorten the period of febrile neutropenia
d. To prevent neutropenia in all patients receiving chemotherapy

4.80 Which of the following is considered to be the *most potent* stimulus for erythropoietin production?

a. Hemoglobin less than 9 g/dL
b. Hypoxia
c. Hematocrit less than 30 g/dL
d. Active bleeding

4.81 Epoetin alfa is contraindicated in patients with which of the following medical conditions?

a. Chronic diarrhea
b. Renal insufficiency
c. Uncontrolled hypertension
d. Glaucoma

4.82 Granulocyte colony-stimulating factor is intended to accomplish all of the following *except*

a. Decrease the duration of neutropenia related to chemotherapy
b. Decrease the number of episodes of neutropenic fever
c. Decrease the number of hospital days in patients receiving chemotherapy
d. Decrease the number of antibiotics given during chemotherapy

4.83 Hematopoietic growth factors are used as supportive therapy for which of the following conditions?

a. A patient undergoing modified radical mastectomy
b. A patient with severe cachexia
c. A patient receiving myelosuppressive therapy or a bone marrow transplantation
d. A patient with iron-deficiency anemia

4.84 Hematopoietic growth factors approved by the U.S. Food and Drug Administration (FDA) include all of the following agents *except*

a. Granulocyte-macrophage colony-stimulating factors
b. Interleukin-2
c. Granulocyte colony-stimulating factors
d. Interleukin-11

4.85 Hematopoietic growth factors (HGFs) are administered not sooner than 24 hours after chemotherapy for which of the following reasons?

a. HGFs could increase cell kill of white blood cell precursor cells if given before 24 hours postchemotherapy.
b. Myalgias and arthralgias are enhanced when HGFs are given before 24 hours post-chemotherapy.
c. HGFs are ineffective when given before 24 hours postchemotherapy.
d. The nadir is prolonged if HGFs are given before 24 hours postchemotherapy.

Antineoplastic Agents

4.86 Your patient is receiving oxaliplatin. He is instructed to avoid cold fluids during therapy and for 5 days after therapy. He also wears gloves and a scarf and covers his mouth when breathing cold air. These precautions are useful to avoid which of the following complications of oxaliplatin?

a. Palmar-plantar erythrodysesthesia
b. Acute neurotoxicity
c. Pancytopenia
d. Nausea and vomiting

4.87 When administering capecitabine (Xeloda) to a patient who is also taking warfarin it is important to frequently monitor the international normalized ratio (INR) or prothrombin time (PT). What is the nature of this drug interaction?

a. Capecitabine interferes with the metabolism of warfarin in the liver.
b. Capecitabine interferes with absorption of warfarin.
c. Clinically significant decreases in PT and INR occur.
d. Clinically significant increases in partial prothrombin time occur.

4.88 All of the following are important teaching points for prostate cancer patients who are receiving ketoconazole therapy *except*

a. Ketoconazole should be taken on an empty stomach with an acidic environment.
b. Ketoconazole should be taken after meals.
c. Ketoconazole blocks the production of male hormones in the testes and the adrenal glands.
d. Antacids and cimetidine interfere with absorption of ketoconazole.

4.89 The metabolic activation and inactivation or catabolism of drugs is carried out primarily by the

a. Liver
b. Spleen
c. Gastrointestinal system
d. Kidneys

4.90 Chemotherapy drug resistance occurs primarily because the cancer cell has the ability to do all of the following *except*

a. Decrease the number of target enzymes
b. Repair DNA lesions
c. Modify target enzymes so as to interfere with binding to antagonistic drugs
d. Increase the number of target enzymes

4.91 Capecitabine is an oral agent used to treat patients with metastatic colorectal or breast cancer. Which of the following statements *best* describes how this drug becomes activated in the body?

a. This drug is activated via the cytochrome P-450 system.
b. This drug undergoes enzymatic changes before becoming 5-FU.
c. Once metabolized in the liver, the metabolic byproducts become cytotoxic.
d. Activation is dependent on the presence of leucovorin to enhance tumoricidal effects.

4.92 While teaching your new patient about capecitabine therapy you note that he is also taking folic acid for a folic acid deficiency, dilantin for a chronic seizure disorder, and low-dose warfarin to maintain patency of his implanted catheter. Patient care would include all of the following *except*

a. Monitoring his international normalized ratio and his prothrombin time due to a potential drug interaction with capecitabine.
b. Monitoring his dilantin levels because capecitabine could cause elevated dilantin levels.
c. Consider increasing the dose of folic acid because it could potentially increase the efficacy of capecitabine.
d. Discontinuing the folic acid to prevent drug interactions.

4.93 Mrs. Collins has breast cancer and is about to begin docetaxel. She has taken her decadron as premedication. As you check her lab tests, you notice her liver function test results are elevated. Which of the following statements is important regarding your course of action?

a. The docetaxel should be delayed until liver function improves.
b. Docetaxel is eliminated by the kidney, so liver function is not important.
c. The docetaxel dose may need to be reduced because of elevated liver function results.
d. The steroid often causes an elevation of liver functions and can be ignored.

4.94 The rationale for the use of preoperative chemotherapy in patients with osteogenic sarcoma includes all *except* which of the following aspects?

a. It treats micrometastases.
b. It decreases the size of the primary tumor, possibly facilitating limb salvage surgery.
c. It enhances the effect of postoperative radiation.
d. It evaluates the effectiveness of the chemotherapy.

4.95 When telling Jeanne about cyclophosphamide, methotrexate, and 5-fluorouracil (CMF), you are careful to give her instructions regarding which of the following potential side effects?

a. Severe thrombocytopenia and bleeding
b. Severe mucositis
c. Symptoms of bladder infection as early signs of hemorrhagic cystitis
d. Transient peripheral neuropathies

4.96 Nursing care of patients receiving capecitabine therapy includes teaching patients to discontinue their drug at the first sign of a grade 2 toxicity. All of the following side effects of capecitabine would warrant discontinuing the drug *except*

a. Four bowel movements over their normal or one nocturnal stool in a 24-hour period
b. Vomiting more than once in a 24-hour period
c. Stomatitis with pain or discomfort
d. Tingling of the fingertips

4.97 Although 5-fluorouracil is the cytotoxic agent of choice for colorectal cancer, it is *most commonly* administered in combination with

a. Floxuridine
b. Capecitabine
c. Leucovorin
d. Oxaliplatin

4.98 Mrs. Otis has been diagnosed with multiple myeloma and will begin therapy with melphalan and prednisone. You will monitor Mrs. Otis closely for adverse drug effects such as

a. Decreased blood urea nitrogen and creatinine
b. Hypercalcemia and bone pain
c. Bone marrow-suppressive effects
d. Stomatitis

4.99 One week into his first treatment with capecitabine, your patient calls to report some redness and slight peeling of the palms of his hands and soles of his feet. He also has some tolerable discomfort. You instruct him to do which of the following?

a. Continue therapy and report any worsening in symptoms.
b. Continue therapy but reduce the dose by one-half.
c. Discontinue therapy until symptoms go away, and resume at full dose.
d. Discontinue therapy until symptoms go away, and resume at 50% dose.

4.100 Chemotherapy agents damage the hair most when it is in which phase of hair growth?

a. Anagen
b. Catagen
c. Telogen
d. Transitional

4.101 Which of the following chemotherapy agents is *least likely* to cause hair loss?

a. Cyclophosphamide
b. Docetaxel
c. Vinorelbine
d. Etoposide

4.102 The primary rationale for the use of corticosteroids in the management of arthralgias and myalgias due to taxane therapy is which of the following?

a. Corticosteroids decrease symptoms of inflammation.
b. Steroids decrease the fever associated with taxane therapy.
c. Steroids suppress muscle enzymes, which cause myalgias.
d. Steroids increase proinflammatory genes.

4.103 Delayed nausea and vomiting occurs *more commonly* with which of the following agents?
a. Carboplatin
b. Mechlorethamine
c. Cisplatin
d. Vincristine

4.104 Which of the following chemotherapy agents is *not* commonly associated with palmar-plantar erythrodysesthesia (hand and foot) syndrome?
a. Topotecan
b. Doxorubicin hydrochloride liposomal
c. Capecitabine
d. Cytarabine

4.105 The *most common* and lethal side effect of chemotherapy is
a. Respiratory distress
b. Electrolyte imbalance from nausea, vomiting, and diarrhea
c. Myelosuppression
d. Increased liver function tests

4.106 Which of the following chemotherapeutic agents is *not* considered to be platelet sparing?
a. Ifosfamide
b. Mitoxantrone
c. Mitomycin
d. Vincristine

4.107 After the administration of doxorubicin, you notice that swelling has occurred at the injection site. The patient complains of some burning. You determine that there is a lack of blood return. These clues alert you that the patient may be experiencing
a. Venous flare
b. Erythema
c. Extravasation
d. Venous streaking

4.108 The signs and symptoms of an extravasation from chemotherapy can be subtle. Which of the following might be considered a definite sign of infiltration of a vesicant agent?
a. A bleb formation at the injection site
b. Redness around the infusion site
c. Loss of a blood return
d. Slowing of infusion flow

4.109 Monique is experiencing hyperpigmentation. You explain to her that this may be a reaction to
a. Asparaginase
b. Bleomycin
c. Paclitaxel
d. Cisplatin

4.110 Which of the following chemotherapy drugs is *not* associated with arthralgias and myalgias?
a. Paclitaxel
b. Docetaxel
c. Ifosfamide
d. Vinorelbine

4.111 Metabolic encephalopathy manifested as blurred vision, seizures, motor system dysfunction, and irreversible coma has been reported in up to 30% of patients receiving which drug?

a. High-dose cisplatin
b. Etoposide continuous infusion
c. Ifosfamide
d. Cytarabine

4.112 Melanie is about to undergo treatment with cyclophosphamide and doxorubicin. She is at risk for developing hemorrhagic cystitis. What preventive measures can be taken?

a. Protection of the bladder focuses on reduced hydration.
b. Intravenous acrolein may produce sulfhydryl complexes and subsequent detoxification.
c. She is instructed to drink 8–10 glasses of fluid a day and void frequently.
d. She should receive amifostine therapy daily.

4.113 The dose-limiting toxicity of 5-fluorouracil when given as a continuous infusion is

a. Myelosuppression
b. Mucositis
c. Nausea and vomiting
d. Cerebellar ataxia

4.114 Which of the following chemotherapy agents is *not* associated with a moderate to high incidence of emesis?

a. Vincristine
b. Methotrexate
c. Doxorubicin
d. Topotecan

4.115 Mr. Johns is undergoing chemotherapy for high-grade testicular cancer. He complains of being jittery, and his lab tests reveal low magnesium, albumin, and calcium. He is *most likely* experiencing which of the following complications of chemotherapy?

a. Anorexia and weakness due to chemotherapy
b. Low magnesium due to cisplatin therapy
c. Low calcium due to uremia syndrome
d. A paraneoplastic syndrome

4.116 Which of the following chemotherapy agents is known to cause fluid retention that may manifest as abdominal ascites, as a pleural effusion, or as a combination?

a. Mitoxantrone
b. Megestrol acetate
c. Docetaxel
d. Paclitaxel

4.117 Chemotherapy-related constipation is associated with which of the following?

a. Colicky abdominal pain
b. Peripheral nerve dysfunction
c. Decreased colonic transit time
d. Reduced rectal emptying due to spinal cord compression

4.118 Physiologically, the etiology of chemotherapy-induced diarrhea involves all of the following *except*
   a. Shortening or denuding of the intestinal villa
   b. The destruction of the actively dividing epithelial cells
   c. Microvilli flattening and reducing the absorptive surface
   d. Decreased gastrointestinal motility

4.119 5-Fluorouracil is commonly given with leucovorin to treat gastrointestinal malignancies. The *best* reason to combine these two drugs is
   a. Combination effects of two chemotherapeutic drugs
   b. To potentiate the effect of 5-fluorouracil
   c. To decrease diarrhea occurrence
   d. To shorten the time of administration

4.120 Which of the following chemotherapy agents is *least likely* to cause diarrhea?
   a. Bleomycin
   b. Irinotecan
   c. Docetaxel
   d. Methotrexate

4.121 Which of the following metabolic disorders is *most common* in patients who receive cisplatin therapy?
   a. Hypokalemia
   b. Hypomagnesemia
   c. Hypophosphatemia
   d. Hypocalcemia

4.122 Which of the following *best* describes the features of chemotherapy-induced pulmonary toxicity?
   a. There is an inflammatory-type reaction in the endothelial cells of the lungs.
   b. It is easily detected on x-ray.
   c. It is common only in patients who smoke.
   d. Pulmonary toxicity is reversible if detected early.

4.123 The earliest symptom of chemotherapy-induced pulmonary toxicity is
   a. Bilateral basilar rales
   b. Hypoxia with hypocapnia
   c. Productive cough
   d. Hyperthermia

4.124 Which of the following chemotherapeutic agents causes anemia by inhibiting the maturation of the erythroid lineage cells in the bone marrow?
   a. Cyclophosphamide
   b. Nitrogen mustard
   c. Cisplatin
   d. Carboplatin

4.125 A number of drugs cause cardiotoxicity, especially the anthracyclines. All of the following statements about cardiotoxicity are true *except*:

a. Acute effects are immediate in onset and resolve quickly without serious complications.
b. Chronic cardiotoxicity occurs weeks or months after administration and effects are nonreversible.
c. Acute effects are dose related and dose reduction prevents further toxicity.
d. Chronic effects are dose related and dose reduction prevents further toxicity.

4.126 Which of the following chemotherapeutic agents is *least likely* to cause constipation?

a. Vinorelbine
b. Vincristine
c. Vinblastine
d. Carmustine

Hematopoietic Stem Cell Transplant

4.127 Allogeneic transplant is *most frequently* indicated for which of the following diagnoses?

a. Breast cancer
b. Non-Hodgkin's lymphoma
c. Acute lymphocytic leukemia
d. Chronic lymphocytic leukemia

4.128 Hematopoietic growth factors (HGFs) are administered to patients undergoing blood cell transplantation just before pheresis. The timing of administration of the HGFs is intended to accomplish which of the following outcomes?

a. Get the patient ready for blood cell transplantation as soon as possible.
b. Stimulate stem cell receptors to make them more vulnerable to cell kill effects.
c. Mobilization, which makes more stem cells available for collection from the circulation.
d. HGFs are administered after pheresis to encourage replacement of the harvested cells.

4.129 After transplantation Ms. Daniels is monitored for complications. Naturally, you will monitor her for possible relapse and any related complications. Besides relapse, what reaction is the *most common* life-threatening complication experienced by stem cell transplantation patients in response to preparative regimen-related toxicity?

a. Renal complication
b. Veno-occlusive disease
c. Congestive heart failure
d. Interstitial pneumonia

4.130 If Ms. Daniels were to acquire chronic graft-versus-host disease (GVHD) as a late complication of hematopoietic stem cell transplantation, which factor is *most likely* to be a causative risk factor?

a. Mismatched donor and recipient
b. Male-to-female transplant
c. Age under 18
d. Failure to receive methotrexate and cyclosporine as chronic GVHD prophylaxis in chronic myelogenous leukemia

4.131 Mr. Jackson is admitted for marrow infusion. He will receive allogeneic stem cell transplantation and is about to undergo total body irradiation (TBI). You tell him that TBI

a. Offers optimal tumor cell kill but without penetrating the central nervous system
b. Is given before marrow infusion to prevent graft rejection by the patient's own immune system
c. Is usually given in single doses to reduce toxicities
d. Should not be given as a booster in any form to patients with bulky disease because of the risk of major organ toxicity

4.132 A patient is first considered for bone marrow transplant. However, the physician selects blood cell transplantation as the treatment of choice, using peripheral pluripotent stem cells and progenitor cells obtained from peripheral blood. This procedure

a. Delays recovery of neutrophils and platelets when progenitor cells are used
b. Enables neutrophils and platelets to recover rapidly
c. Involves collecting committed progenitors that are not as far along the differentiation pathway as the PPSCs harvested from the bone marrow
d. Decreases the risk of graft versus host disease

4.133 Mrs. Adams has diseased marrow as a result of leukemia. Her physician plans a hematopoietic stem cell transplant (HSCT) and chooses autologous rather than allogeneic stem cell transplant. Mrs. Adams tells you, "I've never heard of using a person's own bone marrow cells. Why would anyone do that when I'm the one with the disease?" You explain that autologous stem cell transplant

a. Eliminates the risk of graft-versus-host disease (GVHD) and other toxicities, such as myelosuppression
b. Is less toxic, although there is an increased risk of veno-occlusive disease
c. Reduces the risk of tumor contamination seen in allogeneic stem cell transplants
d. Reduces the risk of the graft-versus-leukemic effect (graft-versus-leukemic effect can increase the risk of relapse)

4.134 Which of the following presents the *best* explanation for why blood-derived cells rather than bone marrow-derived cells are most often used for autologous transplantation?

a. Bone marrow-derived cells are obtained by bone marrow aspiration, and it is more painful.
b. Bone marrow can be contaminated by tumor cells.
c. The procedure of obtaining cells from the bone marrow increases neutropenia.
d. A shortened nadir period is found with blood cell transplant.

4.135 Under which of the following circumstances is administration of platelet concentrate from a single donor or human leukocyte antigen (HLA)-matched donor preferable to that of a random donor platelet concentrate?

a. When the patient is severely immunosuppressed
b. When cost is a major factor
c. When a patient's red blood cell antigens (ABO) are not known
d. When time is a major factor

4.136 A patient is to receive a blood transfusion of two units of packed red blood cells that have been irradiated. Which of the following explains the rationale for irradiating the blood?

a. To kill any possible cancer cells in the blood
b. To prevent the spread of the AIDS virus
c. To prevent graft-versus-host disease
d. To sterilize the blood

4.137 Ms. Daniels, who had an allogeneic stem cell transplant, is about to receive a blood product. You must ensure that the blood has been treated to prevent graft-versus-host disease. This means you will check to be sure that the blood product has been

a. Exposed to alloimmunization and platelet refractoriness
b. Infiltrated with saline solution
c. Treated via plasmapheresis
d. Irradiated

4.138 After a long period of time Ms. Daniels, who had an allogeneic stem cell transplant, develops recurrent varicella zoster virus. What is the *most likely* treatment approach?

a. Cyclosporine
b. Methotrexate
c. Acyclovir
d. Cyclosporine and methotrexate in combination

4.139 Which of the following measures has been found to be *most consistently* effective in preventing infection in the hematopoietic stem cell transplant environment?

a. Meticulous hand washing, scrupulous hygiene, and protective isolation
b. Antimicrobial prophylaxis
c. Bacterial prophylaxis
d. Fungal prophylaxis

4.140 Which of the following agents is used to prevent graft-versus-host disease in hematopoietic stem cell transplant?

a. Medroxyprogesterone acetate
b. Cyclosporine
c. Cyclophosphamide
d. Dexamethasone

4.141 Risk factors for veno-occlusive disease of the liver in hematopoietic stem cell transplant include all of the following *except*

a. Patients with hepatitis
b. Antimicrobial therapy with acyclovir, amphotericin, or vancomycin
c. Cytomegalovirus and fungi
d. Chemotherapy and radiation therapy before transplant

4.142 Trimethoprim-sulfamethoxazole is generally the treatment of choice for *Pneumocystis carinii*. Which of the following is *not* usually a side effect of this drug?

a. Nausea and vomiting
b. Hemolytic anemia
c. Hepatotoxicity
d. Myelosuppression

4.143 Elise develops graft-versus-host disease after undergoing allogeneic stem cell transplant. Which of the following will probably *not* be part of Elise's treatment plan?

a. Systemic immunosuppressive therapy
b. Topical steroids
c. Nonsteroidal anti-inflammatory drugs
d. Antithymocyte globulin

4.144 ***Pneumocystis carinii* is potentially fatal and requires treatment with**

a. Foscarnet
b. Ganciclovir
c. Trimethoprim-sulfamethoxazole
d. An aminoglycoside

4.145 **Numerous acute hepatic complications can arise following hematopoietic cell transplantation (HCT). Which of the following is *not* diagnostic for veno-occlusive disease?**

a. Fluid retention
b. Hyperbilirubinemia
c. Hypernatremia
d. Right-upper quadrant pain

4.146 **Correctly identify the sequence of events in the pathophysiology of veno-occlusive disease:**

1. Cytokine and tumor necrosis factor activation
2. Injury of the endothelial lining of hepatic venules and sinusoids
3. Hypercoagulation and thrombosis
4. Impaired blood flow
5. Renal insufficiency

a. 2, 1, 3, 4, 5
b. 5, 2, 1, 3, 4
c. 2, 4, 1, 5, 3
d. 4, 1, 2, 3, 5

4.147 **A stem cell transplant patient has an oral herpetic lesion and asks you how she could have gotten it. Which of the following statements is *not* accurate concerning oral herpes simplex virus (HSV) infections?**

a. Most oral infections are due to reactivation of latent infections.
b. HSV infections in this population present as soft-tissue ulcerations rather than vesicles.
c. The incidence of HSV infection in this population is about 50%.
d. This population is more at risk for disseminated HSV infection than other immunocompromised patients

UNPROVEN/ALTERNATIVE THERAPIES

4.148 **Homeopathy is *best* described by which of the following?**

a. It is a method of manipulating physical and psychological characteristics of the human body to treat illness.
b. It is a medical system that promotes the healing power of nature.
c. It is a theory that purports that a drug that causes symptoms at full strength will cure those symptoms if it is diluted.
d. It is a medical system that focuses on the relationship between body structure and function.

4.149 **The use of the mind-body technique, or psychic energy, in cancer includes all of the following *except***

a. Healing touch
b. Reflexology
c. Reiki therapy
d. Polarity therapy

4.150 Which of the following is *not* one of the four basic principles involved in the administration of psychiatric drugs to cancer patients?

a. The starting dose of the drug is generally lower than that typically given to healthy individuals.
b. The dosage is increased more slowly.
c. The therapeutic dose may be significantly higher in cancer patients than in healthy individuals.
d. Potential side effects are monitored carefully, as antidepressants often affect the same organs as drugs used in cancer treatment.

4.151 A patient is having trouble sleeping and wants to take a "natural" sleep aid rather than a prescription drug because she is afraid of becoming addicted to sleeping pills. Which of the following statements is *most accurate* concerning the use of herbal agents as sleep aids?

a. Herbal agents are perfectly safe, even if taken for extended periods of time.
b. Herbal agents, especially lavender, can be addicting.
c. There is no integrative therapy that has been sufficiently tested to produce strong evidence supporting its use.
d. Ginseng is an effective sleep aid and can safely be taken with monoamine oxidase inhibitors.

4.152 Homeopathy is defined as a medical approach to care that emphasizes which of the following?

a. Holistic care focuses on the whole person in their environment.
b. Energy techniques correct physical problems with adjustments in energy flow.
c. It is based on the theory of similars, which holds that a drug causing symptoms at full strength will cure those symptoms if it is diluted.
d. Care of the individual and family in their own home using traditional herbal therapies is emphasized.

4.153 The *most optimal* outcome from Cognitive Behavioral Therapy is when

a. There is a good match between the appraisal of the situation and the coping strategy selected.
b. Emotion-focused coping strategies are used when there is little control over the situation.
c. Problem-focused coping strategies are used when there is little control over the situation.
d. There is a good match between the outcome of the situation and the coping strategy selected.

ANSWER RATIONALES

Please note: All page numbers referenced in the Answer Rationales sections refer to the textbook *Cancer Nursing: Principles and Practice, Seventh Edition*, by Connie Henke Yarbro, Debra Wujcik, and Barbara Holmes Gobel (Jones & Bartlett Learning, © 2011).

Major Treatment Modalities

Vascular Access Devices

4.1 The answer is a.
Since she has had chills in the past after chemotherapy she can go home but needs to report any temperature elevation. Systemic infections can be thrombus related or caused by intraluminal catheter colonization with a wide variety of infective organisms. Signs and symptoms include fever and chills, especially following vigorous flushing of the catheter. Blood cultures are taken through each lumen of the device (if applicable) as well as peripherally. Page 424.

4.2 The answer is a.
During a landmark prospective-randomized study in a surgical intensive care unit, researchers evaluated 10% povidone-iodine, 70% isopropyl alcohol, and 2% aqueous chlorhexidine skin disinfection before central venous catheter insertion and for site maintenance every other day. The chlorhexidine treatment group had a significantly decreased incidence of local catheter-related infection and infusion-related bacteremia. Page 423.

4.3 The answer is c.
The peripherally inserted central catheter (PICC) requires daily flushing and central line dressing changes as frequently as every 3–7 days. Although some PICCs have more than one lumen, any lumen can be used for blood withdrawal. The major advantage is that the catheter can be placed by specially trained nurses in the home so the patient can avoid going to the hospital or doctor's office. Page 417–418.

4.4 The answer is b.
In the case of implanted ports, the cause of drug extravasation is usually a misplaced or displaced needle. Another mechanism for drug extravasation from ports involves retrograde subcutaneous leakage from percutaneously inserted catheters obstructed by a fibrin sheath. Page 422.

4.5 The answer is d.
Swelling and pain are signs of catheter malfunction or displacement. In the absence of these and a catheter that flushes easily without evidence of occlusion, the lack of blood return is episodic and likely due to either a fibrin sheath or the tip of the catheter impinging on the vessel wall. Tissue plasminogen activator 2 mg instilled into the catheter following catheter flush usually results in a good blood return at the next visit. Approximately 20% of patients with implanted ports experience withdrawal occlusion periodically throughout the use of the catheter. Page 424.

4.6 The answer is c.
The Ommaya reservoir is surgically implanted through the cranium. It is placed underneath the skin with the catheter extending from the reservoir to the ventricle. It provides permanent intraventricular access for patients in whom repeated translumbar puncture is impractical.

Cerebrospinal fluid is gently aspirated and sent for cytology or laboratory studies. The chemotherapy drug is administered slowly. Page 416.

4.7 **The answer is d.**
PICCs are ideal for short-term access (1 week to several months). Page 417–418.

4.8 **The answer is a.**
Epidural ports are used to administer intrathecal or epidural medications. Epidural ports are flushed with 1–2 ml of sterile preservative-free saline after use. Never flush epidural lines with heparin. Page 421–422.

4.9 **The answer is c.**
Signs and symptoms of a venous thrombosis are related to impaired blood flow and include edema of the neck, face, shoulder, or arm; prominent superficial veins; neck pain; tingling of the neck, shoulder, or arm; and skin color or temperature changes. A venogram with contrast media is used to assess for a venous thrombosis. Page 425.

4.10 **The answer is a.**
When giving a vesicant, it is always better to have a blood return throughout the injection, so a smaller gauge needle is not preferable in that situation. For patients with small veins, choose an angiocatheter that is thin walled with an over-the-needle cannula. Avoid starting the IV below a venipuncture site. Page 405–406.

4.11 **The answer is a.**
A patient undergoing BCT requires a catheter that is stiffer than the traditional central venous catheter used for ABMT because of the need for high volume and pressure during pheresis. Page 421.

4.12 **The answer is c.**
The incidence of catheter-related bacteremia is influenced by specific therapy, degree of catheter use, patient population, catheter insertion technique, and care and maintenance procedures. However, neutropenia remains the primary risk factor for patients with an infection who have a vascular access catheter. Page 423–424.

Surgery

4.13 **The answer is b.**
Radiation is usually indicated if the tumor is found to be invading nearby tissues that cannot be surgically resected. Chemotherapy is used to eliminate micrometastasis. Page 1690–1693.

4.14 **The answer is c.**
Situations lending themselves best to surgical treatment include such factors as slow-growing tumors that consist of cells with prolonged cell cycles. A surgical procedure intended to be curative must involve resection of the entire tumor mass as well as a margin of safety of normal healthy tissue surrounding the tumor. Superficial and encapsulated tumors are more easily resected than those that are embedded in inaccessible or delicate tissues. Page 236–238.

4.15 **The answer is b.**
Regional biopsy involves obtaining several samples of tissue from different locations within a tumor. Regional biopsies are used to diagnose metastatic disease in a defined, but not localized, region of the body. Stereotactic biopsy uses radiographic images to create three-dimensional views of a suspected neoplasm. Page 1108–1109, 1167.

4.16 The answer is a.
Small cell lung cancer invades the submucosa and is thought to arise from neuroendocrine cells that secrete peptide hormones. Squamous cell carcinoma, adenocarcinoma, and large cell carcinoma are all examples of non-small cell lung cancer. Page 1433, 1444, 1447.

4.17 The answer is c.
Because the esophagus is thin walled and draws upward with each swallow, an anastomosis involving the esophagus has more of a tendency to leak than any other area of the gastrointestinal tract. For this reason contrast studies are performed 4–6 days after surgery to check for patency of the anastomosis. Small leaks usually close spontaneously; larger leaks often require surgical approximation. Page 1305.

4.18 The answer is c.
Possible contraindications to major hepatic resection for liver cancer include the following: (1) severe cirrhosis; (2) distant metastases in the lung, bone, or lymph nodes; (3) jaundice, which is often indicative of obstruction of the common bile duct; (4) ascites, which is usually indicative of liver failure and an inability to tolerate a surgical procedure; (5) poor visualization on angiographic studies, which may jeopardize the certainty with which the surgeon resects the tumor; (6) certain biochemical changes that indicate poor liver function and lower the probability of survival; and (7) involvement of the inferior vena cava or portal vein, which would make surgical intervention hazardous. Page 1408–1409.

4.19 The answer is a.
In women a radical cystectomy includes the removal of the bladder, urethra, uterus, ovaries, fallopian tubes, and anterior wall of the vagina. In men the term is synonymous with prostatectomy and includes excision of the bladder with pericystic sac, the attached perineum, the prostate, and the seminal vesicles. Page 1087.

4.20 The answer is b.
Prostate cancer is not cured by TURP. Rather, TURP is used to treat symptoms of bladder outlet obstruction, and in some patients provides pathologic evidence that a cancer, previously unsuspected, is present. Page 1619.

4.21 The answer is b.
Hemorrhage, hypovolemia, and hypotension pose the greatest threats to an individual who has just undergone surgery for cancer of the pancreas. As soon as possible after pancreatectomy, small feedings are started with a diet that is usually bland, low in fat, and high in carbohydrates and protein. Restrictions include caffeine, alcohol, and overindulgence. The stool should be examined daily for the characteristic signs of steatorrhea: frothy foul-smelling stool with fat particles floating in the water. Page 1598–1599.

4.22 The answer is c.
Risk of death is significantly higher in patients who are still smoking within 1 month of pneumonectomy. There is higher morbidity and mortality for smokers who continue to smoke before surgery. Patients who stop smoking within 10 weeks of surgery have the same risk as those who had never smoked. Page 1426, 1443–1444.

4.23 The answer is b.
Lymphedema is a benign iatrogenic problem caused by radical cancer surgery. Arm lymphedema often developed after the most common treatment for all types of breast cancer in the past: radical mastectomy with axillary node dissection followed by radiation. It now occurs much less frequently. Lymphedema of the leg may develop after groin dissection that

is performed for the treatment of metastatic disease from primary tumors. Mechanical interruption (surgical technique) and radiation often produce lymphatic obstruction, the most common cause of lymphedema. Page 1135–1136, 1569–1570.

4.24 The answer is b.
A lymph node dissection stages disease. It is not a therapeutic procedure. Page 1110–1111.

4.25 The answer is b.
Women at risk of lymphedema should always wear a compression garment for air travel and avoid heavy lifting with the affected arm. Page 1135–1136.

Radiation

4.26 The answer is c.
The four *R*s of radiobiology and their influence on dose fractionation is as follows: *R*epair of damaged cells; *R*edistribution of cell age so tumor cells will become more radiosensitive; *R*epopulation, which takes place during cell division; and *R*eoxygenation, which allows the tumor cells that are in a hypoxic or anoxic state to become oxygenated and radiosensitive. Page 257.

4.27 The answer is d.
Whole breast radiotherapy is still used in breast-conserving radiotherapy; however, treatment is changing for patients with early-stage breast cancer to include the concept that partial breast irradiation yields similar control. The MammoSite system delivers high-dose radiation directly to the site of tumor excision and targets the area where the cancer would most likely recur. The Intrabeam system uses a single dose of intraoperative radiotherapy in comparison to the fractionated dosing system of MammoSite. Page 1117.

4.28 The answer is b.
Megavoltage equipment operates at 2–40 million electron volts (MeV), compared to orthovoltage equipment's 40,000–400,000 electron volts (kV). It has the advantages of deeper beam penetration, more homogeneous absorption of radiation (minimizing bone absorption), and greater skin sparing. Megavoltage equipment includes cobalt and cesium units, the linear accelerator, the betatron, and such experimental units as those producing neutron beams, heavy ions, and negative pi-mesons. Page 294.

4.29 The answer is b.
In addition to radioactive implantation, some radioactive isotopes are administered orally or intravenously or by instillation. Liquid sources administered as colloids or solutions are adsorbed or metabolized and present a possibility of contamination of equipment, dressings, and linens, depending on the mode of administration and metabolism. Page 1263.

4.30 The answer is b.
Efforts to improve the therapeutic ratio have resulted in the development of certain compounds that act to increase the radiosensitivity of tumor cells or to protect normal cells from radiation effect. Radiosensitizers are compounds that apparently promote fixation of the free radicals produced by radiation damage at the molecular level. Page 259–260.

4.31 The answer is d.
During a course of radiotherapy, certain treatment-related side effects can be expected to develop, most of which are site specific as well as dependent on volume, dose fractionation, total dose, and individual differences. Many symptoms do not develop until approximately 10–14 days into treatment, and some do not subside until 2 or more weeks after treatments have ended. Page 318–320.

4.32 **The answer is a.**
Simulator machinery may involve the use of diagnostic X-rays, fluoroscopic examination, transverse axial tomography, computed tomography, and ultrasound, with the goal of localizing a tumor and defining the volume to be treated with radiotherapy. Other aspects of treatment planning include the tattooing of the treatment area, installing various restraining and positioning devices to immobilize the person, shaping the field, and determining what structures are to be blocked and protected from radiation. Page 271–274.

4.33 **The answer is a.**
The biologic effects of radiation on humans are the result of a sequence of events that follows the absorption of energy from ionizing radiation and the body's attempt to compensate for this assault. Radiation effect takes place at the cellular level, with consequences in tissues, organs, and the entire body. Page 251–252.

4.34 **The answer is c.**
All of the other choices are opposites of the actual goals of fractionation. Fractionation redistributes cell age within the cell cycle, making tumor cells more radiosensitive. It allows normal cells to repopulate, sparing them from some of the late consequences that occur if new growth is inhibited. It also provides time between treatments for tumor cells to reoxygenate, thus making them more radiosensitive. Page 257.

4.35 **The answer is c.**
Effects of radiation may be acute and immediate (seen within the first 6 months) or may be late (seen after 6 months). Acute effects are due to cell damage in which mitotic activity is altered. If early effects are not reversible, late or permanent tissue changes occur. These late effects are due to the organism's attempt to heal or repair the damage inflicted by ionizing radiation. Page 339–340.

4.36 **The answer is d.**
After insertion of the source, hospitalization lasts until decay of the source is reduced to 30 millicuries or less. A condom should be worn during intercourse for 2 months after implantation, but the patient poses no danger as a radioactive source. Page 1627.

4.37 **The answer is a.**
Exposing women to LED photomodulation can significantly reduce painful treatment-interrupting skin reactions. The process consists of LEDs in a specific array that emits a non-thermal low-energy light at a pulsating frequency. It promotes skin repair. Fibroblasts repair themselves to build up the collagen. Page 280.

4.38 **The answer is c.**
Fatigue associated with radiation therapy may be caused by anemia, an accumulation of cell destruction end products, or increased energy requirements to repair damaged epithelial tissue. Fatigue has been reported to affect 65%–85% of individuals receiving radiation therapy and has been related to length of treatment, pain, depression, and weight loss. Fatigue has not been found to consistently be influenced by age, stage of disease, time since surgery, weight, or length of time since diagnosis. Page 323, 325.

4.39 **The answer is b.**
Radiation therapy can cause sexual and reproductive dysfunction through primary organ failure (e.g., ovarian failure and testicular aplasia), through alterations in organ function (e.g., decreased lubrication and impotence), and through the temporary and permanent effects of therapy associated with reproduction (e.g., diarrhea and fatigue). In addition, radiation therapy

can cause decreases in sexual enjoyment, ability to reach orgasm, libido, and frequency of intercourse and sexual dreams, as well as vaginal stenosis in women. Page 346–347.

4.40 **The answer is a.**
Gentle skin washing with lukewarm water and mild soap should be initiated when treatment begins. Rosa should avoid shaving in the treatment field, avoid lotions in the treatment field, and protect her skin when outside using sunblock products with at least 30 SPF. Page 318–320.

4.41 **The answer is c.**
Factors that determine the degree, onset, and duration of radiation-induced skin reactions include the following, among others: Higher doses given over shorter periods of time to larger volumes result in more severe acute skin reactions; electrons produce greater skin reactions than do photons; and placing tissue-equivalent material on the skin reduces the skin-sparing effect of radiation therapy, allowing for maximum dose at the level of the skin. Finally, when treatment is targeted at areas of skin apposition, increased reaction secondary to warmth and moisture can be expected. Page 318–320.

4.42 **The answer is b.**
Following radiation therapy the skin's ability to protect itself from ultraviolet rays is decreased as a result of destruction of melanocytes in the irradiated epidermis and the slower rate of melanin production in new epidermal cells in the radiation field. Page 319–321.

4.43 **The answer is c.**
Tenderness and soreness remain highly prevalent after SLNB at 3 and 6 months after the procedure. Tenderness, soreness, tightness, and numbness are among the most severe and distressing symptoms associated with both SLNB and axillary lymph node dissection. Page 1110–1111.

4.44 **The answer is a.**
Somnolence syndrome is a cluster of symptoms consisting of excessive sleepiness and drowsiness, lethargy, and fatigue with anorexia. The cause is related to transient demyelination secondary to radiation. Symptoms occur 4–12 weeks after radiation and can last for 2–8 weeks. Patients need reassurance as the syndrome runs its course. Page 330.

4.45 **The answer is d.**
Esophageal fistula, stricture, hemorrhage, radiation pneumonitis, and pericarditis are all possible complications of radiotherapy for esophageal cancer. Side effects to be expected are swallowing difficulties, including burning, pain, dryness, and skin reactions. Page 332.

4.46 **The answer is a.**
Radiation therapy side effects include impotence, urinary incontinence, bone marrow depression, lower extremity edema, cystitis, urethral strictures, diarrhea, proctitis, and rectal bleeding. Diarrhea can be problematic, because a part of the colon and rectum lie within the irradiated pelvic field. Page 1627.

4.47 **The answer is c.**
Constipation is sometimes induced intentionally among patients undergoing brachytherapy for gynecologic or prostate cancers. In these situations a low residue diet and antidiarrheal agents are prescribed to prevent bowel movements while implants are in place. Page 1626–1627.

4.48 **The answer is b.**
The most common injury to the large bowel that occurs after radiotherapy is proctosigmoiditis. Another commonly encountered side effect is increased bowel motility, which creates abdominal cramping and loose watery stools. Page 1227–1228.

4.49 The answer is d.

Alterations in taste are reported during the second week of treatment. Doses in the 50- to 65-Gy range cause maximum taste loss. The most severely affected taste qualities are salt and bitter. Sweet taste is generally least affected. Page 332.

4.50 The answer is d.

Ultimately, 76% of patients who receive mediastinal radiotherapy develop pericardial toxicity. A retrospective review of patients who underwent mediastinal irradiation and required valve replacement concluded that radiation injury was a major factor responsible for the development of mitral valve disease and was a contributing factor in aortic valve disease. Page 1501.

4.51 The answer is d.

Although cardiac complications are much less frequent using current radiotherapy techniques, long-term effects include pericarditis, cardiomyopathy, and congestive heart disease. Page 344–345.

Targeted Therapy

4.52 The answer is c.

The major side effects of gefitinib (Iressa) are skin rash and diarrhea. It rarely causes any allergic type reaction, hypotension, or effect on the bone marrow. Page 571–572.

4.53 The answer is c.

The most common side effects reported by 774 patients are asthenia/malaise, abdominal pain, fever, headache, nausea, vomiting, diarrhea, acneform rash, and others. Nail disorders are rare, but choice *c* is the best answer. Rarely is alopecia or disorientation seen with cetuximab. Page 568–569.

4.54 The answer is b.

Cetuximab (Erbitux) is a monoclonal antibody that attaches to epidermal growth factor receptor on both normal and tumor cells. When cetuximab attaches to the epidermal growth factor receptor, it blocks the signaling agents from attaching and starting the cell dividing process. Page 568–569.

4.55 The answer is a.

Severe infusion reactions are rare with cetuximab, but they do occur. Approximately 90% of severe infusion reactions were associated with the first infusion despite the use of prophylactic antihistamines. These reactions were characterized by the rapid onset of airway obstruction (bronchospasm, stridor, and hoarseness), urticaria, and/or hypotension. Caution must be exercised with every cetuximab infusion because some patients experienced their first severe infusion reaction during later infusions. Severe infusion reactions require the immediate interruption of therapy and permanent discontinuation from further therapy. Page 568–569.

4.56 The answer is d.

Bevacizumab is an antiangiogenic agent that inhibits blood vessel formation, which starves the tumor. In addition, bevacizumab may have an effect of remodeling existing tumor vasculature to improve drug penetration, thereby enhancing antitumor efficacy of chemotherapeutic agents. Page 562, 569.

4.57 The answer is d.

Nitric oxide is a messenger molecule (a molecule that carries signals between cells) that can regulate various physiologic functions, including blood pressure. Some studies suggest that vascular endothelial growth factor increases nitric oxide production, resulting in vasodilation. Reducing nitric oxide production results in vasoconstriction; it has been hypothesized that this process could play a role in hypertension. Page 562, 569.

4.58 **The answer is c.**
Proteinuria can occur with cancer and some cancer therapies. In a clinical setting impairment of the glomeruli that make up the kidney may be a pathologic cause of persistent proteinuria. Inhibition of vascular endothelial growth factor, a key endothelial growth factor, has been shown to impair glomerular endothelial cells that normally filter water and small solutes but not proteins or cells. Page 562, 569.

4.59 **The answer is a.**
Because malignant tumors cannot grow beyond 1–2 mm without establishing a new blood vessel system, agents are being studied that have the capacity to neutralize growth factors, such as vascular endothelial growth factor. Page 567.

4.60 **The answer is b.**
Hypersensitivity reactions are common and are related to the infusion rate. Hypotension, bronchospasm, and angioedema may occur. Stop the infusion if serious cardiac arrhythmias develop. Angina may occur postinfusion, especially in individuals with a prior history. Page 799–780.

4.61 **The answer is c.**
Patients who react to the cetuximab usually react the first time with the loading dose but then not again during subsequent dosing. The patients generally do very well once they have the diphenhydramine and can continue their treatment. Page 795, 799.

4.62 **The answer is c.**
This is not considered an allergic reaction because it is the result of direct interference with the functions of epidermal growth factor receptor's signaling in the skin and is treated locally with steroid cream. Antibiotics are used for pustular lesions. The drug would only be stopped if the rash covered greater than 60% of the body with symptomatic erythroderma or if vesicular eruption or desquamation occurs. Page 572–573.

4.63 **The answer is d.**
High levels of epidermal growth factor receptors (EGFRs) on cells from cancers of the breast and bladder indicate a worse prognosis. High levels of EGFRs are noted on many epithelial carcinomas, and mutant EGFRs have been found on high-grade glioblastomas. Page 565.

4.64 **The answer is a.**
There is an inverse correlation between epidermal growth factor receptors and ER status, with ER-negative tumors tending to have a higher level of epidermal growth factor receptor than ER-positive tumors. Page 1110.

4.65 **The answer is d.**
The angiogenic switch refers to the ability of tumor cells to release angiogenic factors and convert the tumor cell to an angiogenesis inducer. This switch correlates with an increased production of VEGF, which is known to induce angiogenesis. A primary trigger of the angiogenic switch is tumor hypoxia, which turns on the VEGF tyrosine kinase signaling pathway. Page 567.

4.66 **The answer is c.**
Tumor angiogenesis is a complex multistep process that enables tumors to develop a new blood supply from a preexisting vascular network. Page 567.

Biotherapy

4.67 The answer is c.
Cytokines (which include lymphokines) are substances released from activated immune system cells that affect the behavior of other cells. They may alter the growth and metastasis of cancer cells by augmenting the responsiveness of T cells to tumor-associated antigens, enhancing the effectiveness of B-cell activity, or decreasing suppressive functions of the immune system, thereby enhancing immune responsiveness. Included among the cytokines are the interferons and interleukins, tumor necrosis factor, and colony-stimulating factors. Page 29–30.

4.68 The answer is b.
Body temperature is controlled by preoptic anterior hypothalamic brain centers in a feedback mechanism. Pyrogenic pathogens, toxins, or drugs stimulate the release of endogenous pyrogenic cytokines, which act on thermal brain centers via prostaglandin release and create an upward reset of the body's temperature set point. Feedback mechanisms now read the body temperature as cold and initiate heat-producing actions such as involuntary muscular contractions or rigors. Page 545–547.

4.69 The answer is a.
BCG is approved for intravesical instillation as treatment of cancer *in situ* of the bladder. BCG instillation sets off a cytokine cascade that produces a T-cell mediated immune response and a mucosal infection that may last several months. BCG is contraindicated when the patient has an infection (including active tuberculosis), recent surgery (biopsy, transurethral resection) or hypersensitivity to a BCG product. Common side effects of BCG instillation include painful urination and fever. Page 548.

4.70 The answer is a.
Biologic response modifiers can be classified as agents that restore, augment, or modulate host antitumor immune mechanisms; cells or cellular products that have direct antitumor effects; and biologic agents that have other biologic antitumor effects. Agents that bind with cell surface receptors are targeted therapies. Page 531, 562.

4.71 The answer is d.
The interferons (IFNs) are a family of naturally occurring complex proteins that belong to the cytokine family. Each of the three major types in humans—alpha-IFN, beta-IFN, and gamma-IFN—originates from a different cell and has distinct biologic and chemical properties. All three types of IFNs exhibit the cellular effects listed in choices *a–c*. Page 543.

4.72 The answer is d.
The cytokine network is an overlapping, interactive communication pattern within the immune system. Cytokines share many properties, such as mediating and regulating the immune defense functions of the body. They can influence the stimulation of other cytokines to produce synergistic effects, as in a cytokine network, or to antagonize the actions of other cytokines. They do not direct lymphocyte migration. Page 28–29.

4.73 The answer is a.
Although some thinning can occur, true alopecia is rare. Severe itching and pruritus can be intense because of severe skin dryness. Rapid weight gain occurs as a result of capillary leak syndrome. The most severe nausea, vomiting, and diarrhea occur with interleukin-2 therapy, particularly high-dose regimens. Page 536–540.

4.74 The answer is a.
Intense chills and headache generally occur before fever spike and are predictable within the first 2–4 hours of administering biologics. Ways to minimize the severity of the symptoms is

to administer the drug by subcutaneous injection or in the evening so the patient can sleep through the symptoms. Patients should be prepped prophylactically with acetaminophen with or without benzodiazepine to avoid symptoms from becoming so intense they have a negative impact on the patient's quality of life. They should also be informed that these symptoms, including myalgias, arthralgias, and fatigue, are common with flulike syndrome. This syndrome has been identified as one of the most common dose-limiting toxicities associated with therapy with biologics due to its interference with normal activities. Page 536.

4.75 **The answer is b.**
Corticosteroids are usually avoided with biotherapy because they may block the effects of these drugs on the immune system. Corticosteroids inhibit prostaglandin synthesis. Page 540–546.

4.76 **The answer is d.**
Colony-stimulating factors mediate cellular proliferation, differentiation, and metabolism but not programmed cellular death. Page 602.

4.77 **The answer is b.**
Granulocyte and granulocyte-macrophage colony-stimulating factors decrease myelosuppression, febrile episodes, and number of hospital days when given in conjunction with chemotherapy. Both mucositis and anorexia are complications of chemotherapy and have no relationship to biotherapy. Page 605–606.

4.78 **The answer is c.**
HGFs activate the production and maturation of distinctive cell lineages, thereby enhancing the activity of mature neutrophils—phagocytosis, oxidative burst, antibody-dependent cytotoxicity, and chemotaxis. These actions allow the neutrophils to be more aggressive and effective in destroying pathogens. HGFs lessen the duration and severity of neutropenia, but they do not speed the onset. Page 605–606.

4.79 **The answer is d.**
Colony-stimulating factors are appropriate when febrile neutropenia is expected in more than 40% of patients, such as results from high-dose chemotherapy. It is not appropriate as routine prevention of neutropenia. Page 606, 468–469.

4.80 **The answer is b.**
Tissue hypoxia is the single most potent factor in erythropoietin production. In the presence of hypoxia, the kidneys increase production and secretion of endogenous erythropoietin. This in turn stimulates red blood cell production by the bone marrow, thereby correcting hypoxia. Page 603.

4.81 **The answer is c.**
Epoetin alfa is contraindicated in patients with uncontrolled hypertension. Hypertension, associated with rapid increases in hematocrit, rarely has been noted in cancer patients treated with epoetin alfa. Nevertheless, blood pressure should be monitored carefully, particularly in patients with an underlying history of hypertension or cardiovascular disease. Page 603.

4.82 **The answer is d.**
Granulocyte colony-stimulating factor has been shown to decrease the duration of neutropenia, the number of episodes of neutropenic fever, and the number of hospital days in patients receiving chemotherapy. Page 605–606.

4.83 **The answer is c.**
Hematopoietic growth factors are used as supportive therapy for patients receiving myelosuppressive therapy or undergoing a bone marrow transplant. Page 605–606.

4.84 **The answer is b.**
FDA-approved hematopoietic growth factors include granulocyte-macrophage colony-stimulating factors, granuloctye colony-stimulating factors, erythropoietin alfa, and interleukin-11, which prevents thrombocytopenia. Page 604.

4.85 **The answer is a.**
Stimulating the bone marrow to produce white blood cells when chemotherapy is given would enhance cell kill of the white blood cells and potentially cause mutations of myeloid cells and even leukemia. After 24 hours the chemotherapy is generally excreted, and administration of HGFs is deemed to be safe. Page 605–606.

Antineoplastic Agents

4.86 **The answer is b.**
Teach patients that paresthesias may occur in hands, feet, and hypopharynx. Patients should avoid exposure to cold for 1 to 5 days after the drug is given. A scarf wrapped around the neck and mouth prevents inspiration of cold air that could cause pharyngolaryngeal dysesthesia, which is an acute neurotoxicity. Page 374–375.

4.87 **The answer is a.**
For patients receiving capecitabine and warfarin concomitantly, frequent monitoring of INR or PT is recommended. Clinically significant increases in PT and INR have been observed within days to months after starting capecitabine and infrequently within 1 month of stopping capecitabine. The interaction of capecitabine and warfarin is probably due to an inhibition of cytochrome P-450 by capecitabine and/or its metabolites, whereby warfarin is not metabolized properly. Page 431, 1228–1229.

4.88 **The answer is d.**
Ketoconazole is a drug used to treat fungal infections but is also used as a second or third choice hormonal agent to treat prostate cancer. It blocks the production of male hormones in the testes and the adrenal glands, slowing the growth of some prostate cancers. Food, antacids, cimetidine, and rifampin impair absorption, whereas the acidic nature of cola and orange juice has been shown to enhance absorption. Page 737, 1629.

4.89 **The answer is a.**
The metabolic activation and inactivation or catabolism of drugs is carried out primarily by the liver. Page 367–368, 579.

4.90 **The answer is a.**
Cancer cells can overcome the effects of cytotoxic drugs either by increasing the number of target enzymes or by modifying the enzyme so as to interfere with binding to antagonistic drugs. The ability of cells to repair DNA lesions is an important resistance mechanism seen with alkylating agents and cisplatin. Page 559–560.

4.91 **The answer is b.**
Capecitabine is a prodrug, a chemical precursor of 5-FU. It undergoes three enzymatic changes in the body before becoming 5-FU within the body tissues. Page 1228, 1231.

4.92 The answer is c.
Altered coagulation and bleeding have been reported in patients taking capecitabine and anticoagulants concomitantly. These events occurred within several days and up to several months after initiating capecitabine therapy. The mechanism of interaction between dilantin and capecitabine appears to be the inhibition of the CYP2C9 isoenzyme by capecitabine or its metabolite. This interaction results in toxicities associated with elevated dilantin levels. Folic acid should be discontinued in patients receiving capecitabine because it could potentially increase the toxicity of 5-FU. Page 1228, 1231.

4.93 The answer is c.
Docetaxel is metabolized by the liver, and elevated liver functions can interfere with metabolism, causing enhanced toxicity of docetaxel. The dose needs to be reduced. Page 380–381, 491, 493.

4.94 The answer is c.
Chemotherapy currently is given preoperatively. The rationale for preoperative chemotherapy is to treat micrometastasis, to decrease the size of the primary tumor (thereby increasing the likelihood of limb salvage surgery), and to assess the effectiveness of the chemotherapeutic agents for 2–3 months. The route of the chemotherapy is either intravenous or intra-arterial. Page 1176.

4.95 The answer is c.
Side effects associated with CMF include myelosuppression, hair loss, and hemorrhagic cystitis. Page 243.

4.96 The answer is d.
Capecitabine is stopped at the first sign of any of the following grade 2 toxicities:

- Four bowel movements over normal
- Nocturnal stool
- Stomatitis with pain or discomfort
- Vomiting more than once in a 24-hour period
- Hand–foot syndrome with pain or discomfort or affecting activities of daily living
- Nausea, loss of appetite, or decrease in food intake over a 24-hour period
- Unexplained bleeding (especially for those on warfarin) Page 431, 1228.

4.97 The answer is c.
Although 5-fluorouracil is the cytotoxic agent of choice for colorectal cancer, it is most commonly administered in combination with leucovorin. Floxuridine is used in intraportal chemotherapy through the portal vein or hepatic artery into the liver in individuals with metastasis to the liver. Page 366.

4.98 The answer is c.
Patients are monitored closely for signs of renal impairment (increased blood urea nitrogen and creatinine, proteinuria), and the dose of melphalan may need to be reduced based on the severity of renal toxicity. It is also important to closely monitor serial blood counts because the bone marrow-suppressive effects of melphalan may be cumulative in older patients. Hypercalcemia and bone pain are symptoms of the disorder itself rather than adverse effects. Page 1525–1526.

4.99 The answer is c.
On the first occurrence of grade 2 toxicity (hand–foot syndrome with pain or discomfort or affecting activities of daily living) hold therapy until toxicity reaches a grade 0 1, and then restart at 100% dose. On the second occurrence, hold therapy until toxicity reaches grade

0–1, and then restart at 75% dose. Third occurrence, hold therapy until toxicity reaches grade 0–1, and then restart at 50% dose. Fourth occurrence, discontinue therapy. Page 431, 1228.

4.100 **The answer is a.**
Chemotherapy agents affect actively growing (anagen) hairs. Because anagen hair is the most rapidly proliferating cell population in the human body, alopecia is a common toxicity. Page 485–486.

4.101 **The answer is c.**
Chemotherapy agents associated with only mild hair loss include vinorelbine, bleomycin, carmustine, epirubicin, 5-FU, methotrexate, mitoxantrone, and capecitabine. Page 486.

4.102 **The answer is a.**
Arthralgias and myalgias with the taxanes is thought to be due to an inflammatory process. Corticosteroids are effective because of their ability to reduce the symptoms of inflammation and inhibit a variety of proinflammatory genes. Although arthralgias and myalgias are not associated with muscle inflammation per se, corticosteroids are effective in relieving the aches and pains associated with these symptoms. Page 490–491.

4.103 **The answer is c.**
Despite effective antiemetic regimens, 93% of patients receiving a high dose of cisplatin experience delayed nausea and vomiting up to 6–7 days. Page 471.

4.104 **The answer is a.**
The hand–foot syndrome is characterized by an often painful rash and swelling of the palms of the hands and soles of the feet. Patients can have difficulty walking, especially if the cause is capecitabine. Topotecan has similar effects as capecitabine but less dermatologic toxicity. Page 573–574.

4.105 **The answer is c.**
Myelosuppression is the most common and lethal side effect of chemotherapy. Because hematopoietic cells divide rapidly, they are vulnerable to chemotherapy, potentially resulting in dangerously low levels of red blood cells, white blood cells, and platelets. When this occurs, patients are at risk for bleeding, infection, and circulatory compromise. Page 465.

4.106 **The answer is c.**
Mitomycin causes cumulative and often delayed thrombocytopenia. Page 752.

4.107 **The answer is c.**
Symptoms that could indicate extravasation include swelling; stinging, burning, or pain at the injection site (not always present); redness (not often seen initially); and lack of blood return. Lack of blood return alone is not always indicative of an extravasation. An extravasation can occur even if a blood return is present. This patient is presenting the classic signs of extravasation, and the possibility of a flare reaction is inappropriate. Page 405–406.

4.108 **The answer is b.**
The most obvious sign of drug infiltration is a bleb formation at the injection site or swelling that occurs in more deeply accessed veins. The absence of a blood return does not confirm an extravasation. The needle bevel or cannula tip may be positioned against the vein wall, preventing appropriate and obvious blood return. Page 405–406.

4.109 **The answer is b.**
Hyperpigmentation occurs with bleomycin. Other drugs inducing this reaction include cyclophosphamide, busulfan, carmustine, nitrogen mustard, 5-FU, and etoposide. The other

drugs listed as choices in this question have in common hypersensitivity reactions. Page 483–484.

4.110 The answer is c.
Ifosfamide can cause cerebellar and cranial dysfunction but not myalgia or arthralgia. Page 490–491.

4.111 The answer is c.
Neurotoxicity characterized by metabolic encephalopathy manifested as blurred vision, seizures, motor system dysfunction, urinary incontinence, cranial nerve dysfunction, or irreversible coma has been reported in 5–30% of patients treated with ifosfamide. Page 490–491.

4.112 The answer is c.
To help prevent hemorrhagic cystitis during therapy with cyclophosphamide, patients are encouraged to drink 8–10 glasses of fluid a day and to void frequently. Page 496–498.

4.113 The answer is b.
The dose-limiting side effect for 5-FU when given as an intravenous bolus is myelosuppression, but when the drug is given by continuous intravenous infusion the dose-limiting side effect is mucositis. Page 1231–1234.

4.114 The answer is a.
Vincristine has a very low (< 10%) emetogenic potential. Page 470–472.

4.115 The answer is b.
Cisplatin frequently causes hypomagnesemia, which manifests as shaking. Daily magnesium supplementation is indicated during cisplatin therapy, and electrolyte levels should be monitored frequently. Page 438.

4.116 The answer is c.
A side effect of docetaxel is fluid retention. The incidence is related to the cumulative dose, which can be disabling and worsens with higher doses. Fluid retention is exhibited peripherally as abdominal ascites, as a pleural effusion, or as a combination. Page 381.

4.117 The answer is a.
Chemotherapy agents cause constipation as a result of autonomic nerve dysfunction manifested as colicky abdominal pain. Rectal emptying is diminished because nonfunctional afferent and efferent pathways from the sacral cord are interrupted. Page 470.

4.118 The answer is d.
When these cells are destroyed, atrophy of the intestinal mucosa and shortening of the intestinal villa with flattening and reduction of the absorptive surface results in a "slick gut." Thus the intestinal contents move rapidly through the gut, reducing absorption of nutrients. Page 469–470.

4.119 The answer is b.
The leucovorin potentiates the antitumor effect of the 5-fluorouracil, but it also increases the diarrhea. Page 366.

4.120 The answer is a.
Bleomycin can cause some mucositis, but not like the others, which cause mucositis plus potentially severe diarrhea. Page 469–470.

4.121 The answer is b.
Platinum-based chemotherapy can cause a specific nutritional deficiency, resulting in hypomagnesemia. The deficiency is highly specific to the particular drug. Page 438.

4.122 **The answer is a.**
Pulmonary toxicity usually is irreversible and progressive as a result of chemotherapy administration. The initial site of damage seems to be the endothelial cells, with an inflammatory-type reaction resulting in drug-induced pneumonitis. Page 493.

4.123 **The answer is a.**
Pulmonary toxicity usually presents clinically as dyspnea, unproductive cough, bilateral basilar rales, and tachypnea. Page 493.

4.124 **The answer is c.**
Cyclophosphamide and nitrogen mustard are alkylators and quite toxic but generally do not cause significant anemia. Carboplatin is platelet sparing. Page 465–466.

4.125 **The answer is c.**
Acute effects are immediate in onset, resolve quickly without serious complications, and dose reduction is not indicated. Chronic cardiotoxicity occurs weeks or months after administration. Because effects are non reversible, the cumulative dose is monitored and discontinued prior to onset of toxicity. Page 487.

4.126 **The answer is d.**
Vincristine, vinblastine, and vinorelbine are the most common chemotherapy agents to cause neuropathies that can result in constipation. Page 470.

Hematopoietic Stem Cell Transplant

4.127 **The answer is c.**
Allogeneic transplants are indicated for acute myelogenous leukemia, chronic myelogenous leukemia, and acute lymphocytic leukemia. Autologous transplants are indicated for breast cancer predominantly and are used for non-Hodgkin's lymphoma and multiple myeloma. Page 506–507.

4.128 **The answer is c.**
Growth factors, made through recombinant DNA processes, stimulate pluripotent stem cells to differentiate and mature. These products are administered in transplantation and cause the body to overproduce pluripotent stem cells beyond the body's required needs and also induce cell differentiation and maturation. The administration of HGFs takes place right before pheresis so that more cells are available for collection from the circulation. This process is referred to as mobilization. Page 365, 601–602.

4.129 **The answer is b.**
Veno-occlusive disease is almost exclusive to hematopoietic stem cell transplantation and is the most common nonrelapse life-threatening complication of preparative regimen–related toxicity for hematopoietic stem cell transplantation. Page 520, 522.

4.130 **The answer is a.**
Risk factors for late chronic GVHD include, among others, mismatched donor and recipient, female-to-male transplants, positive herpes simplex and cytomegalovirus, patient age over 18 years, prior grade 2–3 acute GVHD, and chronic myelogenous leukemia recipients who received methotrexate and cyclosporine as chronic GVHD prophylaxis. Page 517.

4.131 **The answer is b.**
TBI is given before marrow infusion to prevent graft rejection by the patient's immune system. It offers optimal tumor cell kill because it penetrates the central nervous system and other privileged sites. It is usually given in fractionated doses to reduce toxicities, and it can be given as a booster to patients with bulky disease. Page 505, 264–265.

4.132 The answer is b.

One advantage to using peripheral PPSCs and progenitor cells obtained from peripheral blood is the more rapid recovery of neutrophils and platelets when progenitor cells are used. This is because the committed progenitors collected for blood cell transplant are farther along the differentiation pathway than are the PPSCs harvested from the bone marrow. Another advantage is that no anesthesia is required for blood cell transplant, so there is less risk of complications and fewer medical contraindications than with bone marrow harvest. Page 506–508.

4.133 The answer is a.

The advantages of autologous transplant over allogeneic transplant are the absence of GVHD and fewer toxicities. Autologous transplant is less toxic because there is no veno-occlusive disease or GVHD. However, there is a risk of tumor contamination in the autologous marrow, and there is no benefit of the GVL effect, which can reduce the risk of relapse. Page 506–507.

4.134 The answer is b.

One of the main reasons for using blood rather than bone marrow-derived cells for autologous transplantation is to avoid tumor contamination from bone marrow. Gene-marking experiments have clearly indicated that relapses can originate from tumor cells contaminating the cryopreserved cells. It is true that there is a shortened nadir with blood-derived cells, but it is not the best answer. Page 506–507.

4.135 The answer is a.

A random donor platelet concentrate may expose the recipient to multiple tissue antigens, leading to platelet refractoriness. A single donor platelet concentrate is taken from one donor or one (human leukocyte antigen) HLA-matched donor; patients are therefore not exposed to multiple antigens. This may be important with patients who are severely immunosuppressed, such as those who have undergone stem cell transplantation. Page 750.

4.136 The answer is c.

A serious transfusion complication in patients who are significantly immunosuppressed is the risk of developing graft-versus-host disease. It is generally recommended that all blood products given to the severely immunocompromised host be exposed to pretransfusion irradiation. Blood is irradiated to inhibit proliferation of lymphocytes without impairment of platelets, red cells, or granulocytes. Page 516.

4.137 The answer is d.

Blood products must be irradiated to destroy T lymphocytes, which can cause graft-versus-host disease in the marrow recipient. Patients whose platelets become refractory to random platelet transfusions can receive (human leukocyte antigen) HLA-matched platelets from family or community donors, and platelets that have undergone plasmapheresis from marrow donors yield optimal increments. Alloimmunization and platelet refractoriness contribute to a 1% case fatality rate from hemorrhage complications. Page 516.

4.138 The answer is c.

Aggressive antiviral therapy with intravenous acyclovir is the standard therapy. Page 515.

4.139 The answer is a.

Anecdotal reports and clinical observations suggest that use of masks and garment covers is declining. Cost–benefit analysis does not ensure that such methods eliminate or reduce infection. Hand washing, scrupulous hygiene, and protective isolation may be the most cost-effective and meaningful conventions for infection control. Page 514–516.

4.140 **The answer is b.**
Immunosuppressive medications are aimed at removing or inactivating T lymphocytes that attack target organs. Cyclosporine and methotrexate inhibit T lymphocytes that are believed to be responsible for acute graft-versus-host disease and are the first-line therapy. Page 515.

4.141 **The answer is c.**
Veno-occlusive disease (VOD) is almost exclusive to hematopoietic stem cell transplantation (HSCT) and is the most common nonrelapse life-threatening complication of preparative regimen-related toxicity for HSCT. Patients at risk for VOD include those with hepatitis and infections before HSCT and those who receive repeated doses of chemotherapy before transplant in addition to high-dose irradiation. An additional risk factor is the use of antimicrobial therapy with acyclovir, amphotericin, or vancomycin and mismatched or unrelated allogeneic marrow grafts. Page 515, 520.

4.142 **The answer is b.**
Side effects of trimethoprim include rash, nausea, vomiting, hepatotoxicity, and myelosuppression. Page 514–515.

4.143 **The answer is c.**
Treatment strategies for graft-versus-host disease include systemic immunosuppressive therapy; topical steroids, which may or may not be beneficial; and antithymocyte globulin as a single agent or in combination with steroids. Page 518–519.

4.144 **The answer is c.**
P. carinii is a protozoan that causes infection in children with primary immunodeficiency disorders, persons with AIDS, and those with cancer who are undergoing immunosuppressive therapy. Untreated, *P. carinii* is fatal, and even with therapy mortality is high. The treatment of choice is trimethoprim-sulfamethoxazole. Page 514–515.

4.145 **The answer is c.**
The diagnosis of veno-occlusive disease is based on clinical findings in the first 21 days after HCT. Diagnostic criteria include two or more of the following symptoms: hyperbilirubinemia, hepatomegaly, right-upper quadrant pain, and fluid retention. Page 520.

4.146 **The answer is a.**
The pathophysiology of the syndrome begins with injury of the endothelial lining of hepatic venules and sinusoids. This endothelial injury leads to cytokine and tumor necrosis factor activation, which stimulates coagulation and thrombosis. The resulting impairment of blood flow produces the syndrome of hepatic veno-occlusive disease, which leads to renal insufficiency and, ultimately, to multiorgan failure and death. Page 515.

4.147 **The answer is c.**
The incidence of oral herpes simplex virus infection in cancer patients receiving chemotherapy is approximately 50%. In the hematopoietic stem cell transplantation population, the incidence approaches 80%. Page 515.

Unproven/Alternative Therapies

4.148 The answer is c.
Homeopathy is based upon the theory of similars, which holds that a drug that causes symptoms at full strength will cure those symptoms if it is diluted. Page 629.

4.149 The answer is b.
The mind–body approach can be divided into two different approaches, the use of the mind to overcome dysfunction (i.e., hypnosis) or the use of the psychic energy of the body to overcome problems. The latter approach is embodied in techniques such as healing touch, Reiki therapy, and polarity therapy. Page 627–628.

4.150 The answer is c.
The therapeutic dose may be significantly lower in cancer patients, and tricyclic antidepressants should be taken as scheduled and should not be withdrawn or stopped suddenly. Doing so may risk cholinergic rebound, including nausea and vomiting, headache, diaphoresis, and chills. Page 672.

4.151 The answer is c.
Herbal agents can be harmful if taken over extended periods of time; kava can cause liver damage. Ginseng is a stimulant used for hypersomnia that should not be taken with monoamine oxidase inhibitors or anticoagulants. There is no evidence that lavender is addicting. Page 645.

4.152 The answer is c.
Homeopathy, a medical system developed in the late 18th century, is based on the theory of similars, which holds that a drug that causes symptoms at full strength will cure those symptoms if it is diluted. Page 629.

4.153 The answer is a.
Cognitive Behavior Therapy has the best outcome when there is a good match between the patient's appraisal of the situation and the coping strategy selected. Emotion-focused coping strategies are used when there is little control over the situation, and problems-focused coping strategies are used when there is high control over the situation. Page 678.

CHAPTER 5

Symptom Management

ETIOLOGY AND PATTERNS OF SYMPTOMS

5.1 Mr. James has metastatic prostate cancer, diabetes, and uncontrolled hypertension. He has mild congestive heart failure and is currently receiving two units of packed red blood cells for a hemoglobin of 8 g/dL. Your colleague asks why he is not given erythropoietin alfa rather than risk complications of a fluid overload. Your *most appropriate* response would be which of the following?

a. Erythropoietin alfa injections take 2–6 weeks to be effective.
b. Erythropoietin alfa is contraindicated in patients with uncontrolled hypertension.
c. Erythropoietin alfa can potentially increase his severity of congestive heart failure and stroke.
d. Erythropoietin alfa is only given to anemic patients being treated with myelosuppressive chemotherapy with noncurative intent and who are mildly symptomatic.

5.2 Based on modality of treatment, which of the following patients would you expect to have the *most severe* fatigue?

a. Joe, who is being treated with biologic response modifiers
b. Karen, who is undergoing chemotherapy
c. Martha, who has just had surgery
d. Thomas, who is undergoing radiation treatment

5.3 Alex has undergone allogeneic stem cell transplantation, and it is now day + 30. He is experiencing itching and burning of the skin. Which of the following statements is *true* concerning his symptoms?

a. These symptoms are indicative of acute graft-versus-host disease.
b. These symptoms are indicative of chronic graft-versus-host disease.
c. These symptoms are to be expected and are likely due to the multiple medications he is taking.
d. These symptoms suggest an appropriate immune response.

5.4 Pruritus frequently accompanies jaundice in patients with obstructive biliary disease. Which of the following *best* describes the mechanism of pruritus under these circumstances?

a. Itching is primarily due to dry flaky skin.
b. Itching is caused by irritation of the cutaneous sensory nerve fibers by accumulated bile salts.
c. Itching is due to poor body hygiene and the use of deodorant soaps.
d. Itching is due to the accumulation of cholestyramine.

5.5 Your patient, who is receiving radiation therapy for a malignant brain tumor, complains of increased daytime fatigue and somnolence. To help her understand what might be causing her symptoms, you could say all *except* which of the following?

a. The incidence of sleep disturbances is 50% greater in people who receive radiation therapy to the brain.
b. Somnolence is commonly seen in patients who receive whole brain irradiation.
c. Sleep disturbance occurs 4–12 weeks after radiation is complete.
d. Her symptoms might be related to other medications she is taking, specifically corticosteroids.

5.6 Your patient is receiving paclitaxel on a weekly basis. She commonly experiences nausea and is prescribed the antiemetic granisetron to take if she needs it. She complains that she is having trouble sleeping and often feels agitated at night. Which of the following is a logical explanation for her symptoms?

a. Her difficulty in sleeping is likely due to the decadron she takes to prevent hypersensitivity reactions to the paclitaxel.
b. She is probably feeling agitated due to the granisetron.
c. Adverse neurologic effects, including sleep disruption, are common in patients taking paclitaxel.
d. Insomnia and restlessness are common in anyone undergoing treatment for cancer.

5.7 Your patient has lymphoma and has been tracking his fever for the past week. He has not recently had chemotherapy but does complain of a fever that has been low grade with only a slight spike without returning to normal. He is frequently tachycardic and tachypneic with some periods of extreme fatigue. Given these symptoms his fever pattern is probably indicative of which type of infection?

a. Disseminated fungal infection
b. Viral infection
c. Bacterial infection
d. Gram-negative infection

5.8 Mr. Allen received high-dose methotrexate for sarcoma of his pelvis 6 days ago and is currently at home complaining of a low-grade fever, slight mucositis, and diarrhea (5 to 6 times per day) for the past 2 days. His medications include prophylactic antibiotics and morphine sulfate for pain. Nursing management includes which of the following?

a. Give loperamide 2 mg orally with each loose stool, not to exceed 16 mg per day.
b. Push fluids and oral hygiene. Slight mucositis and diarrhea are expected.
c. Stop the antibiotics because they are probably causing the diarrhea.
d. Get a stool specimen to test for *Clostridium difficile*, which is common in patients receiving prophylactic antibiotics. He is probably neutropenic.

5.9 Management of a febrile nonhemolytic transfusion reaction presenting as fever, chills, headache, hypotension, tachypnea, and dyspnea includes all *except* which of the following?

a. Stop the transfusion, and maintain patent intravenous line with normal saline.
b. Notify physician, and administer acetaminophen for fever, meperidine for chills and rigors, and antihistamine for dyspnea.
c. Place the patient in the Trendelenburg position, and administer a fluid bolus.
d. Assist in ruling out infection.

5.10 Your patient has notified you that she has intense pain across her scalp 2½ weeks after her first dose of chemotherapy. Your advice to her would include all *except* which of the following management strategies?

a. Referral to her doctor because this could indicate skin metastases
b. Anti-inflammatory agents to decrease inflammation
c. Massage the scalp
d. Warm compresses to the scalp

5.11 A 70-year-old patient is receiving cyclophosphamide, doxorubicin, and vincristine for lung cancer. He also is receiving opioid analgesics for pain. He normally has a bowel movement every day. He reports that he has not had a bowel movement in 3 days but does not feel the urge and has not been eating normally. Appropriate nursing assessment and management include which of the following?

a. He has not had a normal routine so it is a good idea to increase fiber and fluids and call if there is no bowel movement in 24 hours.
b. He should take a laxative, such as milk of magnesia, and call if he has no bowel movement in 48 hours.
c. Elderly patients often have a decrease in colonic transit time, and with time he will have results.
d. He should take a laxative and call if there are no results in 24 hours.

5.12 The etiology of anemia of malignancy is complicated, but the two *most common* causes include

a. Tumor secretion of cytokines that affect red blood cell metabolism and anemia of chronic disease
b. Protein-calorie malnutrition and bleeding
c. Increased red blood cell destruction due to chronic hemorrhage and hemolysis
d. Decreased red blood cell production secondary to primary disease and myelosuppressive therapy

5.13 Your patient with leukemia who has recently undergone a stem cell transplant is severely immunosuppressed and is experiencing a coagulopathy. She is also experiencing hemoptysis, dyspnea, and fatigue. She is *most likely* suffering from which of the following?

a. Lung cancer
b. Pneumonia
c. Alveolar hemorrhage
d. Cardiac tamponade

5.14 Management of hemoptysis due to alveolar hemorrhage includes which of the following?

a. Antianxiety medications
b. High-dose corticosteroids
c. Thoracentesis to relieve dyspnea
d. Codeine or hydrocodone for cough suppression

5.15 **A 72-year-old patient with lung cancer complains of extreme fatigue. He is not very active, but with a hemoglobin of 7.7 g/dL the decision is made to bring him into the outpatient infusion center to be transfused with two units of packed red blood cells. The *primary* problem associated with a low hemoglobin count and the reason to transfuse is which of the following?**

a. Risk for hemorrhage
b. Risk for angina
c. Risk for stroke
d. Risk for hypovolemia

5.16 **Emesis is a complex physiologic response to the toxic effects of chemotherapy. Which of the following is *not* considered to be a part of the chemotherapy-induced nausea–vomiting response mechanism?**

a. Stimulation of cells that line the duodenum
b. Serotonin stimulation of the vagal nerve
c. Physical injury to cancer cells
d. Vagal stimulation of the medulla oblongata

5.17 **Which of the following chemotherapy agents is *most likely* to potentiate the problem of esophagitis in patients also receiving radiation therapy to the esophagus?**

a. Dactinomycin
b. 5-Fluorouracil
c. Paclitaxel
d. Procarbazine

5.18 **An elderly woman presents with a thyroid mass and symptoms of dyspnea and dysphagia. Assessment indicates carcinoma of the thyroid with metastases to the lung. Her symptoms of dyspnea and dysphagia are *most likely* to be the result of which of the following?**

a. Involvement of the parathyroid gland and associated hypercalcemia
b. Compressive effects of the tumor on the larynx and esophagus
c. Infection caused by irritation of the oral mucosa
d. A high concentration of iodine in the follicular cells of the thyroid

5.19 **Following a course of high-dose chemotherapy your patient complains of mouth soreness. Upon physical inspection you notice the lining of her mouth to be ulcerated with red patches. Your care recommendations are based on which of the following facts regarding oral care?**

a. She should rinse with granulocyte-macrophage colony-stimulating factor (GM-CSF) mouthwash.
b. She should decrease the frequency of her oral care because the lining of her oral cavity is becoming irritated.
c. She should rinse with a normal saline solution 4× daily.
d. She should rinse with a chlorhexidine solution.

5.20 **Mucositis is observed more often when**

a. Fluorouracil (5-FU) is given alone
b. High-dose methotrexate is given alone
c. Bleomycin is used to abruptly replace 5-FU
d. 5-FU is combined with other mucositis-producing drugs, such as methotrexate and doxorubicin

5.21 Which of the following factors is considered a *major* risk factor for stomatitis with cancer treatment?

a. Dehydration
b. Malnutrition
c. Preexisting dental problems
d. Patients with hematological malignancies.

5.22 Which of the following poses the *greatest* risk of mucositis to a patient receiving radiation to the base of the tongue?

a. Metal tooth fillings
b. Tobacco usage
c. Alcohol consumption
d. Poor oral hygiene

5.23 Which of the following would be considered an example of direct stomatotoxicity?

a. The cytotoxic action of drugs on the cells of the oral basal epithelium causes a decrease in the rate of cell renewal.
b. Bleeding from the gums following flossing in the patient with low platelets.
c. Cellular breakdown is due to high alcohol content in mouthwashes.
d. Pancytopenia and gingivitis occur.

5.24 After radiation treatment, Michelle complains of a dry mouth and within 3 weeks develops thick ropy saliva. What is the side effect Michelle is experiencing?

a. Xerostomia
b. Mucositis
c. Trismus
d. Desquamation

5.25 Four weeks after radiation therapy ends, Mr. Allen complains that the xerostomia is not improving. The physician prescribes oral pilocarpine. Your teaching includes which of the following points?

a. Photosensitivity worsens over time.
b. The pilocarpine is a saliva substitute.
c. The pilocarpine is used to suppress the exocrine gland production.
d. Side effects include diaphoresis, lacrimation, and increased gastric secretion.

5.26 Besides a dry mouth, the *primary* problem with xerostomia is

a. Lack of pH balance in the mouth
b. Enamel decalcification
c. Heightened taste sensation for sweet and sour foods
d. Increased tracheal and esophageal irritation

5.27 Mr. Zahir is receiving cisplatin therapy for testicular cancer and requires a 5-HT_3 receptor antagonist and a corticosteroid daily during his treatment. The rationale for this combination is based on which of the following?

a. The corticosteroid and 5-HT_3 antagonist provide a direct analgesic effect.
b. The corticosteroid is used to boost the immune system.
c. The corticosteroid enhances the antiemetic effect of the serotonin antagonist.
d. The 5-HT_3 receptor antagonist alone is not compatible with cisplatin.

5.28 Which of the following antineoplastic agents is *not* associated with delayed nausea?
a. Cisplatin
b. Paclitaxel
c. Doxorubicin
d. Cyclophosphamide

5.29 Anticipatory nausea and vomiting during the 12-hour period before chemotherapy occurs in approximately what percentage of patients?
a. 15%
b. 20%
c. 25%
d. 30%

5.30 Betty will be having a mastectomy. In planning ahead and helping her to get ready for the surgery, you tell her that
a. Because of the bed rest required in recovery, surgery will decrease her energy requirements.
b. Nutritional problems resulting from her surgery will probably extend well past the immediate perioperative period.
c. Surgery on her breast cancer should not have any direct implication for her nutritional needs.
d. Surgery can increase her energy requirements to 1.5 times what she normally needs.

5.31 Mr. Thomas has pancreatic cancer and feels as if he cannot get out of bed at times and that if he tried he would probably be up for only a few minutes due to an overwhelming loss of strength. This loss of strength is referred to as which of the following?
a. Asthenia
b. Marasmus
c. Protein-calorie malnutrition
d. Anorexia-cachexia syndrome

TOXICITY AND RATING SCALES

5.32 Mr. Allen describes his pain as a 7 on the verbal numeric rating scale. He has no evidence of tachycardia, hypertension, diaphoresis, or pallor. From these observations you conclude which of the following regarding Mr. Allen's pain?
a. He is experiencing acute or intermittent pain.
b. He is experiencing chronic pain.
c. Because he does not appear to be in pain, further assessment is necessary before treating his pain.
d. His pain medication is inadequate.

5.33 Ms. Clay has metastatic breast cancer and is currently undergoing chemotherapy and is receiving an antiemetic regimen of granisetron, dexamethasone, and lorazepam. Her white blood cell count is 3200/mm^3, hemoglobin is 11.2 g/dL, and platelets 72,000/mm^3. Her chief complaint for the week after her treatment is fatigue. She only begins to feel better just before her next treatment. Which of the following *most appropriately* addresses her complaint?
a. Suggest that she stop any exercise as she may become short of breath.
b. Evaluate her antiemetic regimen to determine which drugs might be causing her fatigue.
c. Suggest that she be started on darbepoietin alfa injections.
d. Suggest that she practice meditation for 1 hour each day.

5.34 Which of the following is the *most accurate* measure of dyspnea in the individual with cancer?

a. Respiratory rate
b. Oxygen saturation
c. Arterial blood gas level
d. Patient self-report

5.35 Which of the following chemotherapy agents is *most frequently* associated with moderate to severe hair loss?

a. Doxorubicin
b. Bleomycin
c. Methotrexate
d. Mitoxantrone

5.36 The primary criteria for assessment of depression include all of the following characteristics *except*

a. Characteristics that are a change from previous functioning
b. Characteristics that are persistent
c. Characteristics that were preexistent
d. Characteristics that occur more days than not

5.37 A patient's physical performance classification is established before treatment and is intended to accomplish all *except* which of the following?

a. Determine whether or not the individual is a candidate for a research study.
b. Influence the type of treatment planned.
c. Establish the individual's quality of life using numeric values.
d. Provide prognostic information.

5.38 You are attempting to choose an instrument to gain a more complete diet history from Carlos. He has already told you that he doesn't pay much attention to what he eats, and he has a hard time remembering what he had for lunch (or if he had lunch) yesterday. Carlos is very upset about his recent cancer diagnosis, and this has changed his eating habits considerably. However, he is willing to cooperate with you, and he understands the importance of being honest in the things he tells you. Keeping in mind that Carlos is in the hospital now but he will not be for most of his treatment, you choose

a. A calorie count
b. A 24-hour dietary recall
c. A food frequency record
d. A diet diary

5.39 A proxy rater in quality-of-life studies should be used when

a. The patient is not considered to be a reliable rater.
b. The patient is not likely to give an honest response.
c. The patient does not want to complete a quality-of-life study.
d. The patient has cognitive impairment that makes them unable to complete the rating.

5.40 The Functional Assessment of Cancer Therapy (FACT/FACIT) instrument is used to measure all *except* which of the following dimensions of quality of life?

a. Sexual well-being
b. Physical well-being
c. Emotional well-being
d. Social/family well-being

5.41 Which of the following antiemetic regimens would be *most appropriate* for a cisplatin-based (level-5 emetogenic chemotherapy [> 50 mg/m^2]) regimen?

a. Metoclopromide, 10–20 mg PO QID
b. Ondansetron, 32 mg IV, before chemotherapy
c. Metoclopromide, 1–3 mg/kg/IV, before and q 2–4 hours for 2 additional doses (± dexamethasone, 5–8 mg with first dose), and 10 mg QID PRN ± dexamethasone, 4 mg TID.
d. Metoclopromide, 2–3 mg/kg IV, before and for 1 to 4 additional doses (add IV dexamethasone, 10 to 20 mg, ± lorazepam, 1 to 2 mg, to first dose), + metoclopromide 10 mg PO QID, + dexamethasone, 4 mg TID, or prochlorperazine spansules, 15 to 30 mg q 12 hours, + dexamethasone, 4 mg TID, ± lorazepam, 1 mg q 4 hours PRN

ALTERATIONS IN COMFORT

5.42 Poorly treated or unrelieved pain is a common problem for the individual with cancer. A *common* reason for this is which of the following?

a. Access to health care and appropriate treatment
b. Reluctance of the patient to report pain
c. Failure of the healthcare profession to routinely assess pain and pain relief
d. Difficulty controlling cancer pain and expensive medications

5.43 Your patient recently began oral morphine therapy. He complains of nausea, vomiting, and itching. The best option(s) for managing these symptoms include all *except* which of the following?

a. Switch to tramadol.
b. Switch to fentanyl or oxymorphone.
c. Change the dosing regimen or route of the same drug.
d. Add another drug that counteracts the adverse effects.

5.44 Which of the following statements regarding the use of tricyclic antidepressants (TCAs) in pain management is *true*?

a. TCAs (low dose) are effective for the treatment of neuropathic pain.
b. Concomitant use of opioid analgesics is not problematic because sedation and orthostatic hypotension are uncommon with low-dose TCAs.
c. The dose of TCAs must be increased from the doses used to treat depression to be effective in pain management.
d. TCAs have not been found to be effective in treating neuropathic pain.

5.45 The dimension of pain that encompasses the meaning that the pain experience has for a person is the

a. Behavioral dimension
b. Affective dimension
c. Sensory dimension
d. Cognitive dimension

5.46 Opiate-related daytime sedation is a known side effect of chronic pain management. Which of the following agents has *not* been shown to be an effective treatment for opiate-induced sedation?

a. Lorazepam
b. Methylphenidate
c. Donepezil
d. Dextroamphetamine

5.47 Which of the following is *not* effective treatment for pruritus related to systemic opioids?

a. Meticulous skin hygiene
b. Emollient lotions
c. Naloxone
d. Antihistamines

5.48 In general, dyspnea *most commonly* occurs when which of the following is present?

a. Chronic pain
b. Physiologic parameters indicating altered pulmonary function tests
c. An increase in respiratory effort necessary to overcome obstructive or restrictive disease
d. A decrease in the amount of respiratory muscles required to maintain adequate breathing

5.49 Ms. Howe has persistent productive coughing, which, she says, is exhausting. Which intervention should *not* be used?

a. Inspired air is warmed and humidified.
b. Cigarette smoking is discouraged.
c. Deep breathing and coughing techniques are taught and reinforced.
d. Narcotic medications are used for cough suppression.

5.50 Mrs. James has recently started morphine sulfate to control her pain. She is concerned about the side effects. You assure her that within 1–2 weeks she will become tolerant of all *except* which of the following side effects associated with opioid administration?

a. Constipation
b. Lethargy
c. Nausea
d. Agitation

5.51 Which of the following is considered *appropriate* first-line treatment for dyspnea?

a. Glucocorticoids
b. Benzodiazepines
c. Morphine sulfate
d. Oxygen therapy

5.52 After amputation, Mr. Riley reports pain in the missing lower leg. The nurse should be aware that this phantom limb pain

a. Generally decreases substantially during the first year
b. Is likely to worsen with aging
c. Indicates a patient's inability to cope with loss
d. Usually occurs immediately after surgery

ALTERATIONS IN PROTECTIVE MECHANISMS

5.53 Your patient received chemotherapy 6 days ago and has now called with a fever of 101.8°F and chills. She has a productive cough and, except for not being able to get warm, feels fine. You send her for a complete blood count and learn that her absolute granulocyte count is 500 cells/mm^3. You instruct her to come to the hospital to be admitted. Your decision is based on which of the following?

a. She is at risk for bleeding and severe anemia.
b. She probably has pneumonia and needs to be observed.
c. When the neutrophil count is 500/mm^3 or less, approximately 20% or more of febrile episodes have an associated bacteremia.
d. She is past her nadir, but cultures need to be done to determine the source of a possible infection.

5.54 Your patient has a platelet count of 9000/mm^3 and has had frequent nosebleeds. He has an order for a platelet transfusion, but has acetaminophen, a corticosteroid, and an antihistamine ordered prior to the platelet transfusion. What is the rationale for the premedications prior to the platelet transfusion?

a. To prevent fever in the patient
b. To help make the patient more comfortable
c. To prevent the risk of platelet refractoriness
d. To prevent the risk of a febrile nonhemolytic transfusion reaction

5.55 Mrs. Geoffry has lung cancer that has metastasized to her bones. She has recently completed 3 weeks of radiation to her thoracic spine. She phones you with complaints of recent onset of repeatedly dropping things and radicular pain. Which of the following *best* describes the etiology of her symptoms?

a. Her symptoms are most likely due to delayed effects of radiation.
b. Her symptoms are related to the metastatic disease in her bones.
c. Her symptoms are new and are most likely indicative of spinal cord compression at the level of her thoracic spine.
d. Her symptoms are probably related to metastatic disease in her brain.

5.56 What are the *appropriate* nursing actions for Mrs. Geoffry (see above question) based on her etiology?

a. She should see her physician immediately for evaluation.
b. She should be cautioned against dropping items and instructed to take an analgesic for pain.
c. She should take it easy as she will get better in a few weeks because that is when the radiation has its peak effect.
d. She should be fitted for a spinal brace as the radiation therapy may have weakened her spine.

5.57 Mrs. George has multiple myeloma and has been confined to bed because of a pathological fracture. Her daughter calls the nurse because her mother is sleeping more and is becoming difficult to arouse. The patient's symptoms are most likely *not* due to which of the following?

a. Hyperviscosity syndrome due to multiple myeloma
b. Hypercalcemia due to multiple myeloma
c. Hypocalcemia due to multiple myeloma
d. Steroid psychosis

5.58 Which of the following would *not* be an appropriate therapeutic intervention for chronic phantom limb pain after an above-the-knee amputation?

a. Relaxation to minimize emotional/psychological stress
b. Morphine sulfate with immediate-release morphine as needed
c. Muscle relaxants and tranquilizers
d. Stump shrinker to exert pressure, alternating with heat compresses

5.59 The risk for osteoporosis is increased in men with prostate cancer being treated with androgen-ablative therapy because

a. Osteoblastic bone formation is increased.
b. Osteoclastic activity is decreased.
c. Estrogen therapy increases osteoblasts.
d. Loss of bone mineral density is increased.

5.60 Which of the following *best* describes the therapeutic action of bisphosphonates?

a. Bisphosphonates stimulate osteoclast activity.
b. Bisphosphonates bind to bone to stabilize the bone mineral and inhibit breakdown.
c. Bisphosphonates are natural inhibitors of bone mineralization.
d. Bisphosphonates inhibit osteoblast activity.

5.61 All of the following are goals in the treatment of primary malignant bone cancer *except*

a. Preservation of maximum function
b. Early intervention in children believed to be at high risk
c. Eradication of tumor
d. Avoidance of amputation

5.62 Infection in the neutropenic patient is a serious complication of chemotherapy and can be fatal in what percentage of patients?

a. 15%
b. 30%
c. 60%
d. 75%

5.63 Kate is being treated with chemotherapy for Hodgkin's disease and is monitored weekly for myelosuppression. Her white blood cell count is 4000 cells/mm^3, with 34% segmented neutrophils and 3% bands. What is her absolute neutrophil count (ANC)?

a. 48 cells/mm^3
b. 480 cells/mm^3
c. 1480 cells/mm^3
d. 2480 cells/mm^3

5.64 Based on Kate's ANC the chemotherapy is withheld. What answer *best* describes why the chemotherapy is withheld?

a. Neutropenia is the most common cause of life-threatening infections.
b. Neutropenia is the most common risk factor for the development of oral candidiasis.
c. Neutropenia always precedes the development of anemia, which puts Kate at risk for extreme fatigue.
d. Neutropenia always precedes the development of thrombocytopenia, which puts Kate at risk for bleeding.

5.65 Mr. Mendez, who is receiving high-dose chemotherapy, has developed neutropenia. The usual symptoms of infection will likely be absent or muted in this patient because

a. Most infections are due to organisms that are part of the body's normal flora.
b. The white blood cells drop rapidly, and recovery time is slow.
c. Neutrophils are necessary to produce an inflammatory response.
d. The immunoglobulins are reduced.

5.66 How many days after chemotherapy does neutropenia typically develop, and what is the usual time for recovery?

a. Develops 4–6 days after chemotherapy with recovery in 2 weeks
b. Develops 16–20 days after chemotherapy with recovery in 6 weeks
c. Develops 8–12 days after chemotherapy with recovery in 3–4 weeks
d. Develops 4 weeks after chemotherapy with recovery in 6 weeks

5.67 **The *most common* site of infection in the granulocytopenic patient is which of the following?**

a. Perineal region
b. Respiratory tract
c. Urinary tract
d. Gastrointestinal tract

5.68 **Oral candidiasis can be a serious complication of cancer chemotherapy. Under which of the following circumstances would prophylactic antifungal therapy *not* be indicated?**

a. All neutropenic patients receiving chemotherapy
b. Patients with acute leukemia undergoing chemotherapy
c. Patients undergoing allogeneic hematopoietic stem cell transplantation
d. Afebrile patients with an absolute neutrophil count less than $1000/mm^3$ for more than 1 week

5.69 **The administration of colony-stimulating factors as prophylaxis following highly myelosuppressive chemotherapy is intended to accomplish primarily which of the following?**

a. Prevent pancytopenia.
b. Minimize infection and stomatitis.
c. Maintain white blood cell count above 10,000 cells/mm^3.
d. Decrease the number of days that the white blood cell count is at its nadir.

5.70 **Five days after chemotherapy for lung cancer your 72-year-old patient calls with fever and chills. Blood counts reveal an absolute neutrophil count of $429/mm^3$. Which of the following constitutes *appropriate* management of this patient?**

a. Begin oral antibiotics, and monitor fever.
b. He needs a chest x-ray to rule out pneumonia.
c. Arrange for admission to the hospital, and administer antibiotics immediately.
d. He is at the nadir of the white blood cell count and will gradually improve on his own.

5.71 **The *most common* and lethal side effect of chemotherapy is**

a. Myelosuppression
b. Respiratory distress
c. Increased liver function tests
d. Electrolyte imbalance from nausea, vomiting, and diarrhea

5.72 **Actions of recombinant thrombopoietin include all *except* which of the following?**

a. Reduces the duration of thrombocytopenia
b. Stimulates the proliferation of megakaryocytes into platelets
c. Stimulates the differentiation of megakaryocytes into platelets
d. Stimulates multipotential progenitor cells that result in increased numbers of platelets

5.73 **A cumulative and delayed thrombocytopenia has been associated with all *except* which of the following chemotherapeutic agents?**

a. Lomustine
b. Carmustine
c. Mithramycin
d. Methotrexate

5.74 Mr. Jones has a malignant brain tumor and has been receiving 5-fluorouracil and carmustine every 6 weeks. His blood counts today reveal a white blood cell count of 3000 cells/mm^3, hemoglobin of 10 g/dL, and platelet count of 50,000 cells/mm^3. His treatment is delayed today. The *best* explanation for delaying his treatment is which of the following?

a. He is moderately to severely immunosuppressed.
b. He is moderately anemic.
c. He is at moderate risk for bleeding due to thrombocytopenia.
d. He is at severe risk for bleeding due to thrombocytopenia.

5.75 When platelets decrease to 10,000 cells/mm^3, the patient is *most* at risk for which of the following?

a. Petechiae
b. Epistaxis
c. Concomitant thrombocytopenia
d. Spontaneous central nervous system bleeding

5.76 The *most common* cause of thrombocytopenia in patients with cancer is

a. Infection
b. Hypersplenism
c. Decreased megakaryocytopoiesis
d. Immune-mediated thrombocytopenia

5.77 Jenny has chronic lymphocytic leukemia. She has immature platelets in the bone marrow and a platelet count of 45,000 cells/mm^3. She has evidence of petechiae, purpura, and ecchymosis. Her condition is *most likely* associated with which of the following platelet disorders?

a. Thrombocytopenia
b. Idiopathic thrombocytopenic purpura
c. Thrombocytosis
d. Hypocoagulopathy

5.78 Your patient just started a new regimen of chemotherapy including vincristine and methotrexate 1 week ago. He is elderly and has historically had some problems with constipation. Other significant problems include a platelet count of 20,000 cells/mm^3 and stomatitis. Nursing actions would include which of the following?

a. Rectal exam to rule out impaction
b. Digital disimpaction if he becomes constipated
c. Stool softener and a laxative each day as needed
d. Rectal suppository followed by a tap water enema

5.79 Mr. Czar has an enlarged spleen and has been started on corticosteroid therapy. The primary mechanism of action of this therapy is which of the following?

a. Steroids have a capillary-stabilizing effect.
b. Steroids help to control platelet sequestration.
c. Steroids help to stimulate rapid platelet increases.
d. Steroids alter platelet adhesiveness and allow platelets to be more "sticky".

5.80 Your patient has received multiple transfusions of random-donor platelets and is experiencing no increase in his platelet count. What is this process called?

a. Refraction
b. Alloimmunization
c. Autoimmunization
d. Hyperimmunization

5.81 Which of the following is *not* true regarding radiation-induced skin reactions?

a. Electrons produce greater skin reactions than photons.
b. Higher doses given over shorter periods of time to larger volumes result in more severe acute skin reactions.
c. When treatment is targeted at areas of skin apposition, increased reaction secondary to warmth and moisture can be expected.
d. Placing tissue-equivalent material on the skin creates a skin-sparing effect during radiation therapy, minimizing dose at the level of the skin.

5.82 Monique is experiencing hyperpigmentation. You explain to her that this may be a reaction to

a. Asparaginase
b. Bleomycin
c. Paclitaxel
d. Cisplatin

5.83 Alicia has metastatic cancer with a grade-2 performance status. She returns today for her second course of doxorubicin hydrochloride. Her chief complaint is not being able to eat, fatigue, and a rash that has newly formed on her scalp and spread to her temple just below her left eye. Appropriate nursing actions would include all *except* which of the following?

a. Continue with chemotherapy as ordered because her disease has obviously spread to her scalp.
b. Hold her therapy, and notify the physician immediately.
c. Prevent contact with persons who may be immunocompromised.
d. Teach her to not touch the rash and to wash her hands frequently.

5.84 The consequence of infection with gram-negative organisms that can quickly lead to death is

a. Dehydration
b. Gastrointestinal bleeding
c. Endotoxic shock
d. Anaphylaxis

5.85 *Pneumocystis carinii* pneumonia is potentially fatal and requires treatment with

a. Foscarnet
b. Ganciclovir
c. Trimethoprim-sulfamethoxazole
d. An aminoglycoside

5.86 Risk factors for the development of sepsis in patients with cancer include all *except* which of the following?

a. Skin breakdown
b. Hematologic malignancy
c. Granulocytopenia lasting less than 7 days
d. Low albumin at the onset of symptoms of sepsis

5.87 Which of the following is considered to be the cardinal symptom of infection?
a. Fever
b. Inflammation
c. Pus formation
d. Elevated white blood cell count

5.88 The *primary* cause of infection in cancer patients continues to be
a. Fungal infections
b. Gram-positive organisms
c. Gram-negative organisms
d. Mycobacterial infections

5.89 The body's first line of defense against bacteria, which is commonly altered by cancer therapies, is
a. Granulocytes
b. The skin
c. Macrophages
d. The acid pH of fluid

5.90 The *specific* white blood cell that constitutes 35%–76% of circulating white blood cells and responds quickly to bacterial invasion is the
a. Monocyte
b. Macrophage
c. Lymphocyte
d. Polymorphonuclear neutrophil

5.91 What is the name given to the microbes that normally live in the body and lead to a large percentage of infections in immunocompromised patients?
a. Exogenous organisms
b. Intracellular organisms
c. Extracellular organisms
d. Endogenous organisms

5.92 The single *most important* measure to prevent infection when caring for the patient with granulocytopenia is
a. Promptly instituting empiric antibiotics
b. Washing the hands meticulously
c. Providing optimal nutrition
d. Restricting the presence of live flowers and plants

5.93 The *most important* measure in the early detection of bleeding is
a. Accurate screening, beginning with a platelet count
b. Observation for subtle diagnostic signals, such as skin petechiae
c. A family history, focusing on possible congenital bleeding disorders
d. Diagnostic testing of the complete cardiovascular system

5.94 The *typical* response of the body to a reduction in the platelet count, such as that caused by bleeding, is
a. An increase in the fibrinolytic activity of remaining platelets
b. A release of adenosine diphosphate (ADP) into the bloodstream, which increases the oxygen-carrying capacity of available platelets
c. Sequestering of red blood cells in the spleen
d. Increased production of megakaryocytes in the bone marrow

5.95 Bleeding with cancer is *most often* due either to the mechanical pressure of tumors on organs or to

a. Infection
b. Damage to the spleen
c. Interference with vasculature
d. Hypocoagulability of the blood

5.96 Acute bleeding that occurs as a result of tumor-induced structural damage to the vasculature is *best* managed by

a. Radiotherapy
b. Chemotherapy
c. Oral or parenteral iron supplements to reduce anemia
d. Mechanical pressure (e.g., nasal packing during epistaxis)

5.97 The single *most significant* measure for predicting bleeding in an individual with cancer is

a. Tumor site
b. Platelet count
c. Abnormal platelet function
d. An imbalance in coagulation factors

5.98 You are monitoring Liza, who is receiving chemotherapy for acute myelogenous leukemia, to ensure that she does not develop complications associated with leukocytosis. The *most common* complication is

a. Blast crisis
b. Cerebellar toxicity
c. Tumor lysis syndrome
d. Disseminated intravascular coagulation

5.99 Patients with liver cancer are more at risk for bleeding due to all *except* which of the following?

a. Abnormal platelet function
b. Varices from portal hypertension
c. Decrease in vitamin K absorption
d. Increase in prothrombin time and activated partial thromboplastin time

5.100 Patients with cancers may at times have bleeding, despite normal platelet counts and coagulation factors. An example is bleeding caused by

a. Hypocoagulability
b. Platelet sequestration
c. Decreased platelet adhesiveness
d. Disseminated intravascular coagulation

5.101 Which of the following coagulation factors is necessary for both coagulation and fibrinolysis?

a. Fibrin
b. Thrombin
c. Fibrinogen
d. Prothrombin

ALTERATIONS IN GASTROINTESTINAL FUNCTION

5.102 Your patient experiences intense nausea and vomiting from chemotherapy and is prescribed lorazepam along with her antiemetics at her next chemotherapy treatment. She wants to know why she is given an antianxiety agent when she does not feel anxious. Your explanation would include which of the following?

a. The lorazepam is given to reduce anticipatory nausea and vomiting.
b. Lorazepam can help to prevent motion sickness, which may be contributing to her nausea and vomiting.
c. Lorazepam is given to decrease her anxiety as all patients become anxious while receiving chemotherapy.
d. The lorazepam is given to induce sleep, which is an important strategy for preventing nausea and vomiting with chemotherapy.

5.103 Prolonged diarrhea without adequate management can lead to all of the following *except*

a. Renal failure
b. Dehydration
c. Circulatory collapse
d. Nutritional malabsorption

5.104 A patient is receiving vinorelbine and complains of colicky abdominal pain and abdominal distention. Physiologically, the patient's symptoms are *most likely* caused by

a. Decreased colonic transit time with vinorelbine
b. The effect of the vinorelbine on the gastrointestinal mucosa
c. Cramping and gas pains, which are common with vinorelbine
d. Diminished effectiveness of afferent and efferent nerve pathways

5.105 Twenty-four hours after taking a laxative, a patient calls and complains of nausea and inability to pass gas. He has not had a bowel movement in 4 days. The *most appropriate* approach to this situation includes which of the following?

a. The patient needs to have an enema.
b. A stool softener and a laxative should be recommended.
c. The patient should have a physical exam and a flat plate of the abdomen because he could be obstipated.
d. An oil-retention enema and milk of magnesia should be given and repeated if there are no results in 24 hours.

5.106 Opioids affect the gastrointestinal (GI) tract, contributing to constipation by all of the following mechanisms *except*

a. Activation of opioid receptors in the GI tract and on the central nervous system
b. Increased water absorption due to increased transit time
c. Insensitivity to rectal distention
d. Histamine release

5.107 Opioid-induced constipation is *best* managed by which of the following approaches?

a. Metamucil daily
b. Increase fiber to 3–4 grams per day
c. Increase fluid intake to eight 8-ounce glasses of fluid per day
d. One Senokot tablet plus 100 mg tablet of colace per 30 mg tablet of MS Contin

5.108 Radiation-induced enteritis can cause significant diarrhea. Which of the following interventions is *not* appropriate management of this problem?

a. A liquid diet high in milk and milk products
b. Sandostatin given subcutaneously
c. A low-residue diet
d. Anticholinergics

5.109 A patient is receiving 5-fluorouracil and leucovorin weekly for 4 weeks. He reports abdominal cramping, rectal urgency, and diarrhea that awaken him at night. On questioning he reports four diarrhea stools on each of the past 3 days, each with a volume of about 1 cup. Appropriate nursing action would include which of the following?

a. Encourage him to take loperamide with each loose stool and to push fluids and delay treatment for 1 week.
b. Diarrhea is expected with 5-fluorouracil, and he should receive his chemotherapy with instructions to take loperamide with each loose stool.
c. Myelosuppression is the dose-limiting toxicity of 5-fluorouracil, so if the counts are good he should receive treatment.
d. Assess the patient for dehydration, including orthostatic blood pressures.

5.110 A patient receiving chemotherapy complains of severe diarrhea for 6 days and agrees to come to the outpatient clinic to be evaluated. Appropriate nursing action would include all of the following *except*

a. Monitor fluids and electrolytes.
b. Notify the physician for fluid replacement and evaluation.
c. Monitor the patient for orthostatic hypotension, lethargy, and weakness.
d. Notify the physician for possible administration of an antidiarrheal medication.

5.111 A patient receiving methotrexate complains of a fever of 101.5°F for 1 day and severe diarrhea for 4 days and requests an antidiarrheal medication. Which of the following explanations should be given to the patient regarding the rationale for *not* giving him an antidiarrheal medication?

a. Antidiarrheal agents are only given after 6 days of severe diarrhea.
b. The fever is more important to treat immediately than the diarrhea.
c. Antidiarrheal agents do not work when the diarrhea is caused by an infection.
d. Antidiarrheal agents increase the exposure of the mucosa to the infectious agent.

5.112 Your patient has recurrent intermittent bowel obstruction due to advanced cancer. Which of the following is an *appropriate* option to offer this patient as management strategies for nausea and vomiting due to bowel obstruction?

a. Pain and antinausea medication
b. No treatment as the patient is nearing the end of life
c. Surgical placement of a gastrostomy tube or a percutaneous endoscopic gastrostomy
d. Nasogastric intubation to avoid a surgical procedure in a patient with advanced cancer

5.113 Biliary vomiting is indicative of which of the following?

a. Progressive constipation
b. Obstruction in the lower ileus
c. Intermittent bowel obstruction
d. Obstruction in the upper part of the abdomen

ALTERATIONS IN GENITOURINARY FUNCTION

5.114 Risk factors for urinary incontinence following radical prostatectomy include all *except* which of the following?

a. Age over 65
b. Stage T1a or T1b disease
c. History of bladder spasms
d. Development of anastomatic stricture

5.115 Mr. Frank has undergone a continent/orthoptic urinary diversion. Which of the following statements will help to *best* educate him to avoid nighttime incontinence?

a. Drink at least 8 glasses of fluids throughout the day and evening.
b. Empty the bladder at bedtime (either by voiding or by self-catheterization).
c. Set the alarm to awaken every 2 hours during the night to void or self-catheterize.
d. Wear an adult diaper at night as all patients will experience nighttime incontinence.

5.116 Mr. Benson presents with some pain and frequency of urination. During a rectal palpation, the examiner detects a diffuse enlargement of the prostate. There seems to be no mass, however. With no other information, one might infer that Mr. Benson is *most likely* to have

a. Nephritis
b. Cancer of the prostate
c. Cancer of the bladder
d. Benign prostatic hypertrophy

5.117 Your patient is being prepped for a radical prostatectomy and is concerned about urinary incontinence. Your *best* advice to him is which of the following?

a. He should talk to his doctor about his concerns.
b. Stress incontinence occurs in about 25% of patients but is manageable.
c. Urinary incontinence is a major problem in about 50% of patients.
d. Some 92% of patients achieve urinary control following radical prostatectomy.

5.118 Following transurethral resection of the prostate (TURP) your patient experiences dribbling and stress incontinence. He asks you about his treatment options. The most appropriate response would include all *except* which of the following?

a. The use of a long-term indwelling Foley catheter
b. Surgery to relieve urethral obstruction or stricture
c. Anticholinergic drugs to increase sphincter resistance
d. Kegel exercises to strengthen the pelvic floor muscles

5.119 The primary complications of a cystectomy and urinary diversion are related to all *except* which of the following?

a. Stoma stenosis
b. Wound dehiscence
c. Long-term kidney damage
d. Stoma construction and placement

5.120 A continent urinary diversion is a surgical method substituting bowel to function like the original bladder. Which of the following is *not* a correct description of this procedure?

a. One-way valves prevent urinary reflux.
b. An intra-abdominal pouch is created for storage of urine.
c. A continent urinary diversion provides control of voiding.
d. All continent urinary diversions are constructed from terminal ileum.

5.121 Following a radical cystectomy, the nurse is instructed to irrigate the pouch regularly to maintain patency. The patient expresses dismay, stating that he does not feel he can learn to do this. The nurse's *best* response is which of the following?

a. "Irrigation is necessary to prevent urinary reflux."
b. "Most of the time, the mucus becomes very thin and easy to pass."
c. "Has your doctor told you it will be necessary for you to irrigate the pouch?"
d. "Mucous production will decrease over time, and irrigation will become unnecessary."

5.122 Mr. Makela has an ileal conduit placed following cystectomy for advanced bladder cancer. Which of the following is considered *normal*?

a. A delay of urinary output for 4–5 hours after surgery
b. Protrusion of the stoma 3 inches above the skin surface
c. A stoma that is dark red in color and slightly edematous
d. A small amount of leakage from the appliance

5.123 As you take the history of a patient with nephrotic syndrome, what signs and symptoms would you expect to see or hear reported?

a. Mild hypotension
b. Brown frothy urine
c. Frank blood in the urine
d. Generalized weight loss with anorexia

5.124 Multiple myeloma is associated with renal failure precipitated by numerous factors. Which of the following does *not* contribute to renal failure in multiple myeloma?

a. Infection
b. Dehydration
c. Hypercalcemia
d. Hyperglycemia

5.125 Mr. Prang is at high risk for developing hemorrhagic cystitis in response to high-dose cyclophosphamide therapy for stem cell transplantation. You propose to help prevent this development with the use of

a. Mesna
b. Mannitol
c. Amifostine
d. Amino caproic acid

ALTERATIONS IN RESPIRATORY FUNCTION

5.126 When a patient at the end of life complains of dyspnea, the nurse should *most appropriately* focus on which of the following?

a. Administer bronchodilators as needed.
b. Monitor pulse oximetry to determine need for oxygen.
c. Administer opioids to lessen the sensation of breathlessness.
d. Determine degree of dyspnea by assessing arterial blood gases and pulmonary function tests.

5.127 Which of the following is the *most common* presenting symptom of lung cancer?

a. Cough
b. Sore throat
c. Hoarseness
d. Hemoptysis

5.128 Which of the following sclerosing agents is used *most commonly* to manage recurrent pleural effusions?

a. Bleomycin
b. Doxorubicin
c. Tetracycline
d. Gemcitabine

5.129 Chest x-ray reveals that Mr. Stanton has a large pleural effusion contributing to his dyspnea and difficulty breathing. Once the fluid is drained, the physician instills a sclerosing agent into the pleural space. In preparing your patient for the procedure, you would be certain to mention all *except* which of the following?

a. If the fluid reaccumulates, it can be drained again.
b. The sclerosing agent is given to obliterate the pleural space.
c. The purpose of injecting bleomycin into the pleural space is to kill any cancer cells that might be there.
d. The procedure is painful, and therefore the patient will be given adequate pain medication before the procedure.

5.130 Ms. Daniels, who had an allogeneic stem cell transplantation and is in the postengraftment period, develops a pulmonary infection. You are mindful that because of prolonged periods of immunosuppression caused by her medication, she is at greater risk for developing

a. Interstitial pneumonia
b. Idiopathic pneumonia
c. Cytomegalovirus (CMV) pneumonia
d. Respiratory syncytial virus pneumonia

5.131 The pulmonary function test *most likely* to detect chemotherapy-induced pulmonary toxicity before the onset of clinical symptoms is

a. The carbon monoxide diffusion capacity measurement
b. Pulmonary blood gases
c. CO_2 binding capacity
d. A chest x-ray

5.132 Which of the following factors increases the risk of interstitial pneumonitis, as a late-onset pulmonary complication of stem cell transplant?

a. Viral pneumonia
b. High-dose corticosteroids
c. Previous anthracycline therapy
d. Previous cyclophosphamide therapy

5.133 Malignant pleural effusions are often associated with a poor prognosis. Which of the following is an accurate description of median survival times of patients with malignant pleural effusions?

a. Patients with breast cancer with evidence of a malignant pleural effusion have a median survival time of 5 months.
b. Patients with lung cancer with evidence of a malignant pleural effusion have a median survival time of 1 year.
c. Patients with mesothelioma with evidence of malignant pleural effusion have a median survival time of 3 months.
d. Patients with ovarian cancer with evidence of a malignant pleural effusion have a median survival time of 2 years.

5.134 During a thoracentesis procedure your patient is placed in an upright sitting position. As the fluid is being removed the patient becomes diaphoretic, pale, and appears to be fainting. As you administer care to your patient you realize her symptoms are due to what?
a. Needle phobia
b. Pneumothorax
c. A vasovagal reaction
d. Reexpansion pulmonary edema

5.135 Thoracentesis involves fluid removal from
a. The pleural cavity
b. The spinal column
c. The pericardial sac
d. The abdominal cavity

5.136 The *first and most common* means of obliteration of the pleural cavity in a patient with chronic recurrent malignant pleural effusions is
a. Local radiation
b. Pleural stripping
c. Pleuroperitoneal shunt
d. Pleurodesis with a sclerosing agent

5.137 Cytarabine and mitomycin C can cause diffuse alveolar damage, resulting in which of the following pulmonary disorders?
a. Pneumonia
b. Capillary leak syndrome
c. Obliteration of alveoli
d. Pleural effusion

5.138 What percentage of pleural effusions are malignant?
a. 100%
b. 75%
c. 50%
d. < 25%

5.139 Which of the following differentiates a malignant pleural effusion from a nonmalignant pleural effusion?
a. Malignant effusions are hypocellular.
b. Malignant effusions are almost always clear.
c. Malignant effusions are almost always an exudate.
d. Malignant effusions are almost always a transudate.

ALTERATIONS IN CIRCULATORY FUNCTION

5.140 Which of the following is *not* considered a risk factor for lymphedema?
a. Infection
b. Disease recurrence
c. Axillary irradiation
d. Breast reconstruction

5.141 Prevention of lymphedema in a patient who is at risk for lymphedema includes which of the following strategies?
 a. Education about avoiding obesity
 b. Education about the need to avoid any kind of regular exercise
 c. Education about the use of complete or complex decongestive therapy (CDT)
 d. Education about benefits of strenuous exercise, including weight lifting

5.142 Complex decongestive therapy for the management of lymphedema involves all *except* which of the following?
 a. Exercises
 b. Bandaging
 c. Deep massage
 d. Compression garments

5.143 Following treatment for ovarian cancer, your patient calls to complain that her legs feel heavy, painful, and slightly numb. Nursing management includes which of the following?
 a. Inform her to elevate her legs and restrict fluids.
 b. Instruct her to come into the emergency room to rule out a deep vein thrombosis.
 c. Inform her that her symptoms are likely due to obstruction of lymph drainage in her abdomen, and she needs to be evaluated.
 d. Reassure her that her symptoms are likely due to chemotherapy and will improve over time.

5.144 Cardiotoxicity associated with doxorubicin can be minimized by the administration of which of the following cardioprotective agents?
 a. Digitalis
 b. Amifostine
 c. Calcium gluconate
 d. Dexrazoxane (Zinecard)

5.145 Which of the following is *not* considered to be a significant risk factor for cardiac tamponade?
 a. Lung cancer
 b. Hyperkalemia
 c. Radiation to the pericardium
 d. Pericardial fluid accumulation of 300 cc

5.146 James is starting doxorubicin therapy, without mediastinal radiation. You explain to him that his lifetime total cumulative dose of doxorubicin is
 a. 550 mg
 b. 600 mg
 c. 550 mg/m^2
 d. 450 mg/m^2

5.147 Choose the statement that *most accurately* describes the degree of subjective symptoms produced by malignant pericardial and pleural effusions.
 a. Symptoms tend to be related more to the rate of fluid accumulation than to the volume collected.
 b. Symptoms tend to be related more to the volume of fluid collected than to the rate of the collection.
 c. Symptoms are related more to the underlying disease and length of time the patient has been diagnosed with cancer.
 d. Symptoms correspond directly to whether the metastatic disease is from microscopic seeding of the cavities or from local extension.

5.148 Vaginal cancer is generally treated with surgery and radiation. Complications following treatment include all *except* which of the following?

a. Venous thrombosis and vaginal engorgement
b. Vaginal fibrosis and scarring
c. Constriction in blood supply
d. Loss of vaginal elasticity

5.149 Mr. Archer has had an implanted port for 4 weeks and recently complained of pain in his right neck and shoulder, just above the catheter insertion site. On examination you notice slight swelling over the neck, face, shoulder, and arm. He also complains that his arm is cold at times and there is some tingling in his arm and shoulder. What is the *most appropriate* action to take?

a. Flush the line with heparin to make sure it is not clotted.
b. Notify the physician to examine the patient. A venogram will probably demonstrate a venous thrombosis.
c. Notify the physician to obtain an order for alteplase. The patient probably has a fibrin sheath formation around the tip of the catheter.
d. These symptoms are normal following port placement and should resolve in 2–3 weeks. Have him return to the clinic in a week if he is not better.

5.150 Thromboembolism (TE) is *most frequently* seen with which of the following?

a. Leukemia
b. Soft tissue sarcoma
c. Small cell lung cancer
d. Mucin-secreting bladder carcinoma

5.151 The etiology of thromboembolism is

a. Chronic hemorrhage
b. Bone marrow failure
c. Tumor secretion of cytokines, such as interleukin-1, affecting red cell metabolism
d. The ability of tumor cells to affect systemic activation of coagulation and cause platelet dysfunction

5.152 The prognosis for a patient with colorectal cancer is probably poorest if which of the following exists?

a. High blood pressure
b. Squamous cell involvement
c. Venous and lymph node invasion
d. Location of the tumor above the peritoneal reflection

5.153 The major complication related to thrombocythemia includes all of the following *except*

a. Bleeding
b. Thrombosis
c. Polycythemia vera
d. Pulmonary embolism

ALTERATIONS IN NUTRITION

5.154 Which of the following is considered a contraindication to enteral nutrition?
- a. Diarrhea
- b. Severe weakness
- c. Mechanical obstructions
- d. Functioning gastrointestinal tract

5.155 Which of the following strategies is effective for managing regurgitation with gastrostomy feedings?
- a. Use large-bore tube.
- b. Consider drugs to decrease motility.
- c. Place tube distally into jejunum or duodenum.
- d. Measure residuals and withhold feeding if more than 25–50 cc.

5.156 While receiving parenteral nutrition your patient complains of pain at the site of the catheter. *Appropriate* nursing actions include which of the following?
- a. Stop the infusion, and assess for catheter patency.
- b. Irrigate the catheter with a small-diameter syringe.
- c. Slow the infusion, and observe for swelling.
- d. Do nothing because slight discomfort is normal.

5.157 Which of the following statements regarding enteral and parenteral nutrition is *not* accurate?
- a. Compared to parenteral nutrition, enteral nutrition is associated with more diarrhea.
- b. Compared to parenteral nutrition, enteral nutrition is associated with a higher incidence of metabolic imbalances.
- c. With enteral nutrition, normal enzymatic and mucosal activity is maintained in the gastrointestinal tract.
- d. With parenteral nutrition, there is a higher incidence of infection.

5.158 Mr. Smith, who seems healthy, is scheduled for surgical resection of an esophageal lesion. Which route of administration of nutritional support do you predict is *most likely* to be appropriate for Mr. Smith immediately after surgery?
- a. Enteral nutrition
- b. Home total parenteral nutrition
- c. Total parenteral nutrition for 7–10 days
- d. Parenteral intravenous fluids for 3–5 days

5.159 Which of the following patients would generally *not* be candidates for home parenteral nutrition?
- a. Those with severe enteritis due to radiation
- b. Those patients who are terminally ill and unable to drink fluids
- c. Those patients with significant gastrointestinal malfunction
- d. Head and neck cancer patients who have an upper airway obstruction

5.160 Mr. Cruz is receiving enteral nutrition every 4 hours and complains of diarrhea and cramping. The *least likely* cause of his discomfort is which of the following?
- a. The formula is probably too cold.
- b. The formula probably has too much fiber.
- c. The formula is probably too concentrated.
- d. The formula is probably infused too rapidly.

5.161 Dysphagia is the *most common* presenting symptom of persons with which of the following?

a. Tracheal cancer
b. Epiglottal cancer
c. Laryngeal cancer
d. Esophageal cancer

5.162 A patient has difficulty swallowing without aspirating following a hemilaryngectomy for a supraglottic carcinoma. You consult a swallowing specialist, who recommends which of the following to help the patient relearn swallowing without aspiration?

a. Lean forward for each swallow.
b. Try liquids first and then semisolids.
c. Try crackers or toast followed by a sip of liquid.
d. Before initiating the swallow, have the patient hold his or her breath to close the vocal cords.

5.163 The *primary* difference between primary and secondary cachexia in cancer is which of the following?

a. Secondary cachexia results from voluntary starvation.
b. Secondary cachexia results from chemical toxins and liver failure.
c. Primary cachexia results from tumor-produced metabolic abnormalities.
d. Primary cachexia is where the individual is underweight before cancer.

5.164 Patients with metastatic cancer often have difficulty maintaining their weight because of a lack of appetite. Your patient has just received a prescription for megestrol acetate, 800 mg per day. While discussing her new medication, you are sure to include all *except* which of the following?

a. The purpose of the medication is to treat the cancer.
b. The medication will increase her feeling of well-being.
c. Weight gain is likely to occur due to increase in body fat.
d. She may experience edema, hyperglycemia, and risk of embolism.

5.165 Vinny has started radiation therapy to his left femur for a sarcoma. He complains of diarrhea and slight nausea following his radiation treatment. Your explanation would include which of the following?

a. His feeling of nausea is probably more psychological than real.
b. The waste products of tissue destruction are likely the cause of his symptoms.
c. Because the radiation port does not include his stomach, it is not likely that his symptoms are related to the radiation.
d. The field of radiation may include surrounding pelvic structures that puts him at risk for gastrointestinal changes, such as nausea and diarrhea.

5.166 Anorexia is characterized by all *except* which of the following?

a. Early satiety
b. Cancer cachexia
c. Visceral and lean body mass depletion
d. Abnormalities of carbohydrate, protein, and fat metabolism

5.167 Mary is being treated with chemotherapy for colon cancer and approaches the nurse to tell her that she plans to start on a macrobiotic diet. What is the *most appropriate* response to Mary in regards to this diet?

a. This diet can put her at significant risk for protein-calorie malnutrition.
b. This is a nutritionally sound diet, and it will help her to feel stronger during treatment.
c. Because this diet includes coffee enemas, she should wait to start the diet until her chemotherapy is complete.
d. This diet requires the use of multiple dietary supplements, which may be difficult to manage with her chemotherapy.

5.168 A newly diagnosed patient with unresectable lung cancer complains that he has not had an appetite for many weeks and is concerned because he is losing weight. What is the *most likely* cause of his weight loss?

a. The chemotherapy and radiation cause weight loss.
b. Liver disease is most likely causing his loss of appetite.
c. Anorexia and cachexia are common manifestations of lung cancer.
d. He is probably depressed over his situation and should improve with treatment.

5.169 Which of the following is *not* considered an effective measure to minimize oral stomatitis?

a. Frequent oral hygiene
b. Sucralfate oral suspension
c. Oral cryotherapy during chemotherapy treatment
d. Palifermin during autologous stem cell transplant

5.170 A patient who has been treated with radiation to the mouth and oropharynx has developed mucositis. Effective management of this side effect incorporates all of the following *except*

a. Encouraging the patient to avoid alcohol and cigarettes
b. Removing the plaquelike tissue that forms with mucositis
c. Administering an appropriate systemic analgesic such as morphine
d. Rinsing the mouth with bland mouthwash (such as normal saline) 4 times daily

5.171 Your patient is receiving radiation therapy to the head and neck and complains of a dry mouth and thick ropy saliva. The condition interferes with his appetite and speech. Which of the following is *not* part of your patient education plan regarding this reaction?

a. Xerostomia is a decrease in the quality and quantity of saliva.
b. Saliva substitutes, frequent rinses with ice water, and sugarless gum may provide relief.
c. Xerostomia is a dysfunction of the salivary gland that occurs following chemotherapy or radiation therapy.
d. This reaction is permanent, and, although not life-threatening, it can eventually lead to oral caries and candidal infections.

5.172 Which is *not* part of your treatment plan for the patient experiencing xerostomia?

a. Vitamin C orally as directed
b. Pilocarpine hydrochloride orally as directed
c. Oral care before meals to freshen the mouth and stimulate appetite
d. Increasing fluid intake during meals and snacks helps to lubricate food and ease swallowing

5.173 Xerostomia, a decrease in saliva secretion, is a side effect of

a. Oral surgery
b. Cisplatin administration
c. Head and neck irradiation
d. Stem cell transplantation

5.174 Degree and severity of chemotherapy-induced nausea and vomiting vary based on many factors. Which of the following is *not* considered to be a factor in predicting the degree and severity of chemotherapy-induced nausea and vomiting?

a. History of nausea due to radiation therapy
b. Rate of chemotherapy infusion
c. Drug sequencing
d. Age

5.175 Protracted nausea and vomiting is common following chemotherapy and total body irradiation, but which of the following is *not* responsible for the protracted nature of this problem?

a. Graft-versus-host disease (GVHD)
b. Cytomegalovirus (CMV) esophagitis
c. Gastrointestinal infections
d. Stomatitis

5.176 John has a lung tumor with a single brain lesion for which he has received a full course of radiation therapy. He has been doing well on paclitaxel and carboplatin, until he experienced vomiting that seemed to come on without warning. Select the *most appropriate* advice to give this patient.

a. His vomiting is most likely due to the chemotherapy, and he should take an antiemetic and call back if he does not feel better.
b. He is probably experiencing delayed nausea and vomiting from the combination of the radiation and the chemotherapy. An antiemetic is appropriate.
c. His symptoms could be related to increased intracranial pressure, and he should come to the emergency room as soon as possible.
d. His symptoms could be due to chemotherapy or to increased intracranial pressure, and he should be advised to take dexamethasone, which is appropriate in either case.

5.177 Your patient is beginning radiation therapy to the mandible and is concerned about how this will affect his ability to taste and smell. Your teaching would include all *except* which of the following?

a. Loss of taste is usually permanent.
b. Acidic foods may increase glossodynia.
c. If xerostomia occurs, loss of taste is more likely.
d. Taste acuity is usually restored within 4 months.

5.178 You decide to do some research to find out how and why chemotherapy causes an effect on nutrition. In your reading, you learn all *except* which of the following?

a. Chemotherapy can indirectly cause food aversions.
b. Chemotherapy can alter the intestinal absorptive surface.
c. Chemotherapy does not interfere with specific metabolic reactions.
d. Chemotherapy may cause excitation of the true vomiting center.

5.179 Which of the following is *not* considered to be a cause of altered taste and smell in individuals with cancer?

a. Deficiencies in zinc, copper, nickel, and niacin
b. Direct tumor invasion
c. Hypercalcemia
d. Tumor-associated circulating factors

5.180 Jim complains that food does not taste the same and that everything tastes like cardboard. He especially dislikes the taste of red meat. This is best explained by the fact that persons with cancer commonly experience which of the following?

a. Intolerance to bland foods
b. Difficulty digesting their food
c. An increased threshold for sweet, sour, and salt and a decreased threshold for bitter foods
d. A decreased threshold for sweet, sour, and salt and an increased threshold for bitter foods

5.181 Because of the changed configuration of the aerodigestive tract, the person who has undergone a laryngectomy can expect change in all of the following functions *except*

a. Speaking
b. Eating
c. Taste
d. Smell

5.182 An example of a chemotherapeutic agent that may cause a metallic taste during administration, leading to taste changes, is

a. Etoposide
b. Doxorubicin
c. Dacarbazine
d. Cyclophosphamide

5.183 Which of the following is *not* considered to be a reliable test of protein stores?

a. Midarm muscle circumference
b. Skinfold thickness measurement
c. Serum albumin
d. Serum transtyretin

5.184 Of women who receive adjuvant chemotherapy for breast cancer, many will gain weight and even become obese. What percentage of women on adjuvant chemotherapy for breast cancer gain weight?

a. 15%–25%
b. 30%–40%
c. 40%–100%
d. 60%–90%

5.185 William asks you for an appetite stimulant. Keeping in mind that he is on an extensive chemotherapy regimen, is diabetic, and has not had problems with nausea or vomiting, which of the following drugs is the *best* possible intervention for him?

a. Corticosteroids
b. Megesterol acetate
c. Metoclopramide
d. Tetrahydrocannabinol (THC)

5.186 Cancer-associated nutritional problems, rather than treatment-related nutritional problems, are *best* reversed by

a. Extensive verbal counseling
b. Self-care actions
c. Medications
d. Successful treatment of the tumor

5.187 Charles is one of your patients with lung cancer. Because he is diabetic and already well under his ideal weight, one of your major concerns is to provide Charles with adequate nutrition and prevent cachexia. You are dismayed to learn that he "lost his appetite" when he recently received his diagnosis and almost entirely stopped eating. Which of the following is probably *not* a factor that would have contributed to the loss of appetite?

a. Bombesin
b. Circulating cytokines
c. Cancer-induced sepsis
d. Psychological distress

5.188 Which of the following statements regarding cachexia is *true*?

a. Cachexia is the same as anorexia.
b. Cachexia is due to the tumor consuming the body's nutrients.
c. Cachexia is not reversible with appropriate feeding.
d. Cachexia is the same as starvation.

5.189 Mr. Thomas has been steadily losing weight and progressively deteriorating from his pancreatic cancer. He is experiencing severe muscle wasting and energy loss. The *appropriate* term for this condition is

a. Cancer cachexia
b. Malnutrition
c. Inanition
d. Undernutrition

ALTERATIONS IN NEUROLOGICAL FUNCTION

5.190 Assessment of cerebellar function focuses on all of the following *except*

a. Coordinate movement
b. Maintain normal muscle tone
c. Maintain equilibrium
d. Paralysis

5.191 Which of the following is effective in preventing neurotoxicities associated with cisplatin, paclitaxel, and carboplatin?

a. Pyroxidine (vitamin B_6)
b. Amifostine
c. Nortriptyline
d. Carbamazepine

5.192 Davis is taking vincristine. You are able to discern from his conversation that although he is familiar with some of vincristine's adverse effects, he seems unfamiliar with its neurotoxic effects. Thus, you tell him that vincristine is well known for potential

a. Encephalopathy
b. Peripheral neuropathy
c. Leukoencephalopathy
d. Acute cerebellar dysfunction

5.193 Which of the following chemotherapy agents is *not* associated with peripheral neuropathies?

a. Cytarabine
b. Cisplatin
c. Methotrexate
d. Carboplatin

5.194 A patient receiving paclitaxel has recently complained that she has some trouble walking without stumbling. After examining the patient, the physician changes her chemotherapy. What is the *most logical* explanation for switching her chemotherapy?

a. She probably has a brain tumor, and the chemotherapy is not working.
b. The paclitaxel is causing a cerebellar dysfunction.
c. The paclitaxel could be causing progressive peripheral neuropathy.
d. The cancer could be impinging on the spinal nerves.

5.195 Which of the following chemotherapy drugs is *not* associated with arthralgias and myalgias?

a. Paclitaxel
b. Docetaxel
c. Ifosfamide
d. Vinorelbine

5.196 Which of the following is *not* considered a risk factor for ifosfamide-induced encephalopathy?

a. Hepatic insufficiency
b. Previous taxane therapy
c. Low serum albumin
d. High serum creatinine

5.197 Mr. Rogers has a metastatic cancer of unknown origin. He originally went to his doctor because of ataxia and lower extremity weakness. His doctor described his symptoms as being related to a paraneoplastic syndrome. Which of the following statements *best* describes the cause of the patient's weakness?

a. Cerebellar function is impaired because of the effect of the tumor.
b. The cancer is in the brain and is pressing on the cerebellum.
c. Chemotherapy is the most likely cause of the weakness.
d. Muscle wasting is common in metastatic cancer.

5.198 Your patient has a possible brain tumor involving the frontal lobe. He is unable to coordinate skilled movements but is not paralyzed. This clinical manifestation is called

a. Dysphasia
b. Apraxia
c. Aphasia
d. Dysreflexia

5.199 The cause of peripheral neuropathy as a result of chemotherapy is *best* described by which of the following?

a. Sensory and motor axons are injured.
b. Demyelination reduces nerve conduction velocity.
c. Deep tendon reflexes are lost.
d. Nerve cells are damaged by the cytotoxic effects of the drugs.

5.200 Jonas has finished his last course of chemotherapy including carboplatin and etoposide. He comes for an office visit complaining of colicky abdominal pain, constipation, urinary retention, and impotence. You are concerned because you know that his symptoms are *most likely* due to which of the following?
a. Tumor recurrence
b. A paraneoplastic syndrome
c. Obstipation from chemotherapy
d. The effect of chemotherapy on autonomic fibers

5.201 Annie has just completed her 10 treatments of weekly paclitaxel. Over the last few weeks she has complained of difficulty buttoning her clothes and asks how soon it will get better. Your *most appropriate* response would be which of the following?
a. She cannot receive more paclitaxel.
b. Her symptoms will probably get worse before they get better.
c. Most symptoms will improve 2–3 weeks after treatment ends.
d. Her symptoms will improve but may never completely resolve.

5.202 The risk of ototoxicity from cisplatin therapy is increased by all *except* which of the following?
a. Continuous infusion therapy
b. Aminoglycoside therapy
c. Dehydration
d. Rapid drug delivery

5.203 Mr. Jones is an elderly gentleman who has been receiving 5-fluorouracil and leucovorin weekly as treatment for his colon cancer. His wife phones you to say that he is unsteady on his feet and complains of intermittent double vision. You encourage her to bring him in right away because you suspect which of the following?
a. Acute cerebellar dysfunction due to the 5-fluorouracil
b. Dehydration due to severe diarrhea from the 5-fluorouracil
c. Metastatic disease to the brain causing ataxia and diplopia
d. Leukoencephalopathy from the cumulative effect of the drugs

5.204 After treatment for a brain tumor, Mr. Jessup begins to experience tingling in his extremities on the contralateral side of the tumor as well as progressive motor loss and changes in the level of consciousness. You suspect, therefore, that he *might* have
a. Cerebral ischemia secondary to the tumor
b. Cushing's syndrome, in response to progressive tumor
c. Increased intracranial pressure due to increasing tumor size
d. Intermittent pulmonary failure with cardiac episodes secondary to carotid artery ligation

5.205 A patient who is receiving high-dose cytosine arabinoside for acute myelogenous leukemia (AML) begins to experience slight difficulty with articulation of words. She smiles apologetically and says, "I guess I didn't get enough sleep. My mouth is pretty dry too." Your response is to
a. Withhold her medication, and check her renal function tests.
b. Withhold her chemotherapy dose, and do a neurological evaluation.
c. Do an oral examination, offer mouth care, and continue chemotherapy.
d. Interview the patient to identify factors contributing to sleeplessness, which is also contributing to dry mouth.

5.206 Allison has been on tapering doses of steroids over the past week after the completion of radiation therapy to her brain for metastatic breast cancer. She is now sleeping more and seems confused. The cause of changes in her mental status is *most likely* due to
a. Hypercalcemia
b. Steroid psychosis
c. Tapering of steroids
d. Recurrence of her cancer

5.207 In most instances, the earliest and most sensitive indicator of a central nervous system tumor is a change in
a. Cognitive ability
b. Motor function
c. Sensory function
d. Level of consciousness

ANATOMICAL AND SURGICAL ALTERATIONS

5.208 Which of the following is *not* a typical complication of allograft bone reconstruction?
a. Rejection
b. Infection
c. Fracture
d. Nonunion

5.209 After amputation, Mr. Riley reports pain in the missing lower leg. The nurse should be aware that this phantom limb pain
a. Is likely to worsen with aging
b. Usually occurs immediately after surgery
c. Indicates a patient's inability to cope with loss
d. Generally decreases substantially during the first year

5.210 A graft or flap is *most often* used in the surgical treatment of a nonmelanoma cancer when
a. The lesion is small, superficial, or recurrent.
b. Risks of bleeding are high, and vasculature must be maintained.
c. The lesion is large or located in an area with insufficient tissue for closure.
d. The extent of the tumor must be accurately assessed, and margins are relatively unclear.

5.211 Mr. Jessup, who has a tracheostomy, is having a carotid hemorrhage. Besides controlling the bleeding, what should you do *first* to prevent aspiration of the blood?
a. Inflate the tracheostomy cuff.
b. Suction his throat and oral cavity.
c. Deflate the cuff, and remove the tracheostomy tube to clear the airway.
d. Transport him immediately to the operating room for ligation of the carotid artery.

5.212 The risk of carotid artery rupture after radical neck dissection is associated with all of the following *except*
a. Persistent tumor in the area
b. Infection of the surrounding area
c. A small trickle of blood from the area
d. Coverage of the artery with a skin flap

5.213 An example of a postoperative situation requiring *immediate* nursing intervention is

a. A smooth suture line with no sign of swelling
b. Hematoma formation beneath a skin flap
c. Bleeding on a dressing the size of a quarter
d. Clearing of airway secretions by coughing

5.214 Which of the following procedures will the surgeon *usually* perform when a lesion involves the middle and left transverse colon?

a. A right hemicolectomy that includes the related lymphatic and circulatory channels
b. A one-stage procedure involving resection of the lesion and a primary anastomosis
c. A two-stage procedure involving a temporary colostomy or ileostomy
d. A three-stage procedure involving a diverting colostomy, a resection of the tumor, and take-down of the colostomy

5.215 For upper and midrectal adenocarcinomas, the treatment approach of choice is

a. Prophylactic oophorectomy
b. Abdominoperineal resection with a temporary colostomy
c. Low anterior resection, preserving external anal sphincter control
d. Laser therapy to the tumor bed through a colonoscope or flexible sigmoidoscope

5.216 If the urine passing from a stoma is cloudy, it may be that

a. The patient is dehydrated.
b. Antispasmodics are indicated.
c. The stoma was formed from intestinal tissue.
d. A leak in the stoma pouch has occurred, allowing air and bacteria to enter a sterile area.

5.217 Which of the following postoperative assessments of stoma viability is a matter of concern that should be brought to the surgeon's attention?

a. A dusky or gray stoma
b. Protrusion of the stoma
c. Persistent peristalsis in the bowel
d. Bleeding of the stoma when rubbed

5.218 Postoperative care and teaching of the patient undergoing abdominoperineal resection (APR) for rectal cancer is *most likely* to be influenced by which of the following?

a. The extent of hepatic invasion
b. The type of colostomy to be performed
c. The patient's age, sex, and physical condition
d. The type of closure of the perineal wound to be used

5.219 A patient has recently returned from the operating room with a tracheotomy. He has a high-humidity oxygen collar with orders to suction the trachea every 2 hours as needed. The need for the continuous high-humidity collar is *best explained* by which of the following?

a. The collar protects the airway.
b. The collar provides necessary oxygen to the lungs.
c. The collar provides humidified air to a permanently altered airway.
d. The collar provides humidity to the air normally supplied by the nose.

5.220 After surgery a patient develops aspiration pneumonia. Which of the following symptoms would *not likely* have caused this?

a. Excessive sedation
b. Deep vein thrombosis
c. Difficulty in swallowing
d. Mechanical obstruction from cancer

5.221 In the early postoperative period following pneumonectomy your patient experiences a cardiac arrhythmia. He has a history of a myocardial infarction and is currently on cardiac medications. Nursing actions would include which of the following?

a. Ensure he has received his cardiac medication on schedule.
b. Administer oxygen, and encourage the patient to cough and deep breathe.
c. Arrhythmias are common in the postoperative period and should be monitored.
d. Notify the physician immediately because he may be experiencing atrial fibrillation or another myocardial infarction.

5.222 Your patient is immediate post-op following a right hepatectomy. He is *most* at risk for which of the following non–liver-related complications?

a. Hemorrhage
b. Subphrenic abscess
c. Deep vein thrombosis
d. Pneumonia and pleural effusion

PHARMACOLOGIC INTERVENTIONS

5.223 Contraindications to ambulatory oral antimicrobial therapy for treatment of fever in neutropenic patients include all of the following *except*?

a. Suspected pneumonia
b. Hematologic malignancy
c. Hospital-acquired infection
d. Solid tumors and lymphoma

5.224 After a long period of time Ms. Daniels, who had an allogeneic stem cell transplant, develops recurrent varicella zoster virus. What is the *most likely* treatment approach?

a. Acyclovir
b. Cyclosporine
c. Methotrexate
d. Cyclosporine and methotrexate in combination

5.225 Patients with HIV and neutropenia who have received treatment with corticosteroids or who have had prolonged immunosuppression should be monitored for which of the following?

a. Tuberculosis
b. Second malignancies
c. *Pneumocystis carinii* pneumonia
d. Elevated CD4 lymphocyte count

5.226 Which of the following agents is used to prevent graft-versus-host disease in hematopoietic stem cell transplant patients?
a. Cyclosporine
b. Dexamethasone
c. Cyclophosphamide
d. Medroxyprogesterone acetate

5.227 Risk factors for veno-occlusive disease of the liver in hematopoietic stem cell transplantation include all *except* which of the following?
a. Patients with hepatitis
b. Cytomegalovirus and fungal infections
c. Chemotherapy and radiation therapy before transplant
d. Antimicrobial therapy with acyclovir, amphotericin, or vancomycin

5.228 Trimethoprim-sulfamethoxazole is generally the treatment of choice for *Pneumocystis carinii*. Which of the following is *not* usually a side effect of this drug?
a. Nausea and vomiting
b. Hemolytic anemia
c. Hepatotoxicity
d. Myelosuppression

5.229 A patient diagnosed with candida esophagitis is about to receive her first dose of amphotericin B. Which of the following is *not* a side effect of this drug?
a. Hypertension
b. Bronchospasm
c. Fever and chills
d. Nausea and vomiting

5.230 Prevention of acute side effects of amphotericin B includes all *except* which of the following?
a. Acetaminophen
b. Pepcid intravenously
c. Intravenous meperidine
d. Potassium supplements

5.231 The *primary* rationale for the use of corticosteroids in the management of arthralgias and myalgias due to taxane therapy is which of the following?
a. Corticosteroids decrease symptoms of inflammation.
b. Steroids decrease the fever associated with taxane therapy.
c. Steroids suppress muscle enzymes, which cause myalgias.
d. Steroids increase proinflammatory genes.

5.232 When patients are receiving biotherapy as their primary treatment for cancer, corticosteroids are generally avoided for which of the following reasons?
a. Corticosteroids decrease vascular permeability.
b. Corticosteroids mask a fever that is therapeutic.
c. Corticosteroids promote prostaglandin synthesis.
d. Corticosteroids may block the effects of biotherapy on the immune system.

5.233 Nonsteroidal anti-inflammatory agents (NSAIDs) and acetaminophen are effective in pain management because they facilitate which of the following pharmacologic action(s)?

a. They are antipyretic.
b. They inhibit platelet aggregation.
c. They inhibit prostaglandin synthesis.
d. They facilitate the conversion of arachidonic acid to prostaglandins.

5.234 Corticosteroids and nonsteroidal anti-inflammatory drugs (NSAIDs) are commonly used in the treatment of patients with brain tumors. Which of the following are considered anticipated side effects of this therapy?

a. Hypotension and psychiatric reactions
b. Hypotension and hypoglycemia
c. Hypertension and hypoglycemia
d. Hypertension and gastric ulceration

5.235 Elise develops graft-versus-host disease after undergoing allogeneic stem cell transplant. Which of the following will probably *not* be part of Elise's treatment plan?

a. Steroids
b. Fluoride therapy
c. Systemic immunosuppressive therapy
d. Nonsteroidal anti-inflammatory drugs

5.236 James recently received chemotherapy as treatment for his bladder cancer and has difficulty with myelosuppression. He asks what he should take if he gets a headache. Which among the following is *not* an appropriate response?

a. Aspirin is discouraged because it can cause increased risk of bleeding.
b. Acetaminophen does not interfere with clotting and is safe to use.
c. Acetaminophen's anti-inflammatory properties help headaches.
d. If his platelet count is below 100,000/mm^3, he should avoid taking nonsteroidal anti-inflammatory drugs.

5.237 Zoledronic acid is the most potent bisphosphonate in use in the United States for the treatment of hypercalcemia of malignancy. It is recommended that zoledronic acid be infused over not less than 15 minutes and that the dose not exceed 4 mg every 3–4 weeks. The rationale behind this recommendation is which of the following?

a. Doses higher than 4 mg given in less than 15 minutes increase bone marrow suppression.
b. Doses higher than 4 mg given in less than 15 minutes increase nausea and diarrhea.
c. Doses higher than 4 mg given in less than 15 minutes increase renal toxicity.
d. Doses higher than 4 mg given in less than 15 minutes increase liver toxicity.

5.238 Which of the following drugs is *most commonly* associated with platelet dysfunction?

a. Cimetidine
b. Heparin
c. Aspirin
d. Estrogen

5.239 Which of the following *best* describes the effect that nonsteroidal anti-inflammatory drugs (NSAIDs) have on platelets?

a. NSAIDs inhibit platelet function.
b. NSAIDs inhibit platelet aggregation.
c. NSAIDs enhance the platelet secretory process.
d. NSAIDs increase epinephrine-induced aggregation.

5.240 Nonsteroidal anti-inflammatory drugs (NSAIDs) are known to cause gastrointestinal (GI) side effects. The etiology of these GI effects is *best* explained by which of the following?

a. NSAIDs cause GI side effects only in the presence of pre-existing mucosal irritation, as would occur with chemotherapy.
b. The increased release of prostaglandin increases GI side effects.
c. The drugs directly irritate the GI mucosa, which is why they should be taken with an antacid.
d. The loss of the cytoprotective effect of prostaglandin causes increased GI side effects.

5.241 Aprepitant is indicated for the prevention of delayed nausea and vomiting with highly emetic chemotherapy. Which of the following statements is *true* in regards to its mechanism of action?

a. Aprepitant is a 5-HT_3 receptor antagonist.
b. Aprepitant effectively blocks substance P, a neurokinin-1 receptor.
c. To be effective, aprepitant must be given daily for 5 days with a serotonin antagonist.
d. Aprepitant acts to suppress all major neuroreceptors in the nausea and vomiting process.

5.242 Ms. Jones returns for her third round of high-dose chemotherapy and states that she continues to have unrelenting nausea for a week. Which of the following factor(s) will *most* influence your approach to managing this problem?

a. Ondansetron before chemotherapy will help manage delayed nausea.
b. Neurokinin-1 receptor antagonist on days 1, 2, and 3 will help to manage delayed nausea.
c. Lorazepam is useful on days 1–4 to increase the effectiveness of other agents, and the sedation helps to decrease nausea.
d. Neurokinin-1 receptor antagonist, plus a 5-HT_3 receptor antagonist and dexamethasone, will help manage delayed nausea.

5.243 The *primary* mechanism of action of granisetron and ondansetron as antiemetics is which of the following?

a. Sedation
b. Dopamine antagonist
c. Serotonin antagonist
d. Suppression of autonomic pathways

5.244 The *primary* mechanism of action of dexamethasone as an antiemetic is

a. Anti-inflammatory
b. Dopamine antagonist
c. Histamine receptor antagonist
d. Inhibits prostaglandin synthesis

5.245 Delayed nausea and vomiting occurs more commonly with which of the following agents?

a. Cisplatin
b. Vincristine
c. Carboplatin
d. Mechlorethamine

5.246 Dexamethasone is usually administered along with granisetron or ondansetron. The purpose of the dexamethasone is to do which of the following?

a. To produce euphoria
b. To treat delayed nausea
c. To prevent side effects of granisetron or ondansetron
d. To potentiate the antiemetic effect of the granisetron or ondansetron

5.247 Which of the following is *not* a side effect of the serotonin antagonists?

a. Sedation
b. Dizziness
c. Constipation
d. Extrapyramidal reactions

5.248 When highly emetogenic chemotherapy is to be administered, the patient generally receives a combination of antiemetics rather than a single drug. The rationale for the use of multiple antiemetics is which of the following?

a. The vomiting center is directly activated by multiple pathways.
b. Drugs such as prochlorperizine and granisetron are synergistic in their action.
c. A combination of different antiemetic agents permits the use of lower doses of each agent and is therefore more economical.
d. A combination of different agents allows the care provider to change regimens to different categories.

5.249 The discovery of serotonin has greatly increased the efficacy of antiemetic protocols. Which of the following *best* describes the role of serotonin in nausea and vomiting?

a. Serotonin activates 5-HT_3 receptors on visceral and vagal afferent pathways.
b. Serotonin acts on dopamine receptors in the brain.
c. When serotonin levels are reduced by serotonin antagonists, the patient is more at risk for delayed nausea and vomiting.
d. Serotonin levels are increased when toxic substances such as chemotherapy drugs stimulate the parafollicular cells of the gastrointestinal tract.

5.250 Substance P/neurokinin-1 receptor antagonists are a new class of drugs. Which of the following is an example of these agents and their *appropriate* indication for use?

a. Atovaquone is used to treat taste alterations.
b. Gabapentin is used to treat respiratory congestion in patients with end-stage disease.
c. Aprepitant is used to prevent or reduce acute and delayed nausea and emesis with chemotherapy.
d. Dapsone is used to prevent or treat retrovirus, common in immunosuppressed patients.

5.251 Which of the following opioids is *not* recommended for cancer pain?

a. Demerol
b. Methadone
c. Tramadol
d. Oxycodone

5.252 Patients with metastatic disease to the bone who have little benefit from nonsteroidal anti-inflammatory drugs (NSAIDs) and steroids are *most likely* to benefit from which of the following systemic therapies?

a. Calcitonin
b. Mithramycin
c. Zoledronic acid
d. Saline hydration

5.253 Which of the following statements regarding the transdermal fentanyl system is *not* accurate?

a. Fentanyl is equal to morphine in potency.
b. Approximately 92% of the drug is absorbed into the systemic circulation by 72 hours.
c. Chronic administration in the elderly can lead to toxicity due to saturation of storage sites.
d. Twelve to 16 hours is needed after application of the patch to achieve a therapeutic effect and 18 hours to achieve a steady state in the blood.

5.254 The drug used to treat respiratory depression related to opioid analgesics is
- a. Naproxen
- b. Methadone
- c. Meperidine
- d. Naloxone

5.255 Which of the following is *not* a common side effect of opioids?
- a. Sedation
- b. Constipation
- c. Increased motility
- d. Respiratory depression

5.256 Antidepressants such as amitriptyline may be used to treat pain that is caused by
- a. Tumor infiltration of nerves
- b. Narcotic withdrawal
- c. Brain metastases
- d. Surgery

5.257 Steroids are sometimes used in the management of pain related to
- a. Bowel obstruction
- b. Trigeminal neuralgia
- c. Spinal cord compression
- d. Tumor pressing on a vital organ

5.258 Scheduling of oral analgesics generally should be
- a. As needed
- b. Every 2 hours
- c. At fixed intervals
- d. Related to a patient's activity level

5.259 While caring for a terminally ill patient who is receiving high doses of opioids you notice nocturnal myoclonus. Which of the following constitutes an *appropriate* therapeutic intervention?
- a. Rotate to another opioid.
- b. The opioid dose should be reduced by 25%.
- c. Naloxone should be given to reverse the opioid effect.
- d. Change the opioid, reduce the dose, and add a benzodiazepine.

5.260 Cannabinoids such as dronabinol are generally used as second-line antiemetics. Which of the following is *not* a side effect of cannabinoids?
- a. Amnesia
- b. Dysphoria
- c. Disorientation
- d. Impaired concentration

5.261 The clinical efficacy of antidepressants in persons with cancer is thought to be caused by which of the following?
- a. Antidepressants exert effects on the 5-HT neurotransmission system.
- b. Antidepressants act as stimulants and promote wakefulness.
- c. Antidepressants act to dull awareness of one's situation.
- d. Antidepressants suppress serotonin and norepinephrine.

5.262 Following chemotherapy treatment for her Hodgkin's disease, Allison developed shingles that was successfully treated, but she was instructed to take an antidepressant for approximately 2 weeks. Which of the following explains the purpose of the antidepressant?

a. Treatment for her depression
b. Treatment for her insomnia and fatigue
c. Treatment for itching caused by shingles
d. Treatment to inhibit uptake of the neurotransmitters into nerve terminals

5.263 Lorazepam is commonly used in combination antiemetic therapy. Side effects of this drug include all *except* which of the following?

a. Addiction
b. Drowsiness
c. Amnesia
d. Diarrhea

5.264 Hematopoietic growth factors act on the stem cells to specifically mediate all of the following steps in hematopoiesis *except*

a. Stem cell maturation
b. Cellular proliferation
c. Cellular differentiation
d. Programmed cell death

5.265 Granulocyte and granulocyte-macrophage colony-stimulating factors

a. Decrease myelosuppression
b. Increase febrile episodes
c. Increase mucositis
d. Decrease anorexia

5.266 Epidermal growth factor receptors (EGFRs) are overexpressed in a number of cancers. Of the following statements below regarding EGFRs, which is *not* accurate?

a. EGFRs are expressed in many normal epithelial tissues including skin and hair follicles.
b. EGFR communication is essential for normal cell function.
c. EGFRs are present on hematopoietic cells.
d. EGFRs are a subfamily of the protein tyrosine kinase.

5.267 Hematopoietic growth factors (HGFs) are given to help prevent infection in potentially neutropenic patients. These injections achieve which of the following?

a. Decrease the time from the administration of the drug to the onset of the nadir
b. Decrease the activity of mature cell lineages, thereby preserving them for the period of neutropenia and infection
c. Enhance phagocytosis, antibody-dependent cytotoxicity, and chemotaxis
d. Enhance neutrophil regeneration

5.268 Which of the following is *not* considered a primary reason to administer colony-stimulating factors to patients receiving chemotherapy?

a. To decrease infectious complications
b. To shorten the period of febrile neutropenia
c. To prevent neutropenia in all patients receiving chemotherapy
d. To permit administration of full doses of the chemotherapy agents

5.269 Which of the following is considered to be the *most* potent stimulus for erythropoietin production?

a. Hypoxia
b. Active bleeding
c. Hemoglobin less than 9 g/dL
d. Hematocrit less than 30 g/dL

5.270 Epoetin alfa is contraindicated in patients with which of the following medical conditions?

a. Glaucoma
b. Chronic diarrhea
c. Renal insufficiency
d. Uncontrolled hypertension

5.271 Granulocyte colony-stimulating factor is *not* intended to accomplish which of the following?

a. Decrease the duration of neutropenia related to chemotherapy
b. Decrease the number of episodes of neutropenic fever
c. Decrease the number of hospital days in patients receiving chemotherapy
d. Decrease the duration of thrombocytopenia

5.272 Hematopoietic growth factors are used as supportive therapy for which of the following conditions?

a. A patient with severe cachexia
b. A patient with iron-deficiency anemia
c. A patient undergoing modified radical mastectomy
d. A patient receiving myelosuppressive therapy or a hematopoietic stem cell transplantation

5.273 Hematopoietic growth factors approved by the U.S. Food and Drug Administration (FDA) include all of the following agents *except*

a. Interleukin-2
b. Interleukin-11
c. Granulocyte colony-stimulating factors
d. Granulocyte-macrophage colony-stimulating factors

5.274 Epidermal growth factor receptors have recently been found to be an important prognostic indicator in breast cancer. Which of the following statements regarding the relationship between epidermal growth factor receptors and breast cancer is *false*?

a. The presence of the epidermal growth factor receptor means that a woman is most likely to be estrogen receptor (ER) and progesterone receptor (PR) positive.
b. The presence of the epidermal growth factor receptor means the patient has a poor prognosis.
c. Inhibiting growth factor receptors is therapeutic in women with breast cancer.
d. The presence of the epidermal growth factor has implications for selection of chemotherapy protocols.

NONPHARMACOLOGIC INTERVENTIONS AND COMPLEMENTARY THERAPIES

5.275 Cognitive behavioral therapy is based on the following principles *except*

a. Cognitive reframing
b. Alleviation of symptoms to minimize distress
c. How a patient perceives a situation affects their ability to control it.
d. A patient's ability to control a situation can be improved by changing their perspective.

5.276 The underlying principle of acupuncture in health care includes which of the following?
a. Energy enhances healing by alleviating spiritual blockages.
b. Four secrets of enhancing energy refers to movements that improve health.
c. Stimulation of the appropriate area helps the body correct any imbalance in the flow of energy thereby restoring balance.
d. A therapeutic method that uses pressure to areas or zones that correspond to areas of the body to treat physical disorders.

5.277 Ms. Davis complains of being somewhat depressed and does not want to take traditional antidepressants. She states she would like to try St.-John's-wort. Your *most appropriate* response would be which of the following?
a. She should consider conventional antidepressants.
b. Since she is mildly depressed St.-John's-wort could work for her.
c. She should see a psychiatrist before choosing treatment for her depression.
d. In studies of persons who were severely depressed, St.-John's-wort was not proven to be superior to placebo.

5.278 Janie has ovarian cancer and is beginning her cancer treatment with enthusiasm. In addition to chemotherapy, she wants to begin a macrobiotic diet and take dietary supplements. You want to encourage her and guide her in the right direction. Which of the following is *not* appropriate advice to give this patient?
a. Alternative therapies have not been proved to be effective, and she should not take any vitamins or dietary supplements.
b. Macrobiotic diets tend to be deficient in protein, calories, iron, and vitamin B_{12}.
c. Megadose vitamin supplements tend to be excessively high in the B complex, C, A, D, and E vitamins.
d. Megadose vitamins can cause liver damage, kidney stones, and coagulation abnormalities.

5.279 An example of cutaneous stimulation is
a. Subcutaneous administration of morphine
b. Minor surgery
c. Massage
d. Imagery

5.280 Directing one's attention away from the sensations and emotional reactions produced by pain is known as
a. Distraction
b. Biofeedback
c. Autogenic relaxation
d. Hypnosis

5.281 According to research, which of the following nonpharmacologic measures is *most effective* in relieving fatigue?
a. Exercise
b. Conservation of energy
c. Increasing the number of hours resting or sleeping
d. Motivational strategies to increase self-efficacy beliefs

5.282 Which of the following reasons is *least likely* to explain a decision by a patient with cancer to explore an alternative method of treatment?
a. Pressure from family and friends
b. Valid data on the efficacy of the method
c. Resentment toward an impersonal medical system
d. A desire for greater control over the treatment process

5.283 Rita has lung cancer and wants to try alternative approaches to nutrition to help improve her immune system. She is leaning toward a macrobiotic diet and asks if there are any adverse effects associated with this type of diet. The *major* problem with a macrobiotic diet is which of the following?

a. Constipation
b. Fat deficiency
c. Protein deficiencies
d. Deficiencies in vitamin C

5.284 Mary is being treated with pharmacologic therapy for her cancer-related pain. The physician encourages her to also practice relaxation and guided imagery to help manage her pain. Mary asks you to explain why these interventions for her pain have been recommended. Your *most appropriate* response to her would be:

a. These interventions will interrupt painful sensory input to the brain.
b. These interventions do not help manage pain and should not be used.
c. These interventions may help to decrease patients' emotional response to pain, enabling you to deal with the pain more positively.
d. These interventions help to block the sensation of pain so that eventually pharmacologic interventions will no longer be necessary.

5.285 All of the following nonpharmacological interventions have been identified through research to provide benefit for cancer-related fatigue *except*

a. Exercise
b. Music therapy
c. Energy conservation and activity management (ECAM)
d. Cognitive-behavioral treatment for distressing symptoms

ANSWER RATIONALES

Please note: All page numbers referenced in the Answer Rationales sections refer to the textbook *Cancer Nursing: Principles and Practice, Seventh Edition,* by Connie Henke Yarbro, Debra Wujcik, and Barbara Holmes Gobel (Jones & Bartlett Learning, © 2011).

Etiology and Patterns of Symptoms

5.1 The answer is d.
New guidelines recommend that erythropoietin alfa be given in patients being treated with myelosuppressive chemotherapy with noncurative intent and who are mildly symptomatic. Although results may be seen in 2 weeks, the time required for erythropoiesis and the red blood cell half-life, an interval of 2–6 weeks may occur between the time of a dose adjustment and significant change in hemoglobin. Patients with uncontrolled hypertension should not be treated with erythropoietin alfa. In patients with a history of congestive heart failure, an increase in the rate of rise of the hemoglobin of more than 1 g/dL in any 2-week period was associated with an increase in cardiac arrest and stroke. Page 603–605.

5.2 The answer is a.
Biologic response modifiers tend to produce fatigue that is more severe than that associated with surgery, radiation therapy, and the most commonly used chemotherapy regimens. Page 345.

5.3 The answer is a.
Skin involvement is the most common clinical feature of acute graft-versus-host disease (AGVHD). Chronic graft-versus-host disease can also affect the skin occurring 100 days or longer after stem cell transplant. Symptoms of AGVHD can also occur 100 days after transplant. Page 517, 522.

5.4 The answer is b.
Pruritus, which frequently accompanies jaundice, is precipitated by irritation of the cutaneous sensory nerve fibers by accumulated bile salts. Jaundice and pruritus is evident in patients with obstructive gallbladder cancer. Page 1319, 1327.

5.5 The answer is a.
Radiation therapy is commonly associated with increases in daytime fatigue and somnolence regardless of whether the radiation therapy is for primary brain tumors or for primary tumors in areas other than the brain. Studies indicate that radiation results in less sleep efficiency and a higher level of daytime dysfunction and higher levels of sleep disturbance in patients further along in their radiation treatment protocol. Other medications can disrupt her nighttime sleep, causing her to be more fatigued during the day. Page 330.

5.6 The answer is a.
Corticosteroids are frequently used in antineoplastic drug regimens and in antiemetic drug protocols and commonly cause sleep disruption, insomnia, restlessness, and increased motor activity. Page 475.

5.7 The answer is b.
Viral infections may be characterized by low continuous fevers. Most patients who have infection are tachycardic and tachypneic, except when the infection is so severe as to cause

acidosis. Bacterial infections produce high spiking fevers with periods of return to normal. Disseminated fungal infections usually produce high spiking fevers without any such return to baseline. Subnormal temperatures are associated with gram-negative infections. Page 725.

5.8 **The answer is d.**
The nadir for high-dose methotrexate is 5–7 days, and diarrhea in the presence of neutropenia requires the patient be tested for *C. difficile*, especially if the patient is also receiving antibiotics. This bacteria causes toxin release and is treated with oral vancomycin or metronidazole. Page 449–450, 463.

5.9 **The answer is c.**
Because it is not possible to distinguish an acute hemolytic blood reaction from a non-hemolytic transfusion reaction at the bedside, the reaction should be managed by stopping the transfusion and working the patient up for a possible infection or hemolytic transfusion reaction. Placing the patient in the Trendelenburg position and administering a fluid bolus are not ideal because of the dyspnea. Page 619–620, 767.

5.10 **The answer is a.**
Scalp pain is common approximately 1–2 days prior to hair loss. The bulb of the follicle swells as it is about to release the hair. An anti-inflammatory agent, massage, and/or heat can be helpful. Skin metastases to the scalp rarely cause scalp pain. Page 485–486.

5.11 **The answer is d.**
If a bowel movement does not occur every other day, a laxative must be taken. His risk factors are high for constipation, and it should be emphasized to the patient never to wait more than 3 days without a bowel movement before calling the physician. Page 470.

5.12 **The answer is d.**
Bone marrow failure can occur in heavily treated patients who have received multiple courses of chemotherapy, and, finally, chronic microscopic bleeding in patients with primary or metastatic diseases can result in anemia as a result of chronic hemorrhage. Tumor secretion of cytokines, such as interleukin-1, affect red blood cell metabolism and function and is a factor associated with anemia of malignancy. Patients with protein-caloric malnutrition often have insufficient iron and folic acid stores, leading to anemia. Page 609.

5.13 **The answer is c.**
Patients who are severely immunosuppressed and have a coagulopathy are most likely to bleed into the alveoli. The alveoli fill with blood, prohibiting gas exchange and leading to hypoxia. Diffuse alveolar hemorrhage (DAH) has been reported in as many as 41% of patients who have had hematopoietic stem cell transplant. Page 521.

5.14 **The answer is b.**
High-dose corticosteroids are the primary treatment for diffuse alveolar hemorrhage. If hemoptysis occurs cough suppression might help because coughing is an aggravating factor. For treating substantial hemoptysis, the individual needs to be kept calm and on bed rest, lying on his or her side, with the side of hemorrhage dependent so as not to cause asphyxiation by draining the blood into the other lung. Page 521, 760.

5.15 **The answer is b.**
Anemia manifests as pallor, hypotension, headaches, irritability, and fatigue. Tachycardia and tachypnea may be present due to the hypoxic effects on the heart. Page 609.

5.16 The answer is c.
Emesis occurs through several mechanisms, including stimulation of enterochromaffin cells in the duodenum, leading to release of serotonin. Serotonin binds and stimulates the vagus nerve, which in turn stimulates the spinal cord, medulla oblongata, and then the brain's vomiting center. Page 470–472.

5.17 The answer is a.
Prior or concurrent radiation may augment the severity and extent of mucosal injury. Some drugs, such as dactinomycin and doxorubicin, potentiate radiation injury to the esophagus, and others, including 5-fluorouracil, hydroxyurea, procarbazine, and vinblastine, produce an additive toxic effect with irradiation. Page 334, 483.

5.18 The answer is b.
Because carcinoma of the thyroid can rapidly invade surrounding structures, symptoms may occur that are related to compressive effects of the enlarging mass on adjacent structures. Patients may experience dyspnea or stridor when the trachea is compressed or infiltrated. Compression of the esophagus may cause dysphagia. Hoarseness can result from malignant infiltration or destruction of the laryngeal or vagus nerves. Page 1261.

5.19 The answer is c.
The frequency of oral care should increase with the severity of the symptoms. A basic solution such as sodium bicarbonate or normal saline 4× daily is recommended for practice. Chlorhexidine is not recommended for cancer-treatment related mucositis. Page 815.

5.20 The answer is d.
Mucositis is observed more often with 5-FU when combined with other mucositis-producing drugs such as methotrexate and doxorubicin and when 5-FU is given concurrently with leucovorin to augment its cytotoxicity. Page 479, 811.

5.21 The answer is d.
Stomatitis is 2–3 times higher in patients with hematological malignancies. Page 479.

5.22 The answer is a.
Areas of the oral cavity adjacent to metal tooth fillings are at greatest risk for increased reaction due to radiation scatter from the metal fillings. Mucositis is enhanced and prolonged in patients who have preexisting poor oral or dental hygiene, continue to smoke, use chewing tobacco, consume alcohol, and have poorly fitting dentures. Page 331.

5.23 The answer is a.
Direct stomatotoxicity results from the cytotoxic action of drugs on the cells of the oral basal epithelium, causing a decrease in the rate of cell renewal. The sequelae include a thinned atrophic mucosa and initiation of an inflammatory response (stomatitis). Page 479.

5.24 The answer is a.
Xerostomia is a drying of the oral mucosa resulting from loss of saliva due to damage that occurs to the salivary glands subsequent to radiation therapy to the head and neck; it manifests in a thicker saliva. Mucositis is an inflammatory response of the oral mucosa to radiation therapy. The oral cavity appears inflamed, and white patchy areas may be seen. The patient complains of a sore throat and mouth. Trismus or jaw hypomobility may occur if the posterior mandible is included in the irradiated field. Page 333.

5.25 **The answer is d.**
Oral pilocarpine has been approved for use as a stimulant to the exocrine glands. This results in diaphoresis, salivation, lacrimation, and gastric and pancreatic secretion. Page 333.

5.26 **The answer is b.**
Saliva provides lubrication for oral tissues and protection from bacterial infections. Saliva also inhibits enamel decalcification and provides an important excretory route for blood-borne urea, uric acid, and ammonia. Page 333.

5.27 **The answer is c.**
The 5-HT_3 antagonist plus a corticosteroid is the most effective treatment, providing superior control in patients receiving high-dose cisplatin. Page 438, 476.

5.28 **The answer is b.**
Paclitaxel is not associated with delayed nausea and vomiting. Cisplatin is most commonly associated with delayed nausea; doxorubicin, cyclophosphamide, and ifosfamide can also produce delayed nausea. Page 471.

5.29 **The answer is c.**
Anticipatory nausea and vomiting occurs in 25% of patients as a result of classic operant conditioning from stimuli associated with chemotherapy. Page 471.

5.30 **The answer is d.**
Surgery can increase energy requirements, and she must be assessed prior to surgery in order to address any nutritional deficiencies. Betty can be somewhat reassured that her cancer is not in the aerodigestive or gastrointestinal tract, and she is likely to have nutritional problems resulting from the surgery only in the immediate perioperative period. Page 820.

5.31 **The answer is a.**
Cancer cachexia is characterized by anorexia, weight loss, skeletal muscle atrophy, and asthenia (loss of strength). Marasmus is simple starvation with protein-calorie malnutrition. Page 823–824.

Toxicity and Rating Scales

5.32 **The answer is b.**
Cancer pain may be acute, chronic, or intermittent and often has a definable etiology, usually related to tumor recurrence or treatment. In contrast to acute pain, chronic cancer pain is rarely accompanied by signs of autonomic nervous system (ANS) arousal. The lack of objective signs may prompt the inexperienced clinician to wrongly conclude the patient is not in pain. Answer d is also true, but that is not what the question is asking. Page 686, 689.

5.33 **The answer is b.**
In this situation she is not by definition a candidate for erythropoietin because the National Comprehensive Cancer Network guidelines establish a hemoglobin level of $\leq$ 10 g/dL as the point for initiating therapy with erythropoietin. Also, fatigue due to anemia does not get better on its own; her fatigue is more likely related to the side effects of her antiemetics. Exercise is an appropriate recommendation, especially with the breast cancer population. Page 605, 777–778.

5.34 **The answer is d.**
Respiratory rate, oxygen saturation, and arterial blood gas levels neither correlate with nor measure dyspnea. For example, patients may be hypoxemic but not dyspneic or may be dyspneic

but not hypoxemic. The only reliable indicator of dyspnea in clinical practice is patient self-report. Page 1833.

5.35 The answer is a.
Doxorubicin is frequently associated with moderate to severe hair loss. Bleomycin, methotrexate, and mitoxantrone are associated with mild hair loss. Page 442, 486.

5.36 The answer is c.
Critical to establishing a diagnosis of reactive (situational) depression in cancer patients is the evaluation of selected defining characteristics commonly attributed to depression among the psychiatrically ill. Some common characteristics of depression, however, may also occur in the cancer patient as a result of the disease, its treatment, or its side effects, or they may have existed in the patient before diagnosis. Therefore the primary criteria for assessment of depression are that the characteristics are a change from previous functioning, are persistent, occur for most of the day and on more days than not, and are present for at least 2 weeks. Page 675–676.

5.37 The answer is c.
Performance scales that measure a person's functional status are used frequently in the eligibility criteria for cooperative group clinical trials and also periodically to evaluate the effects of treatment and disease. It may be helpful to interpret a person's quality of life, but it is not a primary objective of performance status. Page 191–192.

5.38 The answer is d.
Because Carlos' eating habits have changed considerably and because he is not going to be staying in the hospital for most of his treatment, both the calorie count method and the 24-hour recall method are inappropriate. Food frequency reporting is not ideal because Carlos has a hard time remembering what he ate. A diet diary would provide an extended record of Carlos' eating habits that would rely on his cooperation and honesty—both of which you believe you can count on. Page 832.

5.39 The answer is d.
There is general agreement that quality of life is best evaluated by the patient, rather than by another observer. There are situations in which the patient may not be able to provide the information such as with cognitive impairment, debilitating fatigue, severe nausea, severe pain, or other symptoms. Page 212.

5.40 The answer is a.
The Functional Assessment of Cancer Therapy (FACT/FACIT) instrument is used to measure the following domains of quality of life: physical, social/family, emotional, functional and overall well-being. Page 208.

5.41 The answer is d.
Cisplatin (> 50 mg/m^2) is considered to be a level-5 emetogenic chemotherapy agent. Level-5 agents cause severe nausea and vomiting. Treatment with level-5 agents require an in-depth emetic history and a preventive action plan with antiemetics. More than one antiemetic agent is required to prevent and manage the nausea and vomiting from level-5 agents, thus adding antiemetics that target different pathways of nausea and vomiting are critical. In addition, for those patients receiving moderately severe to severe emetogenic chemotherapy, antiemetics for delayed nausea and vomiting are needed. Page 471–473, 477.

Alterations in Comfort

5.42 The answer is c.

One of the most common reasons for unrelieved pain in American healthcare systems is the failure of staff to routinely assess pain and pain relief. Many patients silently tolerate unrelieved pain, especially if they are not specifically asked about it. Page 689.

5.43 The answer is a.

Tramadol is a weak opioid receptor agonist not frequently used in cancer care. Changing the dosing regimen or route of the same drug helps to achieve a constant blood level rather than the high peak serum levels that often cause side effects. In general, all strong opioid analgesics have similar side effects, with the exception of fentanyl and oxymorphone, which have little propensity to release histamine, and often causes itching and urticaria. Adding caffeine to counteract sedation or a laxative and nutrition counseling to control constipation or antiemetics for nausea are appropriate to help the patient tolerate the pain medicine. Page 696–697.

5.44 The answer is a.

Low-dose tricyclic antidepressants (TCAs), gabapentin, lidocaine patch 5%, and tramadol are effective agents for the treatment of neuropathic pain, diabetic neuropathy, and postherpetic neuralgia. Sedation and orthostatic hypotension are common, which is why TCAs are given at bedtime and may limit the concomitant use of opioid analgesics. Page 701–702.

5.45 The answer is d.

Of the five dimensions of the cancer pain experience described by Ahles et al., the cognitive dimension relates to the manner in which pain influences a person's thought processes, view of self, and the meaning of the pain. Page 686.

5.46 The answer is a.

Lorazepam is a sedative drug. Methylphenidate and dextroamphetamine are the most common treatments for opiate-induced daytime sedation. Donepezil is an oral acetylcholinesterase inhibitor. This class of agents increases central cholinergic activity and therefore reverses cognitive and sedative side effects of opiate treatment. Page 783–784.

5.47 The answer is c.

Relief from pruritus from any cause may be relieved from meticulous skin care, the use of emollient lotions and antihistamines. The effects of histamine from systemic opioids cannot be reversed with naloxone. Page 485, 697.

5.48 The answer is c.

Dyspnea is described as the "invisible" disease because the patient masks it by resting. So unless the patient has lung cancer, they are rarely asked if they are having any difficulty breathing, and they are reluctant to report this symptom. Dyspnea occurs when an increase in the amount of respiratory effort is needed to overcome obstructive or restrictive disease, an increase (not decrease) in the amount of respiratory muscles is required to maintain adequate breathing, or an increase in ventilator need. Physiologic parameters are rarely present with dyspnea. The pain associated with dyspnea can be a presenting symptom of pulmonary effusion and is generally acute rather than chronic. Page 1833.

5.49 The answer is d.

Although it may be appropriate to suppress a dry, persistent, and debilitating cough, narcotic medications should not be attempted at the expense of removal of secretions. The other strategies suggested promote comfort. Page 1450–1451.

5.50 The answer is a.
The only side effect that patients do not reach a tolerance for is constipation. Agitation is not a side effect of opioids. Lethargy and nausea are common side effects, and patients will become tolerant of these side effects generally within 1–2 weeks. Page 697.

5.51 The answer is c.
Opioids are the first-line therapy in relieving dyspnea, as they decrease the intensity of dyspnea without causing respiratory depression. Benzodiazepines and glucocorticoids, along with oxygen, are useful adjuncts to opioids without fear of respiratory depression, but they are not used alone as first-line therapy for dyspnea. Page 1834.

5.52 The answer is a.
For most individuals, phantom limb pain usually decreases significantly within the first year; however, some may be troubled for years. Although phantom limb sensations (i.e., itching, pressure, tingling) are often experienced shortly after surgery, phantom limb pain (i.e., cramping, throbbing, burning) usually occurs within 1–4 weeks after surgery. Worsening of phantom limb pain may be a sign of a neuroma or of locally recurrent cancer in the stump. Page 1066.

Alterations in Protective Mechanisms

5.53 The answer is c.
When the neutrophil count is less than 500/mm^3, approximately 20% or more of febrile episodes have an associated bacteremia caused principally by aerobic gram-negative bacilli and gram-positive cocci. Page 467, 726, 733.

5.54 The answer is d.
Acetaminophen, corticosteroids, and antihistamines may be given prior to platelet therapy to minimize the chance of a febrile nonhemolytic transfusion reaction. Page 615–616.

5.55 The answer is c.
Individuals with spinal metastasis may have radicular pain, paresthesias, heaviness of limbs, leg buckling, and episodes of dropping items. Based on these symptoms, compression of the spinal cord is likely and needs immediate treatment to prevent progressive neurological injury. Page 983–984.

5.56 The answer is a.
Compression of the spinal cord is likely and needs immediate treatment to prevent progressive neurological injury. Page 983–985.

5.57 The answer is c.
Mental status changes can be an initial sign of hypercalcemia, hyperviscosity syndrome, or drug toxicity. Page 1520, 1527.

5.58 The answer is b.
Phantom limb pain is caused by the nerve pathways that have been transected during surgery. This transection results in the transmission of abnormal impulses. Patients may feel pain, burning, itching, cramping, and throbbing sensations in the limb. These sensations can be exacerbated by stress, fatigue, and emotional stressors. Medications include muscle relaxants and tranquilizers. Simple measures like the use of a stump shrinker that exerts pressure, heat packs, or distraction may reduce the problem. Although narcotics have been used, they are not the best treatment option. Page 1066.

5.59 **The answer is d.**
When patients with prostate cancer receive androgen therapy, osteoblastic bone formation activity is decreased and osteoclastic activity is increased, thereby increasing the loss of bone mineral density and creating an opportunity for osteoporosis to occur. Page 1068.

5.60 **The answer is b.**
Because bisphosphonates inhibit osteoclast activity in bone (causes bone breakdown), they are ideal in the treatment of patients with bone metastases. When bisphosphonates bind to bone, they help to stabilize the bone mineral and inhibit calcium release and further breakdown. Page 955, 1628.

5.61 **The answer is b.**
Avoidance of amputation, preservation of maximum function, and eradication of tumor are all goals in the treatment of primary malignant bone cancer. Although there is evidence of a familial tendency for some of the bone cancers, early intervention in these cases is not common practice. Page 1060–1061.

5.62 **The answer is b.**
Infection in the neutropenic patient is always considered a potentially life-threatening emergency. Mortality rates in individuals with cancer who are neutropenic exceed 30%. Page 714.

5.63 **The answer is c.**
The ANC is calculated by multiplying the total white blood cell count (4000) by the differential proportion of combined segmented neutrophils (34%) and band neutrophils (3%) in a blood sample. ANC = 4000 cells/mm^3 × 0.37% = 1480 cells/mm^3. Page 467.

5.64 **The answer is a.**
Neutropenia is not only the most common dose-limiting side effect of chemotherapy, but it is potentially the most lethal. Page 467.

5.65 **The answer is c.**
The patient with neutropenia is unable to mount an inflammatory response. Fever is usually the first sign of infection. Choices a, b, and d are all true, but they explain why the neutropenic patient is at greater risk for infection rather than why the usual signs and symptoms of infection are often absent. Page 467.

5.66 **The answer is c.**
Neutropenia typically develops in 8–12 days after chemotherapy, with recovery in 3–4 weeks. Page 467.

5.67 **The answer is b.**
The respiratory tract is the most common site of infection in neutropenic patients. A high incidence of pneumonia in immunocompromised patients warrants thorough assessment of the respiratory tract. The mouth and oropharynx are also high incidence sites for infection. Page 723.

5.68 **The answer is a.**
In general, antifungal prophylaxis is not recommended for all neutropenic patients receiving chemotherapy. It is recommended for high-risk patients such as those with acute leukemia receiving chemotherapy or those patients undergoing allogeneic hematopoietic stem cell transplantation. Antifungal prophylaxis is indicated for severely neutropenic afebrile patients with an absolute neutrophil count less than 1000/mm^3 for more than 1 week. Page 731.

5.69 **The answer is d.**
Infections, due to invasion and overgrowth of pathogenic microbes, increase in frequency and severity as the absolute neutrophil count decreases. Risk for severe infections increases when the nadir persists for more than 7–10 days. The purpose of colony-stimulating factors is to reduce the number of days that the nadir is below 500 cells/mm^3. Page 605–606.

5.70 **The answer is c.**
In the setting of neutropenia, the general standard of care is a time frame of 2 hours from fever to administration of the first antimicrobial agent. Chest x-rays are usually ordered, but the yield is relatively low, and this step is considered a lower priority than starting antimicrobial therapy, especially in an elderly patient. Page 731, 740.

5.71 **The answer is a.**
Myelosuppression is the most common and lethal side effect of chemotherapy. Because hematopoietic cells divide rapidly, they are vulnerable to chemotherapy, potentially resulting in dangerously low levels of red blood cells, white blood cells, and platelets. When this occurs, patients are at risk for bleeding, infection, and circulatory compromise. Page 468.

5.72 **The answer is d.**
Thrombopoietin is the factor that stimulates the differentiation and proliferation of megakaryocytes into platelets. It has been shown to reduce the duration of thrombocytopenia. Page 762.

5.73 **The answer is d.**
A cumulative and delayed onset of thrombocytopenia has been observed with carmustine, fludarabine, lomustine, mitomycin C, streptozocin, and thiotepa. Page 466, 752.

5.74 **The answer is c.**
When platelets are lower than 50,000 cells/mm^3, there is a moderate risk of bleeding. As the platelets continue to decrease below 10,000 cells/mm^3, a severe risk exists for fatal bleeding. Page 466, 755.

5.75 **The answer is d.**
Petechiae and epistaxis may occur as the platelet count continues to decrease below 10,000 cells/mm^3, but a severe risk exists for spontaneous central nervous system hemorrhage. Page 466.

5.76 **The answer is c.**
The most common cause of thrombocytopenia in patients with cancer is a disorder involving decreased megakaryocytopoiesis (i.e., platelet production in the bone marrow). Page 749.

5.77 **The answer is b.**
Idiopathic thrombocytopenic purpura occurs most frequently in individuals with lymphoproliferative disorders such as chronic lymphocytic leukemia. It rarely is associated with solid tumors. Page 749.

5.78 **The answer is c.**
Stool softener and a laxative are important for preventing constipation in the patient who is receiving vincristine. Rectal manipulation may place the thrombocytopenic patient at risk for bleeding. The use of suppositories or enemas is contraindicated. Page 760–761.

5.79 **The answer is a.**
Steroids have a capillary-stabilizing effect that is important in minimizing the bleeding potential of thrombocytopenia. Page 763.

5.80 The answer is b.
Platelet survival is greatly decreased when alloimmunization to the platelet transfusion develops. Alloimmunization results when repeated transfusions of platelets fail to provide a therapeutic increment in the platelet count. Page 749–750.

5.81 The answer is d.
Factors that determine the degree, onset, and duration of radiation-induced skin reactions include the following, among others: Higher doses given over shorter periods of time to larger volumes result in more severe acute skin reactions; electrons produce greater skin reactions than photons; and placing tissue-equivalent material on the skin reduces the skin-sparing effect of radiation therapy, allowing for maximum dose at the level of the skin. Finally, when treatment is targeted at areas of skin apposition, increased reaction secondary to warmth and moisture can be expected. Page 319–320.

5.82 The answer is b.
Hyperpigmentation occurs with bleomycin. Other drugs inducing this reaction include cyclophosphamide, busulfan, carmustine, nitrogen mustard, 5-FU, and etoposide. Page 484.

5.83 The answer is a.
Persons who are immunocompromised are at high risk for activation of varicella zoster virus, which once activated spreads down the sensory nerve to skin level. The physician should be notified immediately if the eye is in close proximity because ocular dissemination can result in systemic spread and loss of vision. Therapy is generally held until the extent of the spread is known and treatment is underway. Patients should be taught to wash hands frequently when immunocompromised to minimize the risk of infection. Page 515, 730.

5.84 The answer is c.
The most significant consequence of gram-negative infection is the potential for endotoxic or systemic shock. The release of endotoxins initiates a cascade of events that, unless interrupted, rapidly lead to death for the neutropenic patient. Page 725, 967.

5.85 The answer is c.
Pneumocystis carinii is a protozoan that causes infection in children with primary immunodeficiency disorders, persons with AIDS, and those with cancer who are undergoing immunosuppressive therapy. Untreated, *P. carinii* is fatal, and even with therapy mortality is high. The treatment of choice is trimethoprim-sulfamethoxazole. Page 515, 733, 736.

5.86 The answer is c.
Risk factors for development of sepsis include (but are not limited to) complex polymicrobial infections, granulocytopenia lasting longer than 7 days, skin breakdown (especially in the elderly), hematologic malignancy, shock associated with infection, and low albumin at the onset of symptoms of sepsis. Page 966–967.

5.87 The answer is a.
Fever is the cardinal symptom of infection. The presence of neutropenia masks the classic infection-related symptoms of inflammation, pus formation, and elevated white blood cell counts. Page 725, 967.

5.88 The answer is b.
Gram-positive organisms are responsible for approximately 75% of all infections in patients with cancer. Page 714, 726.

5.89 The answer is b.
The skin is the first line of defense against invading bacteria and subsequent infection. When a break in the skin occurs, environmental microbes and those that normally inhabit hair follicles and sebaceous glands can enter the body and cause infection. Page 718.

5.90 The answer is d.
Polymorphonuclear neutrophils (PMNs) make up 35%–76% of white blood cells and are the first to respond to invading bacteria. The primary function of PMNs is the destruction and elimination of microorganisms through phagocytosis, the process of engulfing and ingesting foreign matter. Page 723.

5.91 The answer is d.
Undisturbed endogenous microbial flora exist as a carefully balanced synergistic microenvironment within the host. Alterations in normal flora predispose persons with cancer to serious opportunistic or nosocomial infection. A large percentage of infections developing in cancer patients arise from endogenous organisms, nearly half of which are acquired during hospitalization. Page 723.

5.92 The answer is b.
Meticulous hand washing, by every person who enters the room or comes in contact with the individual at risk, is the single most important preventive measure against infection in the patient with granulocytopenia. Neutropenic individuals are advised of their risk and are encouraged to remind family, visitors, and staff about hand-washing precautions. Page 467, 730.

5.93 The answer is b.
Because diagnostic signals may be subtle (e.g., skin petechiae that may be noticed while bathing the person, traces of blood during brushing of teeth), it is important for the nurse to be keenly observant. A family history and various screening tests may be valuable in assessment, but they do not substitute for observation. Page 754–755.

5.94 The answer is d.
Megakaryocytes mature in the bone marrow and fragment to form platelets, which are then released into the bloodstream. Under normal circumstances any reduction in platelet count—from bleeding, malignancy, chemotherapy, radiotherapy, or other causes—produces an increase in the production of megakaryocytes and platelets in the bone marrow. This activity is controlled by a regulatory hormone called thrombopoietin. Page 607, 749.

5.95 The answer is c.
Erosion and rupture of vessels precipitated by tumor invasion or pressure is the other major cause of bleeding in persons with cancer. Any tumor involvement of vasculature tissue or any tumor lying in close proximity to major vessels is seen as a threat of bleeding. All the other choices can be factors in bleeding. Bleeding may also be the result of radiotherapy, surgery, or various platelet and coagulation abnormalities. Page 751–754.

5.96 The answer is d.
If acute bleeding does occur, direct methods to halt the hemorrhage should be instituted immediately. Choices *a*, *b*, and *c* are preventive methods. Another example of the use of mechanical pressure to stop acute bleeding is the insertion of an occlusion balloon catheter into the bronchus. Page 763.

5.97 The answer is b.

The platelet count is the single most important factor in predicting bleeding in the individual with cancer. Patients with platelet counts below 20,000 cells/mm^3 have a high risk of bleeding. Low platelet count (thrombocytopenia) is also the most frequent platelet abnormality associated with cancer. Page 746.

5.98 The answer is c.

The presence of leukocytosis (white blood cell count > 30 $\times$ 10^9 cells) is associated with increased treatment death (~50% of cases), most often as a result of tumor lysis syndrome. Page 1391.

5.99 The answer is a.

Patients with liver cancer are more at risk for bleeding because of a decrease in vitamin K absorption, an increase in prothrombin time and partial thromboplastin time, and varices from portal hypertension. Abnormal platelet function resulting in bleeding occurs most frequently in hematologic malignancies. Page 750.

5.100 The answer is c.

Qualitative abnormalities such as choice *c* refer principally to alterations in platelet function, which may include a decreased procoagulant activity of platelets, decreased platelet adhesiveness and decreased aggregation in response to adenosine diphosphate (ADP), thrombocytosis associated with myeloproliferative disorders, and the coating of platelets by fibrin degradation products as a result of the increased activation of coagulation factors. Choices *a* and *d* are coagulation abnormalities; choice *b* is a quantitative abnormality. Page 750, 753.

5.101 The answer is b.

Thrombin, the most powerful of the coagulation enzymes, is required for both coagulation and fibrinolysis. Page 748.

Alterations in Gastrointestinal Function

5.102 The answer is a.

Anticipatory nausea and vomiting are often brought about by the patient's previous experience with uncontrolled nausea and vomiting, and lorazepam has been demonstrated to be effective for anticipatory nausea and vomiting. Lorazepam acts as an antianxiety agent but also has some antinausea effects. Anxiety can occur in patients receiving cancer treatment, but it is not a universal problem for patients with cancer. Page 471, 473.

5.103 The answer is a.

The degree and duration of diarrhea depend on the agent, dose, nadir, and frequency of chemotherapy administration. Patients may experience abdominal cramps and rectal urgency with 5-FU–leucovorin therapy, which can evolve into nocturnal diarrhea or fecal incontinence, leading to lethargy, weakness, orthostatic hypotension, and fluid/electrolyte imbalance. Without adequate management, prolonged diarrhea causes dehydration, nutritional malabsorption, and circulatory collapse. Renal failure does not result from untreated diarrhea. Page 469–470.

5.104 The answer is d.

Rectal emptying is specifically diminished as a result of chemotherapy-induced neuropathies that disrupt the autonomic nervous system. Page 470.

5.105 The answer is c.
The fact that he is nauseated and not passing gas means he could be obstipated and needs to be evaluated immediately. Page 470.

5.106 The answer is d.
Systemic opioids may precipitate histamine release leading to flushing and pruritus. Opioids affect the bowel by activation of specific opioid receptors in both the GI tract and the central nervous system. Increased tone and nonpropulsive motility in the ileum and colon result in increased transit time and water absorption. Morphine-induced insensitivity to rectal distention further contributes to constipation. Page 697.

5.107 The answer is d.
Combining the softening action with the peristaltic stimulant effect lessens constipation. Teaching the patient to increase fiber and fluids will help the action of the senekot and the colace, but will not by themselves help opiate-induced constipation. Metamucil is not recommended for the treatment of opiate-induced constipation. Page 697–698.

5.108 The answer is a.
Management of severe diarrhea in patients with radiation-induced enteritis includes all of these choices except a liquid diet high in milk products. Page 337.

5.109 The answer is d.
Patients may experience abdominal cramps and rectal urgency with 5-fluorouracil, which can evolve into nocturnal diarrhea or fecal incontinence leading to lethargy, weakness, orthostatic hypotension, and fluid/electrolyte imbalance. Page 469.

5.110 The answer is d.
Stool cultures should be obtained prior to administering antidiarrheal medications due to the potential for infection causing the diarrhea. Nocturnal diarrhea or fecal incontinence leads to lethargy, weakness, orthostatic hypotension, and fluid/electrolyte imbalance. Without adequate management, prolonged diarrhea causes dehydration, nutritional malabsorption, and circulatory collapse. Page 469.

5.111 The answer is d.
If a patient has diarrhea that is due to an infectious agent such as *Clostridium difficile*, the use of antidiarrheal agents can increase risk for sepsis by increasing exposure to the mucosa and subsequent absorption of the toxin because antidiarrheal agents decrease colonic transit time. Page 469.

5.112 The answer is c.
If the obstruction continues for more than a few days or is recurrent, a gastrostomy tube is a much more acceptable and well-tolerated route for decompression than nasogastric intubation. Intermittent venting of the gastrostomy tube allows the patient to continue oral intake and maintain an active lifestyle. The two options currently available are surgically placed gastrostomy and percutaneous endoscopic gastrostomy. Pain and antinausea medications may help, but they cannot replace a venting tube. Page 1235.

5.113 The answer is d.
Biliary vomiting is almost odorless and indicates an obstruction in the upper part of the abdomen. Page 1235.

Alterations in Genitourinary Function

5.114 The answer is c.
Risk factors identified for postoperative incontinence following radical prostatectomy include age over 65, development of anastomatic stricture, and T1a or T1b disease. Page 1619.

5.115 The answer is b.
Emptying the bladder at bedtime (either by voiding or by self-catheterization) or setting the alarm to awaken once during the night may help to avoid incontinence. Complete nighttime control returns in approximately 80% of patients who undergo a continent/orthoptic urinary diversion surgery. Page 1087.

5.116 The answer is d.
The normal prostate on palpation is usually a rounded structure about 4 cm in diameter that feels firm. Cancer of the prostate typically appears as a stony hard nodule, whereas benign hypertrophy usually results in a diffuse enlargement of the prostate without masses. Page 1613–1615.

5.117 The answer is d.
After radical prostatectomy, 92% of patients achieve urinary control, 8% experience stress incontinence, and 6% wear one or fewer incontinence pads per day. Approximately 1% of men are incontinent after a transurethral resection of the prostate. Page 1624.

5.118 The answer is a.
Sphincter incompetence presents as dribbling and stress incontinence. Treatment includes anticholinergic drugs and surgery. The drugs increase sphincter resistance. Repeat surgery may be needed to relieve urethral compression or stricture. Kegel exercises help to strengthen pelvic floor muscles that are crucial to maintaining continence. Urinary catheters are not useful for long-term management of incontinence unless no other approach is successful. Page 1624.

5.119 The answer is b.
Wound dehiscence is not primarily related to cystectomy. Complications are related to stoma construction and placement and to the possibility of long-term kidney damage. Other complications include stomal stenosis. Page 1086–1087.

5.120 The answer is d.
There are several types of continent urinary diversions. They differ largely in the specific portion of intestine used to create the pouch. Page 1087.

5.121 The answer is d.
Continent urinary reservoirs and bladder substitutes produce much mucus. They should be irrigated regularly in the early postoperative period to prevent mucous accumulation. Mucous production decreases over time, and irrigation becomes unnecessary. Page 1086–1088.

5.122 The answer is c.
The stoma itself should be a beefy, dark red color. A urinary diversion should produce urine from the time of surgery, and flow should be more or less continuous. Some stomal edema postoperatively is normal, but the edema should not interfere with the stoma function. Leakage from the appliance is abnormal and could lead to skin breakdown. Page 1086.

5.123 The answer is b.
Signs and symptoms of nephrotic syndrome include massive proteinuria and brown frothy urine, as well as facial and peripheral edema, which may progress to anasarca or edema of all

body tissues. The combined water and electrolyte retention may cause mild to moderate hypertension, not hypotension. Page 856–857.

5.124 The answer is d.
Hyperglycemia is not a specific contributing factor to renal failure associated with multiple myeloma. Infection, hypercalcemia, and dehydration are all possible contributing factors to the renal failure associated with multiple myeloma. Page 1519–1520.

5.125 The answer is a.
Prevention of hemorrhagic cystitis is the key to success when administering high-dose cyclophosphamide, including the administration of the uroprotectant mesna as well as aggressive use of hydration and the use of a Foley catheter. Mannitol and amifostine are used to reduce renal toxicity associated with other chemotherapy agents. Amino caproic acid may be used to decrease clotting associated with hemorrhagic cystitis. Page 496–497.

Alterations in Respiratory Function

5.126 The answer is c.
Opioids are the first-line therapy in relieving dyspnea, without causing respiratory depression. Although continuous pulse oximetry is used widely, patients and family members often focus on the monitor, which can increase anxiety and fear. Bronchodilators can relieve bronchospasm but can also increase anxiety. Page 1833–1834.

5.127 The answer is a.
Cough is the most common presenting symptom of lung cancer. Hemoptysis and hoarseness can be presenting signs of lung cancer, but are not as common as cough. Page 1434.

5.128 The answer is a.
Agents used for pleurodesis include bleomycin, talc, doxycycline, and minocycline. Tetracycline, formerly the most frequently used sclerosing agent, is no longer available in the injectable form. Page 868–869.

5.129 The answer is a.
The purpose of the bleomycin is to obliterate the pleural space and prevent reaccumulation of fluid. Bleomycin has antitumor activity, but that is not the primary function when used as a sclerosing agent. Page 868.

5.130 The answer is c.
Cytomegalovirus (CMV) pneumonia is the leading cause of infectious pneumonia during the postengraftment period after stem cell transplantation. The incidence of CMV pneumonia may be higher in allograft-versus-autograph recipients, specifically because of prolonged periods of immunosuppression caused by medication. Page 521.

5.131 The answer is a.
The most sensitive pulmonary function test is the carbon monoxide diffusion capacity measurement that becomes abnormal before the onset of clinical symptoms. Page 493.

5.132 The answer is a.
Infectious processes, most often viral in nature, and prior toxicities related to chemotherapy or radiation therapy are the most common risk factors associated with interstitial pneumonia, as a late-onset pulmonary complication of stem cell transplantation. Previous exposure to anthracyclines and the use of cyclophosphamide can exacerbate the complication of pulmonary edema. Page 521, 524.

5.133 The answer is c.
Median survival times of patients with mesothelioma with evidence of malignant pleural effusion is 3 months. Page 868.

5.134 The answer is c.
Symptoms of a vasovagal reaction include diaphoresis and feeling as if loss of consciousness is imminent. Complications of the thoracentesis may include bleeding, vasovagal reaction, pain from reexpansion of the lung and apposition of pleural surfaces, and, in approximately 5% of cases, pneumothorax requiring tube thoracostomy. Page 868.

5.135 The answer is a.
Thoracentesis involves pleural fluid removal by needle aspiration through the chest wall. Relief of pleural effusion symptoms such as dyspnea, cough, and dull aching chest pain is a short-term treatment goal that is usually achieved when the pleural fluid is mechanically drained. Page 868.

5.136 The answer is d.
Pleurodesis with a sclerosing chemical agent is the most common method used to obliterate the pleural space in patients with malignant pleural effusions. Chemical sclerosing does not prolong the patient's life but may enhance quality of life by relieving symptoms and reducing the time a patient spends in the hospital. Shunts and stripping are surgical methods that become options after other approaches have been tried and the pleural effusion remains uncontrolled. Although external beam radiation may be used as local treatment for mediastinal tumors, hemithoracic radiation is not recommended as a first-line management of malignant pleural effusions because of the hazard of pulmonary fibrosis. Page 868–869.

5.137 The answer is b.
A capillary leak syndrome, involving primarily the lung, occurs 2–21 days after the first dose of cytarabine, resulting in pulmonary edema and respiratory failure. Mitomycin C damage to the lung presents as diffuse alveolar damage with capillary leak and pulmonary edema. Page 493.

5.138 The answer is c.
Approximately 40% to 50% of pleural effusions are due to malignancy. Page 864.

5.139 The answer is c.
Malignant pleural effusions are almost always exudates and are blood-tinged or grossly bloody and hypercellular with leukocytes. Benign effusions are classified as transudates. Page 865–866.

Alterations in Circulatory Function

5.140 The answer is d.
The most common causes of chronic or late lymphedema are prior infection, axillary irradiation, and tumor recurrence or tumor enlargement in the axilla. Page 1135.

5.141 The answer is a.
Evidence suggests that exercise and avoiding obesity can protect against lymphedema. Patients who are at risk for lymphedema should avoid strenuous upper body aerobics or lifting of weights. Complete or complex decongestive therapy is a treatment for lymphedema. Page 1115, 1135.

5.142 The answer is c.
Complex decongestive therapy consists of skin care, manual lymphatic drainage, bandaging, exercises, and wearing a compression garment. Page 1135.

5.143 The answer is c.
Obstruction of lymphatic drainage from the abdomen due to ovarian cancer results in bilateral lower extremity swelling. It can be painful, and the legs feel heavy and painful. Page 1566.

5.144 The answer is d.
Zinecard (dexrazoxane) is currently approved for patients with metastatic breast cancer who have received cumulative doses of 300 mg/m^2 of doxorubicin and are continuing treatment with doxorubicin. Zinecard interferes with the intracellular process responsible for anthracycline-induced cardiomyopathy. Page 487.

5.145 The answer is b.
Hyperkalemia can cause cardiac arrhythmias, but it is not a risk factor for cardiac tamponade. Page 916.

5.146 The answer is c.
The total cumulative dose of doxorubicin is established at 550 mg/m^2, with a decrease in dose to 450 mg/m^2 if mediastinal radiation has been administered. Page 487.

5.147 The answer is a.
Common presenting signs and symptoms of malignant effusions are distressing to most patients. The degree of subjective symptoms produced by a pleural or pericardial effusion depends less on the amount of fluid involved than on the rapidity with which it accumulates. If fluid accumulation is gradual, the heart and lungs can accommodate, but rapid accumulation can trigger an oncologic emergency. Page 865, 871.

5.148 The answer is a.
Venous thrombosis and vaginal engorgement are not complications following surgery or radiation for the treatment of vaginal cancer. For women receiving radiation therapy to the vagina, vaginal fibrosis and scarring with a loss of blood supply and elasticity is a major adverse effect. Page 1735.

5.149 The answer is b.
Signs and symptoms of a venous thrombosis are related to impaired blood flow and include edema of the neck, face, shoulder, or arm; prominent superficial veins; neck pain; tingling of the neck, shoulder, or arm; and skin color or temperature changes. A venogram with contrast media is used to assess for a venous thrombosis. Page 425.

5.150 The answer is c.
The type of cancer most often implicated in incidence of thromboembolism is lung cancer, as well as pancreatic, ovarian, and prostate cancer. Page 854.

5.151 The answer is d.
The etiology of thromboembolism is the ability of tumor cells to affect systemic activation of coagulation and cause platelet dysfunction. Anemia is caused by the other choices given: the tumor secretion of cytokines, such as interleukin-1, affecting red cell metabolism; chronic hemorrhage; and bone marrow failure. Page 854.

5.152 The answer is c.
Staging of disease at presentation is the most important prognostic factor in colon cancer. Poor prognosis has been associated with lymph node involvement, venous invasion, obstructing or perforating carcinomas, occurrence in young people, location of the tumor below the peritoneal reflection, hepatic metastasis, and invasion of the bowel wall. Page 1222.

5.153 The answer is c.
Thrombocythemia occurs in a group of related myeloproliferative disorders that includes polycythemia vera. The major complications related to an increased platelet count are bleeding and thrombosis. Thrombosis may result in symptoms associated with venous thrombosis pulmonary embolism, transient cerebral ischemia, myocardial infarction, and angina. Page 750.

Alterations in Nutrition

5.154 The answer is c.
Additional contraindications to enteral nutrition include severe diarrhea, severe bleeding, malabsorptive conditions, intractable vomiting, gastrointestinal fistulas and inflammatory bowel processes, and overall health prognosis not consistent with aggressive nutritional therapy. Page 838–839.

5.155 The answer is c.
Check tube placement, check residuals, and withhold feeding if more than 100–200 cc remains; keep in Fowler's position; use small-bore tube, and place tube distally; and consider drugs to increase motility. Page 839.

5.156 The answer is a.
Catheter dislodgement is a common problem with parenteral feeding, and the first symptom of this problem is the patient's complaint of pain with infusion. The fluid should be stopped, and the catheter checked for placement. Page 840.

5.157 The answer is b.
Enteral nutrition is much preferred over parenteral nutrition whenever feasible because of the higher incidence of metabolic imbalances and infection with parenteral nutrition. Likewise, enteral nutrition helps to maintain enzymatic and mucosal activity of the gut, which is significantly altered with parenteral nutrition. Page 838, 840.

5.158 The answer is a.
Because Mr. Smith seems to be very healthy otherwise, enteral nutrition is the preferred route, assuming that his gastrointestinal tract is functioning. Total parenteral nutrition (TPN) for brief periods (7–10 days) may be indicated in a severely malnourished patient who cannot be fed via the enteral route. Home TPN or prolonged TPN is indicated only in situations in which enteral feeding is not feasible because of advanced disease or severe toxicities. Page 838–839.

5.159 The answer is b.
Terminally ill patients are not candidates for parenteral nutrition. The largest group of patients with cancer receiving home parenteral nutrition are those with severe enteritis following curative radiation treatment. Patients with head and neck cancer generally have enteral nutrition but may also benefit from total parenteral nutrition. Page 838–839.

5.160 The answer is b.
Adding fiber to the formula helps to prevent diarrhea, as does giving the formula at room temperature, diluting it more, and giving it as a continuous infusion. Page 839.

5.161 The answer is d.
Dysphagia and weight loss are classic symptoms of esophageal carcinoma. Page 1299.

5.162 The answer is d.
To help protect the vocal cords and prevent aspiration, the patient should be taught to hold one's breath before initiating the swallow. Liquids are the most difficult to manage and are

tried last. Semisolids stay together as a bolus and are easier to swallow. These patients do not have a feeding tube, so they must begin a swallowing program as soon as their nasogastric tube is removed. Page 1354–1355.

5.163 The answer is c.
Primary cachexia results from tumor-produced metabolic abnormalities or host responses. Secondary cachexia results from mechanical effects of the tumor or treatment. Page 823–824.

5.164 The answer is a.
Effective doses of megestrol acetate range from 160 to 1600 mg per day, with an optimal dose of 800 mg per day to promote weight gain. Benefits include increased appetite, increased caloric intake, weight gain (due mostly to fat gain), and a sensation of well-being. Side effects include edema and thromboembolic events. It may be used for metastatic breast or endometrial cancer, but the question concerns weight gain. Page 836, 1130.

5.165 The answer is d.
Some fields for radiation of an extremity, such as the hip or femur, include surrounding pelvic structures, thus the patient is at risk for bowel sensitivity such as nausea and diarrhea. Page 338.

5.166 The answer is b.
Anorexia can be an acute reaction to cancer and cancer treatment and may not result in cancer cachexia. Cancer cachexia is one of the most profound nutritional alterations seen in patients with cancer and is characterized by anorexia as well as weight loss, asthenia, and muscle wasting. Anorexia or loss of appetite and declining food intake involves alterations in food perception, taste, and smell that result from the effects of chemotherapy. Abnormalities of carbohydrate, protein, and fat metabolism are central features of anorexia. Visceral and lean body mass depletion are common, along with muscle atrophy, visceral organ atrophy, and hypoalbuminemia. Page 822–823.

5.167 The answer is a.
The macrobiotic diet is low in protein and can lead to protein-calorie malnutrition. This diet has not been studied extensively enough to be able to tell a patient that it is a sound nutritional choice. Page 840–841.

5.168 The answer is c.
Although all the other answers are appropriate, anorexia and cancer cachexia are common manifestations of lung cancer; other factors are contributory. Page 1435.

5.169 The answer is b.
Research has demonstrated that use of sucralfate in patients receiving radiation therapy received no benefit in the treatment of oral mucositis. Page 815.

5.170 The answer is b.
Care should be taken to not dislodge the plaquelike formations of mucositis and cause bleeding. Page 814–816.

5.171 The answer is d.
Xerostomia is a transient dysfunction of the salivary gland that occurs following chemotherapy. It is a decrease in the quality and quantity of saliva. Page 333, 1357–1359.

5.172 The answer is a.
The use of vitamin C is a saliva stimulant and can cause local irritation and demineralization of teeth. Oral care before meals can help to freshen the mouth and stimulate appetite. Increasing fluid intake during meals and snacks helps to lubricate food and ease swallowing.

Data suggest that pilocarpine given orally can reduce the symptoms of postradiation xerostomia. Page 333, 1358–1359.

5.173 The answer is c.
Radiotherapy to the head and neck region destroys taste buds and cells responsible for saliva secretion, resulting in xerostomia. A person who is experiencing this effect produces little saliva, and the saliva that is produced is viscid, acidic, and high in organic content. Affected individuals often complain of decreased taste perception and difficult mastication. Page 333, 1357.

5.174 The answer is c.
Drug sequencing does not predict the degree and severity of nausea and vomiting. Characteristics that affect the occurrence of nausea and vomiting include fatigue, female gender, susceptibility to motion sickness, poor previous emetic control, poor social function, and being young. Page 472.

5.175 The answer is d.
Stomatitis is not a risk factor for protracted nausea and vomiting. Nausea and vomiting following chemotherapy and total body irradiation is a consistent problem. Protracted nausea and vomiting also may be caused by graft-versus-host disease (GVHD), cytomegalovirus (CMV) esophagitis, or gastrointestinal infections. Page 515–516, 518.

5.176 The answer is c.
Vomiting as a sign of increased intracranial pressure may be preceded by nausea, or it may be sudden, unexpected, and projectile. It is not related to food ingestion. Paclitaxel and carboplatin are not usually associated with the sudden onset of nausea and vomiting, especially when it has not been a problem before. Dexamethasone is an appropriate choice for either problem, but the patient's symptoms can progress quickly, and he needs to be evaluated. Page 1156.

5.177 The answer is a.
Taste loss during radiation therapy is expected, given the role of saliva as a mediator of taste. Taste acuity is partially restored within 60 days and is almost completely restored by 4 months postradiation. A burning tongue (glossodynia) is triggered after contact with spicy or acidic foods. Page 332–333, 823.

5.178 The answer is c.
Chemotherapy does interfere with specific metabolic and enzymatic reactions and causes excitation of the true vomiting center, alteration of intestinal absorptive surface, and, indirectly, food aversions. Page 820–821.

5.179 The answer is c.
Altered taste and smell sensors, with loss of taste and olfactory cues, change the normal references that are part of appetite and intake. Changes may be caused by direct tumor invasion; cancer-induced deficiencies in zinc, copper, nickel, vitamin A, and niacin; or cancer-associated circulating factors. Page 823.

5.180 The answer is c.
Physiological increases in the recognition thresholds for sweet, sour, and salt and decreases in the recognition levels for bitter are common. These threshold changes can lead to meat and other food aversions. Page 822.

5.181 The answer is b.
Normal eating is possible after use of a nasogastric tube for nutrition in the immediate postoperative period. Speech is affected by the excision of the vocal cords—esophageal speech or use of a handheld artificial larynx is necessary. Hyposomia and decreased taste acuity are also noted postlaryngectomy. Page 1354–1355.

5.182 The answer is d.
A common complaint during intravenous administration of drugs such as nitrogen mustard, cisplatin, and cyclophosphamide is that they cause a metallic taste. Some individuals become so sensitized to this taste they become nauseated in anticipation of their administration. Page 483.

5.183 The answer is b.
Skinfold thickness measurements are used to determine subcutaneous fat stores. Midarm muscle circumference is used to estimate muscle mass and protein stores. Traditional assessments of nutritional status include serum albumin, thyroxine-binding prealbumin (transtyretin), and transferrin. Page 829–830.

5.184 The answer is c.
From 40% to 100% of women with breast cancer who receive adjuvant chemotherapy gain weight, and some become obese. Page 819.

5.185 The answer is b.
Even though diabetics taking megestrol acetate must monitor themselves closely, the drug is indicated in this case because it increases appetite, causes weight gain, and improves quality of life. Corticosteroids are not indicated in William's case because he is a diabetic, and both metoclopramide and tetrahydrocannabinol are indicated for patients experiencing chemotherapy-induced nausea—which William is not experiencing. Page 836, 839.

5.186 The answer is d.
Cancer-associated nutritional problems are best resolved by successful treatment of the malignancy. Treatment-induced nutritional problems are often successfully handled by medication and self-care actions. Page 833–836.

5.187 The answer is c.
Cancer-induced sepsis initiates an increase of energy needs, which may or may not bring about an increase of appetite but which would not contribute to loss of appetite. All of the rest of these factors—bombesin, cytokines, and psychological distress—could produce a loss of appetite. Page 823–824.

5.188 The answer is c.
Cachexia is not reversible with appropriate feeding. Anorexia leads to cachexia; it is not the same thing. Cachexia does not result from the tumor preferentially consuming the ingested nutrients, and the degree of cachexia is unrelated to tumor burden. Page 823–824, 835.

5.189 The answer is c.
Inanition is progressive deterioration with muscle wasting and energy loss. Cachexia is a general term meaning ill health. It can occur in nonneoplastic diseases but is characterized by anorexia, weight loss, skeletal muscle atrophy, and asthenia. Page 819.

Alterations in Neurological Function

5.190 The answer is d.
Damage to the peripheral nervous system produces paralysis or loss of movement and sensation to those areas affected by the particular nerve. Assessment of cerebellar function focuses on the ability to coordinate movement and to maintain normal muscle tone and equilibrium. Page 490.

5.191 The answer is b.
Amifostine is used to prevent neurotoxicities associated with cisplatin, paclitaxel, and carboplatin. Patients must be pretreated with an antiemetic, dexamethasone, and intravenous hydration. Nortriptyline and carbamazepine are used to manage symptoms rather than to prevent them. Page 491–492.

5.192 The answer is b.
Vincristine is well known for causing potential peripheral neuropathy. Page 490.

5.193 The answer is c.
Methotrexate is associated with cerebellar dysfunction, such as unsteady gait and seizures, but not with peripheral neuropathies. Cytarabine, cisplatin, and carboplatin are all associated with peripheral neuropathies, particularly at higher doses. Page 490–492.

5.194 The answer is c.
Paclitaxel can produce profound peripheral neuropathy. Symptoms are progressive and include paresthesia, numbness, loss of sensory qualities, and a decrease in deep-tendon reflexes. Page 491–492.

5.195 The answer is c.
Ifosfamide can cause cerebellar and cranial dysfunction but not myalgia or arthralgia. Page 490, 492.

5.196 The answer is b.
Risk factors associated with ifosfamide encephalopathy include duration of administration, hepatic insufficiency, previous cisplatin use, presence of bulky disease, low serum albumin, and high serum creatinine. Page 490.

5.197 The answer is a.
Paraneoplastic cerebellar degeneration (PCD) is a group of paraneoplastic neurologic disorders caused by antibodies that attack nerve cells, such as Purkinje cells, resulting in this neurologic syndrome. Page 847.

5.198 The answer is b.
Apraxia is the condition in which an individual cannot coordinate skilled movements but is not paralyzed. Page 1155.

5.199 The answer is d.
The cause of peripheral neuropathy is the effect of the drug on the microtubules in the axon transport system that results in axonal degeneration. Page 490.

5.200 The answer is d.
Damage to the autonomic fibers can occur from chemotherapy and cause dizziness, constipation, abdominal colicky pain, ileus, impotence, urinary retention, and syndrome of inappropriate antidiuretic hormone. Page 490, 1006.

5.201 The answer is d.

Although mild symptoms may appear 1–3 days after high-dose paclitaxel of 250 mg/m^2 or greater, resolving 3–6 months after drug discontinuance, more severe symptoms, such as loss of fine motor movements, may resolve only partially. Page 491.

5.202 The answer is a.

Rapid drug delivery, simultaneous administration of aminoglycosides, and dehydration seem to increase the potential for ototoxicity. Page 490.

5.203 The answer is a.

5-Fluorouracil may cause an acute cerebellar dysfunction, which is usually more common in the elderly. It is characterized by rapid onset of gait ataxia, limb incoordination, dysarthria, nystagmus, and diplopia. Page 490.

5.204 The answer is c.

Numbness or tingling of the extremities on the contralateral side of the tumor, progressive motor loss, and changes in the level of consciousness alert the nurse to possible increased intracranial pressure related to tumor growth. Page 1155–1156.

5.205 The answer is b.

The cytosine arabinoside should be withheld because dysarthria is a symptom of cerebellar toxicity from the drug. High-dose cytosine arabinoside can cause cerebellar toxicities that may be irreversible. A full neurological examination should be done before each dose, even in the absence of symptoms. Page 439, 490, 492.

5.206 The answer is c.

The purpose of the steroids is to minimize swelling of the brain tissue caused initially by the tumor and the radiation. When steroids are tapered or stopped, the swelling may resume, and the patient can become more somnolent. Page 329–330.

5.207 The answer is d.

In most instances the first, earliest, and most sensitive indicator of dysfunction is a change in the level of consciousness. Mental status and cognitive ability, as well as motor and sensory function and cranial nerve function, are also assessed. Page 1147, 1156.

Anatomical and Surgical Alterations

5.208 The answer is a.

The bone is freeze-dried and irradiated, which decreases the bacteria of the graft. Bone allograft recipients do not require immunosuppressive agents. Page 1064.

5.209 The answer is d.

For most individuals, phantom limb pain decreases substantially during the first year; however, some may be troubled for years. Although phantom limb sensations (i.e., itching, pressure, tingling) are often experienced shortly after surgery, phantom limb pain (i.e., cramping, throbbing, burning) usually occurs within 1–4 weeks after surgery. This worsening may be a sign of a neuroma or of locally recurrent cancer in the stump. Page 1066.

5.210 The answer is c.

A graft or flap is indicated when a lesion is large or located in an area in which insufficient tissue for primary closure would result in deformity, for example, after excision of large carcinomas of the eyelid and lip. Function is preserved in this manner. A skin flap consists of skin and subcutaneous tissue that are transferred from one area of the body to another. A flap contains its own blood supply, whereas a graft is avascular and depends on the blood supply of the recipient site for its survival. Page 238, 1674.

5.211 **The answer is a.**
The nursing actions during a carotid hemorrhage focus on maintenance of the airway and control of bleeding. If the patient has a tracheostomy, the cuff should be inflated to prevent aspiration. Firm pressure should be applied to the neck using a towel or dressing material. If an internal carotid bleed is suspected, a vaginal pack or fluff dressing should be used to tightly pack the oral cavity and oropharynx. The patient is then transported to the operating room for ligation of the carotid artery. Page 1347, 1360–1361.

5.212 **The answer is d.**
Skin flaps are usually made to cover and protect the carotid artery. However, skin flap necrosis would leave the artery unprotected, and infection and persistent tumor raise the risk of rupture. Carotid artery rupture usually is preceded by a small trickle of blood from the area. Page 1347–1348.

5.213 **The answer is b.**
Hematoma formation can adversely affect the adherence of skin flaps, resulting in flap necrosis. Excessive bleeding may require a return to the operating room for ligation of the bleeding vessel. Choices *a* and *d* are positive surgical outcomes; as for choice *c*, bleeding is expected postoperatively. The area is observed and noted but requires no immediate action. Page 238.

5.214 **The answer is b.**
When a malignant lesion involves the middle and left transverse colon, the standard procedure involves resection of the lesion and a primary anastomosis. The two- and three-step procedures are riskier and less often performed. A right hemicolectomy is performed on the cecum or ascending colon. Page 1224–1225.

5.215 **The answer is c.**
For upper and midrectal adenocarcinomas, the treatment approach of choice is low anterior resection. This preserves external anal sphincter control, thus eliminating the need for a permanent colostomy. Abdominoperineal resection is usually used for poorly differentiated adenocarcinoma and more advanced disease. Laser therapy to the tumor bed through a colonoscope or flexible sigmoidoscope is used for smaller tumors of the colon and rectum, and prophylactic oophorectomy is recommended for only some women diagnosed with adenocarcinoma of the colon and rectum. Page 1242–1243.

5.216 **The answer is c.**
The intestine normally produces mucus, and mucus is almost always present in diversions using segments of the bowel, causing the urine to appear cloudy. Excessive mucous may clog the urinary appliance outlet, and if this occurs an appliance with a larger outlet may be used. Page 1086–1087.

5.217 **The answer is a.**
An important postoperative nursing function is assessment of stoma viability to identify early signs of compromised circulation to the stoma. A stoma that is dusky, gray, or black indicates an inadequate blood supply and is documented and brought to the surgeon's attention. A stoma with necroses sloughs and generally leads to stomal stenosis. Page 1086.

5.218 **The answer is d.**
Because APR requires a combined surgical approach through the abdomen and perineum, a major complication of APR is the occurrence of perineal and abdominal wound infections.

The type of closure used—primary closure, partial closure with an incisional drain, or leaving the wound open and packing it—determines the necessary postoperative care and teaching. Page 1243–1244.

5.219 The answer is d.
Patients with a tracheotomy have lost the functions of the nose in warming, moistening, and filtering the air when breathing. A tracheotomy is not permanent. Page 1360.

5.220 The answer is b.
Aspiration pneumonia in the surgical oncology patient may be caused by difficulty in swallowing, mechanical obstruction from the cancer, or excessive sedation. Page 240.

5.221 The answer is d.
Atrial arrhythmias are common in the patient who has undergone a lung resection because of irritation to the vagus nerve. Stroke is a complication of atrial fibrillation. Patients are monitored closely during the postoperative period, and beta-blockers are initiated if atrial fibrillation persists. Patients who have had a myocardial infarction within 3 months of resection are at risk of another one, and the mortality from this complication rises with increasing age. Page 1443–1444.

5.222 The answer is d.
Pleural effusion is common following liver resection and is most often seen after right hepatectomy. Page 1411.

Pharmacologic Interventions

5.223 The answer is d.
Contraindications to ambulatory oral antimicrobial therapy for treatment of fever in neutropenic patients include hematologic malignancy, blood and marrow transplantation, suspected pneumonia, history of invasive fungal infection, active malignant disease, serious comorbid health conditions, and hospital-acquired infections. Page 740.

5.224 The answer is a.
Aggressive antiviral therapy with intravenous acyclovir is commonly used for a full year following transplant. Page 515.

5.225 The answer is c.
Patients with HIV and neutropenia, who have had prolonged treatment with corticosteroids, or who have had prolonged immunosuppression should be assessed for the development of *Pneumocystis carinii*. Because symptoms are insidious, a prolonged fever that is unresponsive to antibiotics and associated with a nonproductive cough and dyspnea on exertion may indicate infection. Page 521, 731, 733.

5.226 The answer is a.
Immunosuppressive medications are aimed at removing or inactivating T lymphocytes that attack target organs. Cyclosporine and methotrexate inhibit T lymphocytes that are believed to be responsible for acute graft-versus-host disease and are the first-line therapy. Page 515.

5.227 The answer is b.
Veno-occlusive disease (VOD) is almost exclusive to hematopoietic stem cell transplantation (HSCT) and is the most common nonrelapse life-threatening complication of preparative regimen-related toxicity for HSCT. Fungal and virus infections arise in the liver posttransplant as infections not as VOD. Patients at risk for developing VOD include those with hepatitis and infections before HSCT and those who receive repeated doses of chemotherapy

before transplant in addition to high-dose irradiation in pretransplant conditioning regimens. An additional risk factor is the use of antimicrobial therapy with acyclovir, amphotericin, or vancomycin and mismatched or unrelated allogeneic marrow grafts. Page 515, 520, 522.

5.228 The answer is b.
Hemolytic anemia is not a side effect of trimethoprim. Side effects of trimethoprim include rash, nausea, vomiting, hepatotoxicity, and myelosuppression. Page 515, 736.

5.229 The answer is d.
Amphotericin B is the drug of choice for treatment of systemic fungal infections. However, it is associated with significant side effects and toxicity, including fever, chills, rigors, hypotension/hypertension, bronchospasms, and occasionally seizures. Page 737.

5.230 The answer is b.
Premedication with acetaminophen may help to reduce the fever associated with the amphotericin B. Intravenous meperidine can be used to ameliorate fever and chills that frequently accompany the initial administration of amphotericin. Potassium supplements are needed as renal excretion of potassium is enhanced with amphotericin B. Page 737

5.231 The answer is a.
Arthralgias and myalgias with the taxanes are thought to be due to an inflammatory process. Corticosteroids are effective because of their ability to reduce the symptoms of inflammation and inhibit a variety of proinflammatory genes. Although arthralgias and myalgias are not associated with muscle inflammation per se, corticosteroids are effective in relieving the aches and pains associated with these symptoms. Page 381, 452, 702.

5.232 The answer is d.
Corticosteroids are usually avoided with biotherapy because they may block the effects of these drugs on the immune system. Corticosteroids inhibit prostaglandin synthesis and halt the inflammatory process. Page 536, 803.

5.233 The answer is c.
NSAIDs interfere with the synthesis of the enzyme prostaglandin that blocks the conversion of arachidonic acid to prostaglandins. Prostaglandins are known to sensitize tissues to the effects of inflammatory mediators such as bradykinin. Inhibition of prostaglandin synthesis leads to relief of inflammation and pain. These agents are also antipyretic. Page 701.

5.234 The answer is d.
Adverse effects of corticosteroids and NSAIDs together include hypertension, hyperglycemia, immunosuppression, and psychiatric reactions. Although corticosteroids were previously believed to cause peptic ulcers, this effect probably occurs more with the concomitant use of NSAIDs. Page 475, 701–702.

5.235 The answer is d.
Treatment strategies for graft-versus-host disease include systemic immunosuppressive therapy, steroids, and fluoride therapy for patients at risk for caries secondary to xerostomia. Page 518–519, 521–522.

5.236 The answer is c.
Acetaminophen does not have anti-inflammatory properties. Aspirin has been demonstrated to increase the risk of bleeding. The clinical risk for bleeding associated with nonsteroidal anti-inflammatory drugs is much less than that for aspirin; however, they should be used cautiously in patients with already low platelet counts. Page 701, 764.

5.237 The answer is c.
Because shorter infusion times and higher doses of bisphosphonates correlate with a higher incidence of renal adverse events, doses of zoledronic acid higher than 4 mg and infusion times less than 15 minutes are not recommended. Page 957.

5.238 The answer is c.
Medications such as phenothiazines, tricyclic antidepressants, heparin, cimetidine, thiazide diuretics, and estrogen may suppress platelet activity, but aspirin is the medication most commonly associated with platelet dysfunction. Page 700–701, 764.

5.239 The answer is b.
NSAIDs inhibit platelet aggregation, thus inhibits platelet function. Page 701.

5.240 The answer is d.
The NSAIDs inhibit cyclooxygenase in peripheral tissues, which prevents arachidonic acid from converting to prostaglandin. The loss of the cytoprotective effect of prostaglandin on the GI epithelium causes the occurrence of the GI side effects. Page 701.

5.241 The answer is b.
Substance P is the neurotransmitter that acts at neurokinin-1 receptors centrally in the brain and in the peripheral nervous system. Substance P has been shown clinically to play a role in both acute and delayed nausea and vomiting after highly emetic chemotherapy. Aprepitant effectively blocks these receptors, thereby preventing substance P from binding to the neurokinin-1 receptor sites in the medulla, resulting in inhibition of emesis. Page 477–478.

5.242 The answer is d.
Delayed nausea and/or vomiting occurs more than 24 hours after chemotherapy administration. It often peaks 48–72 hours after chemotherapy and can last 6–7 days. Serotonin receptor antagonists are effective on days 1–3, but after that serotonin levels drop and substance P, the neurotransmitter that acts at neurokinin-1 receptors, becomes the dominant mediator of nausea and vomiting. Page 471, 477.

5.243 The answer is c.
The addition of the serotonin inhibitors has improved the management of chemotherapy-induced nausea and vomiting. The serotonin antagonists have a different mechanism of action (compared to the dopamine antagonists such as prochlorperazine) so they are ideal to use in combination antiemetic therapy. Successful antiemetic regimens interrupt the stimulation of the vomiting center. Combination regimens must be individualized and developed according to the emetic potential of the chemotherapy regimen, expected duration of the nausea and vomiting, and current pattern of symptoms. Page 476.

5.244 The answer is d.
The mechanism of nausea and vomiting is unclear, but prostaglandin synthesis appears to play a role. Dexamethasone appears to inhibit prostaglandin synthesis and therefore helps to prevent nausea and vomiting. Page 475.

5.245 The answer is a.
Despite effective antiemetic regimens, 93% of patients receiving a high dose of cisplatin experience delayed nausea and vomiting up to 6–7 days. Page 437–438, 471.

5.246 The answer is d.
The combinations of dopamine antagonists with steroids have been found to provide complete control of nausea and vomiting in up to 100% of patients undergoing high-dose cisplatin-based

regimens. The combination of ondansetron and dexamethasone has been found to be more efficacious than ondansetron alone in controlling emesis. Page 476.

5.247 **The answer is d.**
Serotonin antagonists and dopamine antagonists have different side effects, which make them ideal for combination therapy to prevent nausea and vomiting. One of the primary side effects of dopamine antagonists is extrapyramidal reactions. Page 475–476.

5.248 **The answer is a.**
The vomiting center lies close to the respiratory center on the floor of the fourth ventricle and is directly activated by the visceral and vagal afferent pathways from the gastrointestinal tract, chemoreceptor trigger zone, vestibular apparatus, and cerebral cortex. Page 470–472.

5.249 **The answer is a.**
Serotonin is released from the enterochromaffin cells in the small intestine. Serotonin activates 5-HT_3 receptors on visceral and vagal afferents, sending a message to the chemotherapy trigger zone and the vomiting center. Page 472, 476.

5.250 **The answer is c.**
Aprepitant is an example of a new class of agents called substance P/neurokinin-1 receptor antagonists, which are used in combination with other antiemetics to prevent acute and delayed chemotherapy-induced nausea and vomiting. Page 477.

5.251 **The answer is a.**
Demerol is not recommended for the treatment of chronic cancer pain. Even though its use has declined considerably, some clinicians are not aware of its risk for producing serious toxic side effects such as agitation, tremors, myoclonus, and seizures. Page 694–696.

5.252 **The answer is c.**
Bisphosphonates such as zoledronic acid and pamidronate effectively palliate pain in patients who have metastatic disease, especially in situations where NSAIDs and steroids are no longer effective. Zoledronic acid has been found to be more effective than pamidronate. Page 702.

5.253 **The answer is a.**
Fentanyl is 75–100 times more potent than morphine. Page 696.

5.254 **The answer is d.**
Naloxone is the drug of choice in the treatment of respiratory depression related to opioid overdosing. The amount of naloxone a patient receives should be titrated to changes in respiratory rate. Rapid injections of naloxone should be avoided in opioid-tolerant patients, so as not to precipitate an abstinence syndrome that may include intense pain. Page 696.

5.255 **The answer is c.**
All these are common side effects, except increased motility; opioids commonly decrease motility. Page 697.

5.256 **The answer is a.**
Antidepressants (e.g., amitriptyline, desipramine, imipramine) control pain by inhibiting the uptake of neurotransmitters into nerve terminals. They are used in the treatment of many types of nonmalignant pain, such as migraine headaches, but are also believed to be useful in neuropathic pain that is due to tumor infiltration of nerves, often described as having a continuous burning quality. Page 701.

5.257 The answer is c.
Steroids are extremely efficacious for managing the pain caused by epidural cord compression. Some side effects of steroid use, such as mood elevation and increased appetite, may also be desirable in some patients. However, the use of these drugs as adjuvant analgesics early in the course of a patient's pain problem is not recommended. Page 987.

5.258 The answer is c.
Except in a few circumstances, oral pain medication should be on a fixed-interval basis. Although the evidence is not conclusive, most caregivers agree that round-the-clock scheduling is most effective in treating pain. Page 688, 700.

5.259 The answer is d.
The opioid dose should be changed, dose reduced by 25% to 50%, and a benzodiazepine added. This toxicity is usually due to neuroexcitatory metabolites of the opioids. Naloxone is not effective in reversing this toxicity. Page 1832.

5.260 The answer is a.
Amnesia is a side effect of the benzodiazepines. Cannabinoids have significant side effects, including dysphoria, disorientation, and impaired concentration, especially in the elderly. Page 474.

5.261 The answer is d.
Antidepressants exert their clinical effects primarily through the increased availability or reduced degradation of neurotransmitters integral to the regulation of mood states. Several tricyclic antidepressants exhibit varying levels of serotonin and norepinephrine inhibition. Page 701.

5.262 The answer is d.
Antidepressants are useful for patients with a neuropathic component to their pain. These drugs act by inhibiting the uptake of neurotransmitters into nerve terminals. Page 701.

5.263 The answer is d.
Lorazepam does not cause diarrhea but can cause sedation, amnesia and confusion. Page 474.

5.264 The answer is d.
Hematopoietic growth factors do not cause programmed cell death. Page 606–607.

5.265 The answer is a.
Granulocyte and granulocyte-macrophage colony-stimulating factors decrease myelosuppression, febrile episodes, and number of hospital days when given in conjunction with chemotherapy. Both mucositis and anorexia are complications of chemotherapy and have no relationship to biotherapy. Page 606–607.

5.266 The answer is c.
EGFRs are not present on hematopoietic cells. Page 562–564.

5.267 The answer is c.
HGFs activate the production and maturation of distinctive cell lineages, thereby enhancing the activity of mature neutrophils—phagocytosis, oxidative burst, antibody-dependent cytotoxicity, and chemotaxis. These actions allow the neutrophils to be more aggressive and effective in destroying pathogens. HGFs lessen the duration and severity of neutropenia, but they do not speed the onset. Page 601–603.

5.268 The answer is c.
Colony-stimulating factors are appropriate when the risk for febrile neutropenia is greater than 20%, such as results from high-dose chemotherapy. It is not appropriate as routine prevention of neutropenia. Page 606.

5.269 The answer is a.
Tissue hypoxia is the single most potent factor in erythropoietin production. In the presence of hypoxia, the kidneys increase production and secretion of endogenous erythropoietin. This in turn stimulates red blood cell production by the bone marrow, thereby correcting hypoxia. Page 603.

5.270. The answer is d.
Epoietin alfa is contraindicated in patients with uncontrolled hypertension. Hypertension, associated with rapid increases in hematocrit, rarely has been noted in cancer patients treated with erythropoietin alfa. Nevertheless, blood pressure should be monitored carefully, particularly in patients with an underlying history of hypertension or cardiovascular disease. Page 603.

5.271 The answer is d.
Granulocyte colony-stimulating factor has been shown to decrease the duration of neutropenia, the number of episodes of neutropenic fever, and the number of hospital days in patients receiving chemotherapy, but it has no effect on the platelets. Page 606.

5.272 The answer is d.
Hematopoietic growth factors are used as supportive therapy for patients receiving myelosuppressive therapy or undergoing a hematopoietic stem cell transplant. Page 605.

5.273 The answer is a.
FDA-approved hematopoietic growth factors include granulocyte-macrophage colony-stimulating factors, granuloctye colony-stimulating factors, erythropoietin alfa, and interleukin-11, which prevents thrombocytopenia. Page 604–605.

5.274 The answer is a.
There is an inverse correlation between epidermal growth factor receptors and ER status, with ER-negative tumors tending to have a higher level of epidermal growth factor receptor than ER-positive tumors. Page 1111.

Nonpharmacologic Interventions and Complementary Therapies

5.275 The answer is b.
Patients' attitudes regarding symptoms (patients' belief in their ability to manage symptoms or their knowledge of which factors are causing specific symptoms) will affect their ability to manage symptoms. Cognitive behavioral therapy is based on the idea that the manner in which patients perceive a situation affects their behavior and beliefs regarding their ability to control it. Patients can change the way they perceive a situation (cognitive reframing), and their ability to control a situation effectively can be improved by changing their perspective. Page 678.

5.276 The answer is c.
The underlying principle of acupuncture is that qi (pronounced *chee* and translated as meaning "energy") is present at birth and maintained throughout life. Health is a balance of yin and yang. Disease is a result of imbalance. Acupuncture results in correcting any imbalance in the flow of energy, thus restoring balance. The four secrets of qi gong means energy cultivation and refers to movement that are believed to improve health, longevity, and harmony. Reiki refers to the creation of energy that alleviates physical, emotional, and spiritual blockages. Reflexology is a therapeutic method that uses manual pressure applied to certain

areas of the feet, hands, or ears that are believed to correspond to areas of the body, in order to relieve stress and prevent and/or treat physical disorders. Page 639.

5.277 **The answer is b.**
Little is known about many complementary therapies that the patient may wish to use. One of the few exceptions was a randomized, controlled trial evaluating St.-John's-wort (SJW) versus placebo in individuals with severe depressive illness. Unfortunately, SJW was not proven to be superior to placebo in this setting. However, this supplement could be effective in treating mild to moderate depression. As monotherapy, SJW has a safety profile considered superior to conventional antidepressants. Page 643.

5.278 **The answer is a.**
Complementary and alternative therapies are being studied and used more extensively. Nurses and doctors need to teach patients about the importance of moderation, given that patients will pursue alternative approaches. Page 633.

5.279 **The answer is c.**
Cutaneous stimulation (e.g., massage, heat or cold therapy, transcutaneous electrical nerve stimulation) is thought to help relieve pain or make pain more tolerable by somehow physiologically altering the transmission of nociceptive stimuli. Page 633, 708.

5.280 **The answer is a.**
Distraction (e.g., conversation, imagery, breathing exercises, watching television) directs attention away from the sensations and emotional reactions produced by pain and blocks awareness of the pain stimulus and its effects. It can be very helpful in reducing pain, but caregivers must remember that simply because a patient is effectively distracted from the pain does not mean that he or she is pain free. Page 708.

5.281 **The answer is a.**
Meta-analyses of randomized trials support the benefit of exercise in the management of fatigue during and following cancer treatment for patients with breast cancer, solid tumors, and those patients undergoing hematopoietic stem cell transplantation. Page 777–778.

5.282 **The answer is b.**
In theory, valid data on the efficacy of an alternative method are the best reason for a patient to choose that method, but then the method would no longer be "alternative." While the number of cancer complementary and alternative methods (CAM) clinical trials are increasing in number and expanding in design, many of these alternative methods have not stood up to scientific scrutiny, especially the requirement of proven efficacy in human subjects. The reasons stated in the other choices are among the most likely to motivate the patient with cancer to seek an alternative therapy. Page 629, 647.

5.283 **The answer is c.**
Although properly constructed diets are adequate, many alternative approaches to nutrition do not provide balanced diets. Potential hazards of macrobiotic diets include protein, calorie, iron, vitamin D, and vitamin B_{12} deficiencies. Colitis, not constipation, is more common with a macrobiotic diet. Page 841.

5.284 **The answer is b.**
Music therapy has not been found through research to improve the symptom of cancer-related fatigue. Several meta-analyses or systematic reviews have demonstrated improvement in cancer-related fatigue related to exercise. Energy conservation and activity management

(ECAM) and cognitive-behavioral treatment for distressing symptoms such as insomnia and depression have also been found through research to benefit the problem of cancer-related fatigue. Page 777–779, 781.

5.285 **The answer is c.**
Nonpharmacologic interventions such as relaxation and guided imagery do not generally affect the underlying pathology causing the pain or alter the perception of pain, but may help to decrease her emotional response to pain, enabling her to deal with the pain more positively and proactively. Nonpharmacologic interventions for pain management are best used as adjuvants to pharmacologic therapies, and should not be used as substitutes for pharmacologic therapies. Pages 692, 707–708.

CHAPTER 6

Psychosocial Dimensions of Care

CULTURAL, SPIRITUAL, AND RELIGIOUS DIVERSITY

6.1 **In the Asian culture, illnesses such as cancer are believed to be due to the following factors *except***
   a. An imbalance between yin and yang
   b. A curse by a spirit or a spiritual imbalance
   c. An obstruction of chi (an essential life energy)
   d. An action that should not have been performed

6.2 **Respect for cultures other than one's own and for people's specific beliefs and behaviors that emanate from their cultural background is known as**
   a. Multiculturalism
   b. Cultural sensitivity
   c. Ethnoculturalism
   d. Developing rapport

6.3 **The *first* line of treatment in Hispanic cultures is the use of**
   a. Home remedies
   b. Prayer
   c. Conventional Western medicine
   d. Holistic medicine

6.4 **The *major* high-risk behavior in the Hispanic population is**
   a. Obesity
   b. Heavy over-the-counter and street drug use
   c. Voodoo practices
   d. Cigarette smoking

6.5 In Native American cultures, the singers are those healers who

a. Can transform themselves into other forms of life to maintain cultural integration at a time of great cultural stress
b. Diagnose the cause of disharmony and may indicate a cure; their primary interest is care for souls
c. Treat illnesses and disharmony by laying on of hands, massage, sweat baths, the use of herbs and roots, and chanting
d. Are spiritualists who received the gift from God to heal incurable diseases

6.6 In a culture plagued by poverty, secondary prevention may be absent because of

a. A lack of insurance
b. A present orientation where survival needs take precedence over screening and early detection
c. Limited care access
d. Inability to pay for service

6.7 Spirituality refers to that dimension of being human that

a. Represents and expresses one's life principle
b. Prompts individuals to make sense of their universe and to relate harmoniously with self, nature, and others
c. Involves reflecting systematically about right conduct and how to live as a good person
d. Represents one's religion and world beliefs

6.8 Regardless of one's beliefs about religion, studies have shown which of the following activities is *most directly* correlated with spiritual well-being?

a. Church-related activities
b. Meditation
c. Prayer (personal and from others)
d. Spiritual imagery

6.9 Helping patients find meaning in cancer through spirituality is *best* accomplished by which of the following?

a. Help patients to accept their diagnosis and prognosis
b. Recognize positive outcomes from negative experiences
c. Counsel patients and families to find spiritual support
d. Promote religiosity among patients and families

6.10 Which of the following is *not* considered to be a central aspect of spirituality?

a. An integrating energy
b. Religiosity
c. A life principle
d. An innate human quality

6.11 Research into spirituality and death reveals many aspects of the relationship between spiritual issues and preparation for death. Which of the following assumptions regarding spirituality and preparation for death is *false*?

a. There is a direct relationship between spirituality and imminence of death.
b. The closer an individual gets to death, the more she or he will become aware of personal spirituality.
c. Individuals with advanced cancer who believed in divine intervention were more apt to have an advanced directive.
d. Religious or spiritual coping was associated with greater desire for life-sustaining measures.

6.12 Mr. Allen is distressed over his wife's apparent anger and rejection of God due to the recent discovery that her breast cancer has recurred. Your efforts to counsel him are based on which of the following cognitive strategies?

a. Individuals assume that traumatic events such as cancer strengthen one's belief that there is meaning and worth.
b. Individuals whose world is shattered will work to reconstruct their world view so that it includes a rationale for God's failings.
c. Individuals use strategies such as making comparisons to another situation to make the event meaningful.
d. The nurse helps to construct for the individual a possible meaning for this event.

6.13 Spirituality is *best* defined by which of the following components?

a. Meaning and motivation
b. Religious beliefs and dogma
c. Ethics and religiosity
d. Self-transcendence and beneficence

FINANCIAL CONCERNS

6.14 Of the following factors regarding economic disruption in the lives of family caregivers, which is *not* true?

a. African Americans and Hispanic caregivers are more likely to experience economic disruption.
b. Between 20% and 77% of family caregivers miss work or quit jobs to provide care.
c. The Family Medical Leave Act of 1993 provides financial support for family caregiving.
d. More than 40% of the families dealing with a devastating illness reported great economic hardship.

6.15 The widespread use of diagnostic-related groups, prospective payment, and increased out-of-pocket medical expenses for consumers have all combined to create the following demands in healthcare delivery *except*

a. A shift to a type of socialized medicine
b. A shift from hospital-based care to outpatient and home care settings
c. A shift of the responsibility for managing treatment side effects from the healthcare providers to patients and their families
d. Regulatory bodies that have assumed increased jurisdiction over where patients will be treated

6.16 Anna has worked as a clerk at a local grocery store for 12 years and has recently been let go because the owner states the cost of health care for all 11 employees is too costly. She has metastatic cancer and is afraid she cannot afford to pay for her own insurance. Your advice to her is based on which of the following?

a. She qualifies for protection from the Americans with Disabilities Act (ADA) and the Family Medical Leave Act (FMLA) and should apply for assistance.
b. She should apply for long-term disability and Medicaid.
c. She should sue her employer for discrimination.
d. The ADA and FMLA apply only to employers with more than 15 and 50 employees, respectively.

6.17 According to the Americans with Disabilities Act (ADA) an employer is required to do which of the following?

a. Change the individual's schedule to permit chemotherapy treatment.
b. Convert the individual's full-time job to a part-time job.
c. Provide insurance coverage for a period of 6 months after termination.
d. Provide paid leave of absence during treatment.

6.18 Individuals with low annual incomes

a. Are more likely to die of cancer than those with high annual incomes
b. Rarely experience a definable difference in survivorship or treatment outcome based solely on their economic status
c. Are twice as likely to experience recurrence, treatment failure, or death as those with higher annual incomes
d. Are less likely to receive curative therapy

6.19 The differences in incidence, mortality, and survival among various ethnic groups has been studied, and it has been determined that poverty, not race, accounts for the lower survival rate. Poverty lowers the survival rate among the many ethnic groups by

a. 5%–10%
b. 10%–15%
c. 15%–20%
d. 20%–25%

6.20 A *primary* barrier to cancer care for many of the ethnic minority population is

a. Inability to pay for services
b. Language barrier
c. Cultural differences
d. Access to care

PSYCHOSOCIAL DISTURBANCES OR ALTERATIONS

6.21 A 68-year-old woman recently diagnosed with metastatic cancer confesses that she has no one to talk to and feels extremely depressed. She has a history of depressive disorder but is currently not taking any medication. Which of the following is *not* a diagnostic criteria for major depressive disorder?

a. Disorientation, impaired memory, rapid heartbeat, elevated blood pressure
b. Depressed mood most of the day or every day
c. Recurrent thoughts of death or suicide
d. Insomnia or hypersomnia nearly every day

6.22 Cancer patients who are most likely to exhibit psychosocial distress include all of the following *except*

a. Those who have been unsuccessful in resolving past stress situations
b. Those who are dealing with stressors simultaneously
c. Those who perceive minimal social support in the situation
d. Those who cope principally through adaptive defense mechanisms

6.23 Your patient seems detached from decision making and tends to shy away from social situations. He says he is depressed regarding his diagnosis. After talking to him for a while about this you conclude that which of the following could be an *appropriate* approach to management?

a. Pharmacologic intervention for his depression is a logical approach.
b. Reassure him that depression is expected and will improve with time without medication.
c. Ignore his symptoms because talking about it could make it worse.
d. Encourage the doctor to place him on suicide precautions.

6.24 Unlike anxiety and depression, which of the following statements is *true* of hopelessness as a response of patients to the cancer experience?

a. It involves a combination of affective, behavioral, and cognitive responses.
b. It has not been implicated in the development of cancer or in the quantity and quality of life after diagnosis of cancer.
c. It can be clearly distinguished from other similar concepts using the accepted defining characteristics.
d. It appears to wax and wane with perceived changes in the patient's life.

6.25 What is one *major* reason that a diagnosis of depression among patients with cancer is often complicated?

a. Some cancer patients had preexisting depressive symptoms before the diagnosis of cancer.
b. Instruments have yet to be developed to measure depression among cancer patients.
c. Symptoms of depression are often identical to those of anxiety.
d. The signs and symptoms of cancer are markedly different from those of depression.

6.26 A nursing intervention for the treatment of patients with cancer-related distress that deals with the patient's affective responses is

a. Negotiating goals for increasing independence in self-care and decision making
b. Giving permission to safely discuss thoughts and feelings
c. Contracting short-term goals of care that the patient can achieve
d. Encouraging physical mobility

6.27 Laryngectomy patients have been reported to be at increased risk of psychosocial stressors, depression, and suicide. A *major* reason for this is which of the following?

a. Functional impairment of chewing and swallowing
b. Speech intelligibility
c. Mobility disorders
d. Inability to cope with day-to-day living

ANXIETY, LOSS AND GRIEF, AND DEPRESSION

6.28 For the person with cancer who is experiencing anxiety, which of the following interventions is *most commonly* used?

a. Problem-focused or emotion-focused coping strategies
b. A prescription for an antianxiety agent
c. Relaxation tapes and exercises
d. Referral to a psychiatrist specializing in behavioral disorders

6.29 **Which of the following symptoms is *least* diagnostic of anxiety in the person with cancer?**
a. Anorexia
b. Distractibility
c. Worry
d. Restlessness

6.30 **When standardized psychiatric interviews and research diagnostic criteria are used, the prevalence of anxiety among patients with cancer is approximately which of the following?**
a. 0.5%–10%
b. 10%–30%
c. 30%–50%
d. 50%–70%

6.31 **Anxiety is defined operationally as an increased level of arousal associated with vague, unpleasant, and uneasy feelings that occur in response to a perceived threat. What is the source of this perceived threat?**
a. A nonspecific external stimulus
b. A specific external stimulus, often a physical threat
c. A nonspecific internal or external stimulus
d. A specific internal stimulus, usually pain or inflammation

6.32 **Why are cognitive and behavioral techniques such as hypnosis, biofeedback, progressive muscle relaxation, or music therapy helpful in the treatment of anxiety related to cancer?**
a. These techniques restore or enhance a sense of self-control.
b. They provide temporary emotional distraction from the reality of the situation.
c. Channeling anger makes it less threatening.
d. Cognitive techniques promote effective denial.

6.33 **As an individual patient with cancer faces imminent death, certain losses and changes are experienced. The individual's response to these losses and changes is usually due to which of the following?**
a. Search for immortality
b. Search for meaning
c. Search for acceptance
d. Search for forgiveness

6.34 **In a discussion of the patient's prognosis for which the patient has requested, the patient and her husband begin to sob softly. Your *most appropriate* nursing action would be which of the following?**
a. Ask them if you have said something that is upsetting to them.
b. To facilitate hope you encourage them not to cry because there are options available and describe what those are.
c. Stop talking, temporarily allowing them to express their grief.
d. Reschedule the appointment because they are not prepared for what you have to say.

6.35 **On his most recent visit, your patient, who is suffering from lung cancer, appears anxious but denies difficulty breathing. He complains of inability to sleep and believes this is due to depression related to his illness. The *most appropriate* pharmacologic intervention for him might be which of the following?**
a. Chlordiazepoxide (Librium)
b. Selective serotonin-norepinephrine reuptake inhibitors (SSNRIs)
c. SSNRI plus a short-acting benzodiazepine
d. Lorazepam (Ativan)

6.36 **Which of the following statements regarding risk factors for depression in the cancer patient is *inaccurate*?**
a. A history of substance abuse increases risk for depression.
b. Adaptation to illness tends to be greater in younger persons than in older persons.
c. Times of treatment failure and recurrence of disease increase risk of depression.
d. Medications commonly prescribed for cancer patients have depression as a side effect.

6.37 **When assessing patients for depression, it is important to be aware of certain misconceptions regarding psychological distress in the patient with cancer. Which of the following statements is a myth and unsubstantiated by empirical data?**
a. Depression is a natural by-product of the cancer experience.
b. Patients with cancer hide their negative emotions to protect their family.
c. Obtaining psychological counseling is regarded by cancer patients as an indication of their inability to cope.
d. Depression affects the course of cancer by increasing morbidity and hospital stays.

6.38 **When screening for depression in individuals with cancer, which of the following questions has the *highest* sensitivity and specificity for correctly identifying depression?**
a. "Are you depressed most of the day nearly every day?"
b. "Have you lost interest in all or almost all activities?"
c. "Do you often feel sad or low?"
d. "How is your distress on a scale of 0 to 10?"

ALTERED BODY IMAGE

6.39 **Most empirical studies dealing with the relationship of cancer to body image and quality of life have focused on**
a. The total self-appraisal of cancer patients, both men and women
b. The effects of various treatments on relationships of cancer patients with significant others
c. Women with gynecologic or breast cancer or males with testicular or prostate cancer
d. The interaction of variables such as age, depression, and activity status on the psychosocial aspects of sexual health

6.40 **Albert is about to undergo chemotherapy that is known to cause significant hair loss. Which of the following will *not* be part of your patient education plan for Albert?**
a. Chemotherapy-induced alopecia occurs slowly and may not occur for several months after the treatment.
b. Once chemotherapy is complete, regrowth is visible in 4–6 weeks.
c. Complete regrowth of hair may take 1–2 years.
d. In situations involving very high doses of alkylating agents, hair may not regrow.

6.41 **Following four courses of chemotherapy, Albert shows you that his fingernails have developed transverse white lines or grooves. You explain to Albert that this symptom**
a. Is a response to doxorubicin because pigmentation has been deposited at the base of the nail
b. Indicates a reduction or cessation of nail growth in response to cytotoxic therapy
c. Reflects a cytotoxic reaction to cyclophosphamide
d. Is a partial separation of the nail plate called onycholysis and is a reaction to fluorouracil (5-FU) therapy

6.42 Because of the staging of her cancer, the size of the tumor, and a number of other factors, Marcia will undergo immediate breast reconstruction after her surgery. Her surgeon has explained that the procedure most likely to be used in her case is the TRAM flap. You explain to Marcia that this will involve removing tissue from her _________ and tunneling it to the mastectomy site.

a. Abdominal muscle
b. Latissimus dorsi muscle
c. Lower abdomen
d. Buttocks

6.43 Sally asks you if there is anything she can do to prevent hair loss with chemotherapy. Which of the following would *not* be an appropriate response?

a. Use a wide tooth comb, and allow hair to dry naturally.
b. Avoid daily shampooing.
c. Use vitamin E to help prevent hair loss.
d. Use only protein-based shampoos and conditioners.

6.44 An individual's body image is affected by all of the following *except*

a. Feedback from significant others and fear of rejection
b. What one perceives as an "ideal" body or image
c. How one's body actually looks and functions
d. The various elements that refer to psychological self

6.45 A woman with breast cancer is being treated with six courses of oral cyclophosphamide for 14 days and methotrexate and 5-fluorouracil injections on days 1 and 8 every 28 days. She is very upset about the possibility of losing her hair. The *most appropriate* response to her concerns regarding hair loss would include which of the following?

a. Reassure her that although she will have significant hair loss, it will grow back.
b. Assure her that it is likely she will not lose any hair at all.
c. Inform her that hair loss is gradual over the next 2 months, and she will require a wig sooner rather than later.
d. Let her know that her hair will likely thin, but she will probably not require a wig.

6.46 A patient being treated with radiation to an abdominal field is concerned about hair loss that she expects to experience following radiotherapy. You can best reassure her by telling her that

a. Hair follicles are relatively radioresistant due to their low rate of growth and mitotic activity.
b. Radiation response is seen mostly in tissues and organs that are within the treatment field.
c. Alopecia is permanent only when radiation is administered in low doses over an extended period of time.
d. Alopecia is more closely associated with brachytherapy than with teletherapy.

LOSS OF PERSONAL CONTROL

6.47 A person who experiences cancer-related symptoms processes information about these symptoms in which of the following ways?

a. By evaluating the symptom and obtaining feedback
b. Cognitively and emotionally
c. Intellectually and socially
d. By its presentation and controllability

6.48 **Which of the following "directions" provides patients who are at risk for loss of decision-making ability the *best* chance of having their healthcare wishes carried out?**

a. Power of attorney for health care
b. Verbal instructions to the attending physician
c. A living will
d. A do-not-intubate/ventilate order on admission

6.49 **The federal Patient Self-Determination Act, enacted in 1991, was intended to accomplish which of the following?**

a. Provide all patients with information about the patient's bill of rights.
b. Provide all patients with information for a living will.
c. Require patients to execute advance directives.
d. Enable healthcare agencies to provide patients with information about their right to accept or refuse treatment and specify their wishes.

6.50 **Mr. Jones expresses reluctance to return to work because he feels he is being discriminated against because of his diagnosis of cancer. Your advice to him would include all *except* which of the following?**

a. Consider legal action sooner rather than later.
b. In an objective manner write down any events that occurred.
c. Talk to your supervisor or human resources manager to be sure they know you have cancer.
d. Cite the law, and encourage him to get help from cancer survivor organizations.

6.51 **Which of the following statements regarding decision making in reference to treatment decisions is *correct*?**

a. Patients who take a passive role in making the final selection of treatment cope better with side effects.
b. Patients who actively participate in decisions have improved function, sense of well-being, and perform effective self-care.
c. Patients whose family controls decision making have improved quality of life.
d. Patients who allow the physician to make the final treatment decisions have improved quality of life.

PATIENT AND FAMILY SUPPORT GROUPS

6.52 **It is not uncommon for the spouse of a patient with cancer to be unwilling to discuss his or her concerns with the patient because of fears that it might be distressing to the patient. This type of communication is referred to as**

a. Privileged communication
b. Filtered communication
c. Balanced communication
d. Protective buffering communication

6.53 **Several decades of research have associated levels of social support with individual coping capabilities. The *most beneficial* finding of all these studies was**

a. Attendance and use of support groups
b. Cognitive-emotional therapy and relaxation therapy
c. Opportunity to discuss thoughts and feelings with an attentive, empathetic, professional listener
d. Supportive-expressive group therapy

6.54 There are barriers that can limit family members' ability to obtain information and support from nurses and other health professionals. The *most common* barrier is

a. Lack of clarity about who is responsible for helping family members
b. Lack of value placed on the support of the family in the care of the patient
c. Lack of effective professional–family communication
d. Lack of time and the constraints that exist in the healthcare system

6.55 When providing support for Ms. Wiggins, a 47-year-old African American, who was just diagnosed with breast cancer, which of the following considerations is *most important*?

a. The woman of the family is generally charged with the responsibility for protecting the health of family members.
b. The family exerts an extremely powerful force in the patient's life, and the needs of the patient are often secondary.
c. Patients may not give consent for treatment until permission is obtained from the mother, grandmother, or aunt.
d. The nuclear family is very important, and men assume dominant roles and decision making.

6.56 The *major* purpose of patient navigator programs is

a. To determine the economic costs of cancer disparities
b. To provide personal assistance in eliminating any barriers to patients obtaining timely and adequate diagnosis and treatment
c. To identify trusted information sources or channels in the community
d. To monitor treatment equity according to established standards of care to diminish bias in the provision of health care

LEARNING STYLES AND BARRIERS TO LEARNING

6.57 Susan has been assigned to teach nursing students the importance of family caregivers. As a part of her class she reviews the key reasons why families of patients with cancer need help and support. Of the reasons below, which is the *most important* reason that they need our support?

a. They lack preparation for the complex care that they are expected to provide.
b. To reduce the burden of care and help them maintain their well-being.
c. Long-term care is most often provided in the home by family caregivers.
d. Lack of effective professional–family communication in healthcare settings

6.58 Strategies for designing effective culturally sensitive patient education programs include which of the following?

a. Consulting with key members of the cultural community in designing the program
b. Limiting involvement of members of the community in program development
c. Presenting the program to the community leaders for their support
d. Teaching educational programs in high school

6.59 Helen is preparing to discuss options with a patient who speaks only Spanish. Helen speaks only English. If given a choice, Helen will probably want to choose the use of

a. A professional interpreter
b. A family member as interpreter because the family is an integral part of treatment delivery and involvement in most Hispanic cultures
c. A friend as interpreter because of the emotional support friends lend in a Hispanic extended family social structure and because a friend is more likely than family to relay the complete message
d. Any of the above, as long as the interpreter is fluent in both languages

6.60 The *most common* means of reducing uncertainty for patients and their family members is

a. Providing preparatory information and education
b. Referring him or her to a professional therapist
c. Protecting the individual from all negative information
d. Encouraging them to maintain an optimistic outlook

6.61 It is important to evaluate the reading grade level of educational materials before giving them to a patient because it has been shown that over 20% of Americans read at or below which grade level?

a. Third grade
b. Fifth grade
c. Seventh grade
d. Eighth grade

6.62 Research concerning cognitive changes associated with systemic cancer treatment demonstrates that people who received systemic cancer treatment demonstrated impairment in which of the following areas?

a. Information processing
b. Spatial skill
c. Verbal memory
d. Attention deficit

SOCIAL RELATIONSHIPS

6.63 The basic unit of society is the

a. Family
b. Social structure
c. Religious structure
d. Relationship of ethnicity and culture to role assignment

6.64 During the initial family assessment, which of the following is *least likely* to be considered during the evaluation?

a. What is the pattern of communication?
b. Who is the primary caregiver?
c. What are the social obligations of family members?
d. What support mechanisms are available to the patient and family?

6.65 On conducting a family assessment, the nurse identifies conflict among the family members caring for the patient. Upon inquiry, the nurse learns that the conflict is "not new" and has existed "for years." Using this information, the nurse establishes a plan of care that

a. Attempts to change the behavior among the family members because the patient is upset by the conflict
b. Involves having psychological services counsel the "conflicting members"
c. Schedules family meetings about how the conflict is affecting the patient and what can be done to resolve it
d. Is sensitive to the feelings of the members in conflict but does not attempt to treat the causes of the conflict

6.66 The psychosocial dimension of cancer care focuses on both the unique needs of the individual at risk for or with cancer and the

a. Unique needs of other individuals in society
b. Clinical training of healthcare professionals
c. Social groups affected by that individual
d. Role of specific therapies in cancer treatment

6.67 Which of the following is *not* a strategy for family caregivers?

a. Family-level teaching with respect to the disease, treatment, rehabilitation, and/or prognosis
b. Anticipatory guidance, positive reframing, and planning
c. Mobilization of community resources such as support groups
d. The provision of intensive family therapy to all families of cancer patients

COPING MECHANISMS AND SKILLS

6.68 Deterioration in communication patterns between individuals with cancer and their family is *most* predictable under which of the following circumstances?

a. When the cancer is first diagnosed
b. When the individual is reluctant to discuss prognosis
c. When the professionals give most information to the patient and not the family
d. When professionals give more information to the family than the patient

6.69 Among the nursing interventions shown to be effective with cancer patients experiencing anxiety are all of the following *except*

a. Helping the patient learn new coping strategies through anxiety-reducing role playing
b. Helping the patient focus on the perceived threat and appraise the stimuli in a different way, thus reducing anxiety
c. Helping the patient identify stimuli that have resulted in a loss of self-esteem
d. Exploring perceived patient concerns and helping patients evaluate these concerns

6.70 You are working with Mr. Gunther and his family, who have just discovered not only that his lung cancer has recurred, but also that it is terminal this time. Which is *not* likely to be true regarding Mr. Gunther's psychosocial needs?

a. When coping with a difficult disease like lung cancer, it is the discovery of meaning in the disease that gives one a sense of mastery.
b. The recurrence of lung cancer can be a greater crisis than the initial diagnosis.
c. Often the fear of dying is not as profound as the fear of suffering in the process.
d. Patients who are allowed to indulge excessively in expressing their fears, concerns, and wishes regarding death are more prone to morbid depression.

6.71 Which of the following statements about effective coping and healthy lifestyle behavior is *true*?

a. Use of denial or behavior disengagement as coping strategies is associated with a poorer psychological well-being.
b. Psychosocial responses to cancer can be clearly identified as either adaptive or maladaptive.
c. A perception of uncertainty in a situation results in an appraisal of danger.
d. Distancing behaviors of health professionals are helpful in preventing overinvolvement.

6.72 Which of the following statements *most accurately* describes the relationship between family responses to a diagnosis of cancer and the responses of patients themselves?

a. Family responses are similar to patient responses.
b. Responses of anxiety and depression are less common among family members than among patients.
c. Responses of hopelessness and altered sexual health are less common among family members than among patients.
d. Family responses generally are not similar to patient responses.

ANSWER RATIONALES

Please note: All page numbers referenced in the Answer Rationales sections refer to the textbook *Cancer Nursing: Principles and Practice, Seventh Edition,* by Connie Henke Yarbro, Debra Wujcik, and Barbara Holmes Gobel (Jones & Bartlett Learning, © 2011).

Cultural, Spiritual, and Religious Diversity

6.1 The answer is d.
American Indians believe that illness is due to an action that should not have been performed, where as among Asian groups, health is a state of harmony in body, mind, and spirit with nature and the universe. A balance between hot (yang) and cold (yin) is essential for good health. Other explanations for illness include an imbalance of humoral elements, an obstruction of chi, a curse, a punishment for immoral behavior, or an imbalance in the body caused by exposure to wind or air. Page 78, 84.

6.2 The answer is b.
Cultural sensitivity is having respect for cultures—and the beliefs connected with those cultures—other than your own. Page 72.

6.3 The answer is a.
Home remedies are first-line treatment in Hispanic cultures. To cure a hot or cold imbalance, the opposite quality of the causative agent is applied. Page 81.

6.4 The answer is a.
Obesity is the major high-risk behavior in the Hispanic population along with alcohol consumption and sexual practices. Smoking is on the rise in adolescents. Page 83.

6.5 The answer is c.
In Native American cultures, the singers (medicine men) are healers who treat illnesses and disharmony by laying on of hands, massage, sweat baths, use of herbs and roots, and chanting. Page 85.

6.6 The answer is b.
In a culture of poverty, secondary prevention may be absent because of an orientation in which survival needs take precedence over screening and early detection. Delayed tertiary prevention is due to a lack of insurance, inability to pay for service, or limited care access. Page 87.

6.7 The answer is b.
Spirituality refers to that dimension of being human that motivates meaning-making and self-transcendence—or intra-, inter-, and transpersonal connectedness. Spirituality prompts individuals to make sense of their universe and to relate harmoniously with self, nature, and others, including any god(s) (as conceptualized by each person). Religion is the representation and expression of spirituality. Ethics involves reflecting systematically about right conduct and how to live as a good person. Page 1798.

6.8 The answer is c.
Regardless of one's beliefs about religion, studies have shown that prayer (personal and from others) more directly correlated with spiritual well-being. Other activities include church-related activities, meditation, spiritual imagery, and spiritual ceremonies. Page 1802.

6.9 The answer is b.
The process of deriving meaning in illness has been described as assisting individuals with recognizing positive outcomes from negative experiences, such as seeing the positive changes in life that may result from a cancer diagnosis. Page 1807.

6.10 The answer is b.
In nursing literature that defines related terms such as spiritual distress, need, or well-being, spirituality is described as an integrating energy, a life principle, an innate human quality. In contrast to spirituality, religiosity often is viewed as a narrower concept. Page 1798.

6.11 The answer is c.
Individuals with advanced cancer who believed in divine intervention and had strong spiritual well-being were less apt to have an advanced directive. Page 1803.

6.12 The answer is c.
Individuals assume that the world is meaningful and that they have worth. Traumatic events such as a cancer diagnosis can shatter these assumptions. When this happens, people work to reconstruct their worldview so it includes assumptions about the event that are wiser and more mature. Cognitive strategies that individuals use for reconstructing the assumptions include making comparisons—for example, "It could be worse." The individuals must construe their own meanings for life's traumas—the nurse cannot do this cognitive work for them. Page 1807.

6.13 The answer is a.
Spirituality prompts individuals to make sense of their universe and to relate harmoniously with self and others. It motivates meaning-making for one's life. Page 1798.

Financial Concerns

6.14 The answer is c.
The Family Medical Leave Act of 1993 guarantees only unpaid leave to care for a seriously ill spouse, son, daughter, or parent. Page 1787.

6.15 The answer is a.
Because of shifts in healthcare delivery from inpatient to outpatient due to the increased restrictions of payment, cost-control measures by other insurers, and increased out-of-pocket expenses, patients and their families must assume responsibility for self-care. Page 460.

6.16 The answer is d.
Because she works for a small business owner with fewer than 15 employees, she is not protected at the workplace by the ADA and the FMLA. She would not win a suit against her employer given these conditions. She should probably apply for Medicaid, for which she qualifies. Page 1750.

6.17 The answer is a.
Because cancer is considered a disability under the ADA, employers must make reasonable accommodations. Scheduling changes are considered reasonable, but turning a full-time job into a part-time job is not required. Employers are not required to provide paid leave of absences during treatment or insurance for individuals who are no longer employees. Page 1750.

6.18 The answer is a.
Individuals with low annual incomes are three to seven times more likely to die of cancer than those with high annual incomes. Page 56, 87.

6.19 The answer is b.
In the late 1970s the question of the role of poverty in the differences in incidence, mortality, and survival of different ethnic groups was first raised. The disproportionate number of African Americans in the lower socioeconomic strata accounted for the increased incidence. However, a landmark report by Freeman concluded that poverty, not race, accounted for the 10–15% lower survival rate from cancer in many ethnic groups. Page 87.

6.20 The answer is d.
A primary barrier to cancer care for many ethnic minority populations is access to health care, especially among the socioeconomically disadvantaged. Many programs focus on providing effective cancer screening for ethnic minority populations using culturally sensitive strategies. Page 88.

Psychosocial Disturbances or Alterations

6.21 The answer is a.
Disorientation, impaired memory, rapid heartbeat, and elevated blood pressure are not a part of the Diagnostic Criteria for Major Depressive Disorder. Page 675–676.

6.22 The answer is d.
According to stress theory, individuals come to the cancer experience with a history of stress responses. Those who have been unsuccessful in resolving past stress situations, who are dealing with several stressors simultaneously, and who perceive minimal social support in the situations are at higher risk for psychosocial distress. Page 669, 1782.

6.23 The answer is a.
The idea that depression is to be expected in cancer patients is not supported by empirical data. Cancer patients are no more likely to develop depression than other medical-surgical patients. People with cancer who also suffer from depression are as likely to benefit from its treatment as anyone else. It is a myth that suicide is a logical choice for all cancer patients. With attention to the problems such as depression, unmanaged pain, or other symptoms, suicide is not common. Page 679.

6.24 The answer is d.
Hopelessness appears not to pervade the experience of the cancer patient, unlike anxiety and depression. Rather, it waxes and wanes with changes in perceived health, relationships, and spirituality. Patients need encouragement to be optimistic and to accept negative feelings as a normal part of the cancer experience, as well as continue to find ways to restore and maintain hope. Page 1791–1792.

6.25 The answer is a.
In addition, the coexistence of signs and symptoms of disease and treatment that are similar to those of depression make the diagnosis of cancer-related distress difficult. Page 671, 675.

6.26 The answer is b.
The other interventions listed are cognitive or behavioral in approach. Before these interventions are attempted, it is important for the nurse to acknowledge the patient's feelings associated with depression, including hopelessness, despair, anger, and guilt. The nurse can do this in many ways, starting with giving the patient permission to discuss those feelings and then demonstrating acceptance of them by attentive listening and by exploring methods for the patient to deal positively with them. Page 678–679.

6.27 The answer is d.
Healthcare providers commonly perceive disfigurement, loss of voice, and disease control as the most relevant issues postoperatively. However, patients may be able to meet rehabilitation goals (talk and eat) but cannot cope with day-to-day living (relationships, finances, work, and performance). Page 1362–1363.

Anxiety, Loss and Grief, and Depression

6.28 The answer is a.
There is robust evidence that cognitive behavioral interventions targeting either problem-focused or emotion-focused coping strategies are effective for depression and anxiety. Page 678.

6.29 The answer is a.
The diagnosis of anxiety in healthy persons is made based on somatic symptoms, including anorexia, fatigue, and weight loss, which in cancer are often symptoms of the disease itself and its treatment. The symptoms of worry, distractibility, restlessness, and fearfulness are more important for diagnosing anxiety among cancer patients. Page 676.

6.30 The answer is b.
There is a wide range in estimates of prevalence for anxiety in the cancer population. However, when standardized psychiatric interviews and research diagnostic criteria are used, the range is more typically 10%–30%. Page 675.

6.31 The answer is c.
Anxiety is most likely to occur when an individual experiences a nonspecific internal or external stimulus that is perceived as a threat to certain beliefs, values, and conditions essential to a secure existence. Page 676.

6.32 The answer is a.
Cognitive and behavioral techniques are well suited to the treatment of anxiety because the techniques are often effective not only in symptom control but also in restoring or enhancing a sense of self-control. Page 678.

6.33 The answer is b.
Social psychologists theorize that significant losses and changes cause individuals to search for meaning as a way of trying to make sense of such a negative experience. Page 1787, 1801.

6.34 The answer is c.
Allow the patient or family members the opportunity to express their emotional response to bad news. Allow the patient or family member to cry and wait for them to stop on their own. This may be an appropriate time for silence. It is important to acknowledge their grief, and tears are an appropriate expression of grief. Only if crying is protracted or hysterical should you consider resuming your discussion at a later time. Page 1788–1792.

6.35 The answer is c.
SSNRIs target a second neurotransmitter, norepinephrine, that plays a role in triggering the fight-or-flight reaction. These medications work well for those patients who have anxiety with an overlay of depression. Because these medications take up to 2 weeks to work, the short-acting benzodiazepines may be used until they take effect. Page 679.

6.36 The answer is b.
Overall adaptations to illness tends to be poorer in younger persons than in older persons. The elderly may cope with chronic illness better than younger patients; however, the elderly

are less likely to report distress. Advanced stage of disease, relapse or progression, unrelieved symptoms, medications, and body image problems have all been associated with depression. An individual or family history of depression or a history of substance abuse places the person with cancer at greater risk of depression as does disease recurrence, medications, and unrelieved symptoms. Page 671.

6.37 The answer is a.

Patients with cancer often believe that depression is normal in those with cancer, which is erroneous. Studies have documented that depression affects the course of cancer by increasing morbidity and hospital stays and negatively impacts treatment compliance and possibly prognosis and mortality. Patients feel a need to protect the family by masking their negative emotions; counseling is viewed as an indication of weakness and inability to cope. Page 670, 675.

6.38 The answer is d.

The distress of all patients with cancer should be assessed by asking "How is your distress on a scale of 0 to 10?" The Distress Management assessment tool developed by the National Comprehensive Cancer Network is a useful resource to assess distress in the patient with cancer. Page 671, 673.

Altered Body Image

6.39 The answer is c.

Most empirical studies dealing with the relationship of cancer to body image and quality of life have focused on women with gynecologic or breast cancer or on men with testicular or prostate cancer. Additional empirical data are needed on the issues of perception of significant others' responses to the physical and psychological sequelae of cancer; the interaction of other variables, such as age, depression, and activity status; and the physical as well as psychosocial aspects of sexual health. Page 203, 880–886.

6.40 The answer is a.

Chemotherapy-induced alopecia occurs rapidly and usually starts 2–3 weeks following a dose of chemotherapy. After discontinuation of the epilating drugs, regrowth is visible in 4–6 weeks, but complete regrowth may take 1–2 years. In situations involving very high doses of alkylating agents, hair may not regrow. Page 485–486.

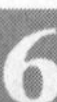

6.41 The answer is b.

Beau's lines indicate a reduction in or cessation of nail growth in response to cytotoxic therapy. Page 486–487.

6.42 The answer is a.

The TRAM flap procedure is sometimes known as the "tummy tuck" because the muscle and fat are tunneled from the abdominal muscle to the mastectomy site. Page 1118–1119.

6.43 The answer is c.

Recommendations to minimize hair loss include using mild protein-based shampoos with conditioners, avoiding daily shampooing, allowing hair to dry naturally, and grooming hair with a wide-toothed comb. Vitamin E has not been shown to prevent hair loss. Page 486.

6.44 The answer is d.

Body image includes those elements that refer to the physical self, including how we perceive our bodies, how our bodies actually look and how they function, the impact of sensory inputs (e.g., pain), and what we perceive as an "ideal" body or image. Page 1245.

6.45 **The answer is d.**
Cyclophosphamide, 5-fluorouracil, and methotrexate commonly cause hair thinning rather than a dramatic loss of hair. The patient may not require a wig over the 6 months of treatment depending on the amount of hair the patient has to begin with. Page 432, 485–486.

6.46 **The answer is b.**
Radiation response is seen mostly in tissues and organs that are within or adjacent to the treatment field (i.e., they are site specific). Thus an individual treated in the abdominal field does not lose scalp hair from radiation. Page 328.

Loss of Personal Control

6.47 **The answer is b.**
Patients process information about their symptoms in two ways. They process cognitively, using a problem-focused approach, which assists in their making a plan for addressing the symptom. They also process information emotionally. Emotional processing can affect planning for self-care. Page 672.

6.48 **The answer is a.**
A living will may be applicable only when it pertains to a terminal illness but not for a patient whose health is declining for medical reasons other than those that can be classified as terminal or if the patient is in a vegetative state. In general, the power of attorney for health care is more useful than the living will. The living will does not identify another person who can act as the agent for a disabled patient. Verbal instructions are of little value if a family member or anyone else chooses to argue against what has been reportedly communicated verbally. Written instructions are necessary. An order that instructs not to intubate does not address any other interventions that might be suggested. Page 1822.

6.49 **The answer is d.**
The purpose of this legislation is to ensure that patients' wishes are carried out in the event they become mentally incapacitated or are incapable of making or communicating their decisions. Page 1822.

6.50 **The answer is a.**
If a patient feels discriminated against it is important to take action sooner rather than later; however, experts advise thinking about legal action only as a last resort. Other steps that should be tried first include documenting the incidents, talking to a supervisor or human resources, speaking to other coworkers who have tread this path before, and citing the law. The individual may be covered by the Americans with Disabilities Act. Also, get help from organizations that regularly help cancer survivors (Cancer Care: 800-813-HOPE). Page 1751.

6.51 **The answer is b.**
Patients who actively participate in treatment decisions have improved functional status, sense of well-being, and perform effective self-care. Including the family as a part of the decision-making process promotes better communication and mutual support. Page 460.

Patient and Family Support Groups

6.52 **The answer is d.**
This communication is referred to as protective buffering, where the family member attempts to keep the patient from incurring further distress. Privileged, balanced, and filtered are additional types of communication between healthcare providers, patient, and family caregivers. Page 1785, 1789.

6.53 The answer is c.
Central to the beneficial findings in research associated with levels of social support with individual coping capabilities is the opportunity for patients to safely discuss thoughts and feelings with an attentive, empathetic, professional listener. Cognitive-emotional therapy, relaxation therapy, aromatherapy, and support groups are important as well. Page 679.

6.54 The answer is d.
The most common barrier to helping families of patients with cancer is the time constraints in the healthcare setting. Page 1781–1782.

6.55 The answer is a.
African American women are generally charged with the responsibility for protecting the health of family members. Whereas the family of Asians or Pacific Islanders exerts an extremely powerful force in the patient's life and the needs of the patient are often secondary, Native Americans may not give consent for treatment until permission is obtained from the mother, grandmother, or aunt. The nuclear family is very important in Hispanics, and men assume dominant roles and decision making. Page 76–84.

6.56 The answer is b.
The major purpose of patient navigator programs is to provide personal assistance in eliminating any barriers to patients obtaining timely and adequate diagnosis and treatment. Page 87.

Learning Styles and Barriers to Learning

6.57 The answer is c.
Families are the bedrock of chronic care in the United States with over 44 million informal family caregivers. Patients are leaving the hospital sicker and sooner than ever before and their long-term care is most often provided in the home by family caregivers who assume multiple roles. Page 1781.

6.58 The answer is a.
Make linkages with key members of the target community, involving members of the community in the development of educational materials, programs, and community outreach strategies. Page 88.

6.59 The answer is a.
The use of professional interpreters, if available, is the optimal choice. Family and friends may be used, but the correct or complete message may not be relayed. Page 89.

6.60 The answer is a.
Education assists patients and family members in reducing their sense of helplessness and inadequacy. The most common means of reducing uncertainty is to provide preparatory information about the specific aspects of the cancer experience faced by the individual. Preparatory information also prevents or alleviates treatment-related symptoms. Page 1791.

6.61 The answer is b.
One aspect of printed patient educational materials that has received considerable attention in the nursing literature is reading level. It is estimated that the majority of Americans read at or below the eighth-grade level. A fifth-grade reading level has been identified as the minimum reading level for making good use of basic written material. Page 88.

6.62 The answer is c.
Individuals who received systemic cancer treatment were impaired in executive functioning, verbal memory, and motor functioning. Page 211, 674.

Social Relationships

6.63 The answer is a.
The basic unit of society is the family. Cultural values can determine communication with the family, the norm for the family size, and the roles of specific family members. Page 1781.

6.64 The answer is c.
A detailed family assessment is important, particularly with regard to the functional abilities of the caregiver, pattern of authority, and support mechanisms available. Families are categorized as supportive, ambivalent, or hostile, and they generally continue to act as they did in previous crises. Page 1788.

6.65 The answer is d.
Family units can be identified as supportive, hostile, or ambivalent, with their behavior described in terms of cohesion, adaptability, and communication. When crisis occurs or families are faced with the serious and difficult implications of cancer and its treatment, their behavior usually does not change and in some cases can intensify. Therefore, if a family were dysfunctional, hostile, or in conflict, it is very likely that their behavior will continue. The home healthcare nurse's primary concern is to support and care for the patient. The chances are high that the home healthcare nurse will be unable to change the behavior of the family members in conflict. Page 1790–1792.

6.66 The answer is c.
Each individual brings to the cancer experience unique personality traits and a personal socialization pattern different from all others. Understanding the uniqueness of the individual is achieved only through study of the commonalities of the personality and social psychological (psychosocial) aspects of illness. Page 207.

6.67 The answer is d.
Intensive family therapy may be helpful in selected situations. However, most cancer patients and family caregivers facing care are well adjusted without the need for intensive intervention. Active coping strategies such as emotional support, planning, and positive reframing are associated with higher psychologic well-being. Page 1792.

Coping Mechanisms and Skills

6.68 The answer is d.
Communication deteriorates the most when information is given to the family but not the patient; this is privileged communication. When communication is just to the patient and not the family, it can be misinterpreted when the patient passes it to the family; this is filtered communication. The family receives the information, but the best communication is balanced communication when the health professional communicate with both the patient and family. Page 1789–1790.

6.69 The answer is c.
Loss of self-esteem is more commonly a symptom of depression. In general, nursing interventions that focus on anxiety are based on helping the patient to recognize various manifestations of anxiety, determining whether the patient desires to do anything about the response, and activating coping strategies to control anxiety levels. Page 676–679.

6.70 The answer is d.
The patient should be allowed to express his fears, concerns, and wishes regarding death; this can provide comfort and emotional healing. When coping with a difficult disease such as

lung cancer, it is the discovery of meaning in the disease that gives one a sense of mastery. The recurrence of lung cancer can be a greater crisis than the initial diagnosis. Often, the fear of dying is not as profound as the fear of suffering in the process. Page 1745–1746, 1784.

6.71 The answer is a.

Denial or behavior disengagement are avoidant coping strategies that are associated with poorer psychologic well-being. Psychosocial responses cannot be clearly identified as either adaptive or maladaptive; this depends largely on the situation and on the adaptive potential of the particular response in that situation. A perception of uncertainty can result in an appraisal of danger or opportunity, depending on the individual's definition of the situation. Distancing behaviors by health professionals enhance patients' sense of loneliness and fear. Overinvolvement with patients can be countered through supportive collegial relationships. Page 1792.

6.72 The answer is a.

Family responses of anxiety, depression, hopelessness, and altered sexual health in response to a diagnosis of cancer have been shown to be similar to those of the patients themselves. Page 783–787.

CHAPTER 7

Oncologic Emergencies

METABOLIC

7.1 **Sepsis is a common cause of disseminated intravascular coagulation (DIC). Which of the following conditions *most accurately* describes how sepsis causes DIC?**
  a. Sepsis causes viruses to thrive, and viruses cause DIC.
  b. Endotoxins released from bacteria activate the coagulation cascade.
  c. Sepsis and bleeding occur simultaneously in patients who are immunosuppressed.
  d. Antiangiogenesis factors are released during periods of sepsis, which leads to DIC.

7.2 **The symptoms of DIC seem paradoxical because**
  a. DIC may be both the cause and effect of malignancy.
  b. Thrombosis and hemorrhage may occur simultaneously.
  c. Both platelet function and platelet numbers are implicated in DIC.
  d. Patients may experience fever at the same time their bodies are hypothermic.

7.3 **Therapy for DIC often involves the administration of several substances. Which of the following is *not* a common treatment for DIC?**
  a. Heparin
  b. Vitamin K
  c. Platelet replacement
  d. Epsilon-amino caproic acid (EACA or Amicar)

7.4 **Patients with cancer may have bleeding, despite normal platelet counts and coagulation factors. An example of this problem is bleeding caused by**
  a. DIC
  b. Hypocoagulability
  c. Platelet sequestration
  d. Decreased platelet adhesiveness

7.5 Which of the following statements *best* describes the physiologic characteristics of DIC?

a. All clotting factors are prolonged.

b. In contrast to what would be expected, the international normalized ratio, prothrombin time, and PTT are elevated.

c. The platelet count is decreased, the plasma fibrinogen is low because of consumption of fibrinogen by the clotting cascade, and the prothrombin time is prolonged.

d. There is an absence of coagulation, and therefore there is widespread hemorrhage.

7.6 Which of the following tests are specific and sensitive for the presence of DIC?

a. Fibrinogen level and platelet count

b. International normalized ratio (INR)

c. Plasminogen level and plasmin α-2-antiplasmin level

d. D-dimer assay and Fibrin Degradation Product (FDP) titer

7.7 The *most common* cause of acute DIC associated with cancer is

a. Anaphylaxis

b. Tumor products

c. Thrombopoiesis

d. Infection and sepsis

7.8 The *only* definitive treatment for DIC is

a. Aggressive antibiotic therapy

b. Treatment of the underlying cancer

c. Administration of platelets and fresh frozen plasma

d. Reversing the clotting cascade by the administration of heparin

7.9 Which of the following drugs has been found to be effective in the treatment of the syndrome of inappropriate antidiuretic hormone secretion (SIADH)?

a. Docetaxel

b. Demeclocycline

c. Arginine sulfide

d. Immunoglobulin

7.10 Which of the following is *not* considered diagnostic for SIADH?

a. Absence of edema

b. Serum sodium less than 135 mEq/L

c. Normal renal, adrenal, and thyroid function

d. Increased levels of blood urea nitrogen, uric acid, creatinine, and albumin

7.11 Mr. Bradford, a patient with small cell lung cancer, develops anorexia, weakness, and fatigue. At first these are attributed to the cancer itself. As his condition worsens Mr. Bradford's wife, who is caring for him through a hospice arrangement, calls you in tears, reporting that he has suddenly become combative. You tell her that he must have a serum chemistry as soon as possible because you suspect

a. Hypercalcemia

b. Hyponatremia

c. End-stage cancer

d. Paraneoplastic adrenotropic hormone (pACTH) syndrome

7.12 Which of the following is indicative of SIADH?

a. Increased plasma sodium and decreased urine output
b. Hyponatremia with high serum osmolality and high urine osmolality
c. Hypernatremia with high serum osmolality and high urine osmolality
d. Hyponatremia with low serum osmolality, high urine sodium, and high urine osmolality

7.13 The problem with ectopic antidiuretic hormone (ADH) secretion as a paraneoplastic syndrome in cancer compared to normal ADH secretion is which of the following?

a. Ectopic ADH is not regulated.
b. Ectopic ADH acts on cardiac tissue.
c. Ectopic ADH does not respond to dehydration.
d. Ectopic ADH is not related to mental status changes.

7.14 Mr. Lindy has a history of small cell lung cancer and returns for his 6-month checkup. He has felt well except for some nausea, weakness, and, at times, confusion, headache, and lethargy. His lab values reveal hypokalemia, hyponatremia, low blood urea nitrogen, and low creatinine. His clinical symptoms are suspicious for which of the following?

a. SIADH secretion
b. Adrenal insufficiency
c. Metastatic disease to the liver
d. Metastatic disease to the brain

7.15 Which of the following is *not* considered a therapeutic approach to the management of SIADH?

a. Bisphosphonates
b. Demeclocycline
c. Hypertonic saline infusions
d. Water restriction to less than 1000 mL/day

7.16 Which of the following is considered the *most important* prognostic indicator for septic shock?

a. Prolonged neutropenia
b. Polymicrobial infections
c. Sepsis-induced hypotension
d. The presence of multiple organ dysfunction syndrome

7.17 Major fluid volume depletion occurs in patients with septic shock. Which of the following pathophysiological mechanisms of fluid volume depletion is *not* characteristic of shock?

a. Third spacing of fluid
b. Vascular pooling and capillary leak
c. Decreased venous tone
d. Arterial vasoconstriction

7.18 Which of the following variables does *not* influence the incidence of sepsis?

a. Duration of granulocytopenia
b. Length of myelosuppressive therapy
c. Concurrent radiotherapy and chemotherapy
d. Absolute granulocyte count less than $500/mm^3$

7.19 What is the single *most important* risk factor for sepsis in individuals with cancer?
a. Age less than 1
b. Age less than 65
c. Chronic illness
d. Granulocytopenia

7.20 Septic shock ultimately causes death due to which of the following?
a. Fever
b. Coagulopathy
c. Tissue ischemia
d. Hypotension

7.21 Jason was just admitted to the hospital via the emergency department with suspected sepsis. He has a history of Hodgkin's disease. What is the *most important* intervention to initiate immediately?
a. Steroid therapy
b. Oxygen therapy
c. Antibiotic therapy
d. Intravenous therapy

7.22 Acute tumor lysis syndrome (ATLS) is *least likely* to be seen in which of the following cases?
a. Colon cancer
b. Lymphoma
c. Acute myelogenous leukemia
d. Non-Hodgkin's lymphoma

7.23 Patients with non-Hodgkin's lymphoma with big, bulky, high-grade disease are at high risk for acute TLS. One important aspect of the nursing care for such patients is
a. Monitoring urine output for signs of renal failure
b. Looking for signs of motor incoordination and cognitive deficits
c. Discontinuing vinca alkaloid treatment if signs of severe jaw pain occur
d. Providing oral or intravenous agents that keep blood and urine acidic

7.24 Mr. James has chronic myelogenous leukemia in blastic transformation. He is considered to have a high tumor burden and has evidence of lymphadenopathy and splenomegaly. Which of the following laboratory tests indicate that he is experiencing acute TLS?
a. Hypokalemia
b. Hypercalcemia
c. Hypophosphatemia
d. Acute hyperuricemia

7.25 A primary physiologic complication of acute tumor lysis syndrome (ATLS) is
a. Liver failure caused by a veno-occlusive disease
b. Tumor lysis, causing release of tissue, which produces pulmonary emboli
c. Uric acid crystallization in the renal tubules, causing obstruction and acute renal failure
d. Tumor cell obstruction of microvasculature, causing disseminated intravascular coagulation

7.26 TLS results in a release of a large amount of phosphorus into the blood and a proportional decrease in what other serum electrolyte?
a. Magnesium
b. Calcium
c. Potassium
d. Sodium

7.27 Which of the following is *not* a key element in the prevention of tumor lysis syndrome?

a. Diuresis
b. Allopurinol
c. Fluid restriction
d. Aggressive hydration

7.28 Mr. Clay has lymphoma and received chemotherapy 4 days ago. He has been doing well but comes in complaining of fatigue, dizziness, and a "fluttering" feeling in his chest. Chemistries reveal potassium, 6 mEq/L; creatinine, 2.7 mg/dL; and calcium, 6 mg/dL. Your assessment is which of the following?

a. He is dehydrated and needs fluids.
b. He could have a life-threatening arrhythmia and should be admitted.
c. He is probably anemic and needs blood.
d. He is losing calcium and needs magnesium.

7.29 Mr. Stevens has just begun his first treatment with rituximab. One hour into the infusion he complains of fever, chills, rigors, and nausea. Appropriate nursing action is based on which of the following?

a. The symptoms are expected and will lessen with each subsequent treatment.
b. This is an anaphylactic reaction, and the medication should be permanently discontinued.
c. The infusion should be maintained; these symptoms are expected and signal a good response to therapy.
d. Monitor the blood pressure because rituximab can significantly raise the blood pressure, requiring the drug to be discontinued.

7.30 Measures to prevent a hypersensitivity reaction to a monoclonal antibody include all *except* which of the following?

a. Administer an antipyretic.
b. Administer a corticosteroid before the infusion.
c. Administer an antihistamine before the infusion.
d. Speed up the infusion to decrease the amount of time the infusion takes.

7.31 Mrs. Howe has just arrived for her first treatment with trastuzumab, a monoclonal antibody. As you plan her teaching about her medication, you are careful to include all *except* which of the following?

a. If she has fever, chills, or rigors, the infusion will be turned off, and she will not receive this medication in the future.
b. She should report any difficulty breathing, chills, or cough because her medication could cause an anaphylactic reaction.
c. If she does have a reaction, the medication will be stopped temporarily and restarted after her symptoms subside.
d. Diphenhydramine and acetaminophen are often given before the first infusion to minimize risk of an infusion-related reaction.

7.32 Alex has an infection of his vascular access device and is beginning vancomycin therapy. Twenty minutes into a 60-minute infusion, you notice his face and upper torso are flushed and warm to touch. Appropriate nursing action includes which of the following?

a. Slow the infusion, and administer morphine.
b. Administer decadron and diphenhydramine immediately.
c. Stop the infusion; he is having an allergic reaction.
d. This is not an antigen antibody reaction; slow the infusion to 90 minutes.

7.33 **Which of the following drugs is *not* commonly associated with a hypersensitivity reaction?**
a. Paclitaxel
b. Cytarabine
c. L-asparaginase
d. Docetaxel

7.34 **Which of the following types of malignancies is *least likely* to be associated with hypercalcemia?**
a. Lung cancer
b. Colon cancer
c. Breast cancer
d. Multiple myeloma

7.35 **Among the common early symptoms in hypercalcemic patients are all of the following *except***
a. Polyuria
b. Diarrhea
c. Drowsiness
d. Nausea and vomiting

7.36 **The *most important* initial treatment for hypercalcemia is**
a. Inhibiting bone resorption
b. Treating the primary tumor
c. Inhibiting osteoclast function
d. Improving renal calcium excretion

7.37 **The pathophysiology of hypercalcemia involves a combination of two factors: bone resorption and**
a. Increased osteoclast activity
b. Increased glomerular function
c. Decreased renal calcium clearance
d. Decreased availability of ionized calcium

7.38 **Factors produced by tumors have been implicated in malignancy-associated hypercalcemia. Probably the *most important* of these humoral circulating factors is**
a. Prostaglandin
b. Bisphosphonate
c. Osteoclast-activating factor
d. Parathyroid hormone-related factor

7.39 **A patient is found to have a large tumor mass associated with high levels of parathyroid hormone-related protein but normal levels of 1,25-dihydroxyvitamin D and normal intestinal absorption rates. Bone absorption is found to exceed bone formation. The *most likely* diagnosis is**
a. Hodgkin's disease
b. Multiple myeloma
c. Primary hyperparathyroidism
d. Humoral hypercalcemia of malignancy (HHM)

7.40 The symptoms of hypercalcemia in patients with cancer are best described as
a. Numerous, vague, and nonspecific
b. Easily identified but difficult to treat
c. Similar to those of acute renal failure
d. Distinct from those of end-stage disease

7.41 A patient develops confusion, disorientation, and hallucinations with an elevated serum calcium and occasional bradycardia. Therapeutic interventions include all of the following *except*
a. Saline diuresis
b. Thiazide diuretics
c. Intravenous pamidronate
d. Aggressive cancer therapy

7.42 Florence is being treated for acute promyelocytic leukemia. On the second day of her chemotherapy she complains of shortness of breath, and you note that she has new bleeding from her peripherally inserted central catheter (PICC) as well as hematuria. Her white blood cell count is 80,000 mm^3, hemoglobin is 9 g/dL, and platelets are 20,000 mm^3. What oncologic emergency is she *most likely* to be experiencing?
a. Anaphylaxis
b. Hypercalcemia
c. Tumor lysis syndrome
d. Disseminated intravascular coagulation (DIC)

7.43 The metabolic abnormalities that are characteristic in tumor lysis syndrome include
a. Hypocalcemia, hypouricemia, hypophosphatemia, and hypokalemia
b. Hypocalcemia, hyperuricemia, hyperphosphatemia, and hyperkalemia
c. Hypercalcemia, hyperuricemia, hypophosphatemia, and hyperkalemia
d. Hypercalcemia, hyperuricemia, hyperphosphatemia, and hyperkalemia

7.44 Jack is receiving his first infusion of paclitaxel. Ten minutes into the infusion he complains of tightness in his chest and shortness of breath, and begins to experience wheezing. What are the *most important* nursing actions to take?
a. Slow the infusion, and monitor the patient closely.
b. Decrease the infusion by half the initial rate, and treat his symptoms.
c. Stop the infusion, maintain a patent intravenous line, and prepare for CPR as necessary.
d. Stop the infusion, maintain a patent intravenous line, and restart the drug when the patient stabilizes.

7.45 Frances is admitted to the hospital for treatment of Burkitt's lymphoma. Her lab values on admission to the hospital demonstrate a potassium of 4 mEq/L, phosphorus of 3.5 mg/dL, calcium of 9 mg/dL, and a uric acid of 9.5 mg/dL. Which of the following medications would you anticipate being ordered initially to help manage Frances?
a. Kayexalate
b. Allopurinol
c. Rasburicase
d. Doxycycline

7.46 Which of the following is *not* used in the treatment of hypercalcemia?
a. Hydration
b. Allopurinol
c. Forced diuresis
d. Bisphosphonate therapy

7.47 Appropriate measures to help prevent hypercalcemia in the at-risk patient include all *except* which of the following?
a. Increasing fluid intake to 3 L per day
b. Promotion of bed rest to prevent bone fractures
c. Promotion of ambulation and weight-bearing activities
d. Controlling nausea and vomiting to prevent dehydration

7.48 The purpose of the Modified Early Warning Score (MEWS) related to sepsis is
a. To act as an algorithm of care
b. To alert physicians when patients are at risk of sepsis
c. To identify the presence of sepsis in patients with cancer
d. To facilitate prompt communication between healthcare providers about early deterioration in a patient's condition

7.49 J.A. is being treated with chemotherapy for small cell lung cancer. His recent lab values demonstrate a serum sodium of 132 mEq/L. What is the likely *initial* treatment for his low sodium?
a. Administer chemotherapy
b. Hypertonic (3%) saline infusions
c. Administration of intravenous furosemide
d. Free-water restriction to 500 to 1000 mL/day

STRUCTURAL

7.50 Malignant pericardial effusions
a. Are extremely rare
b. Are not easily detected because many patients are asymptomatic
c. Are easily detected by tachycardia, low blood pressure, and shortness of breath
d. Occur in 50% of all patients with cancer, especially the hematologic malignancies

7.51 Possible early signs of cardiac tamponade include
a. Hypotension, bradycardia, and fatigue
b. Tachycardia, fatigue, and shortness of breath
c. Hypotension, cough, and narrowing pulse pressure
d. Hypertension, bradycardia, and widening pulse pressure

7.52 Which of the following tumor types is *not* commonly associated with pericardial effusion and tamponade?
a. Leukemia
b. Lung cancer
c. Breast cancer
d. Gastrointestinal cancer

7.53 Your patient is suspected to have a cardiac tamponade. What test is considered to be the *most sensitive* method for diagnosing this oncologic emergency?
a. Chest radiograph
b. Electrocardiogram
c. Magnetic resonance imaging
d. Two-dimensional echocardiogram

7.54 **You will soon begin work in a clinic that specializes in the detection and treatment of spinal cord tumors. You are aware that the *most common* presenting symptom of a spinal cord tumor is**

a. Pain
b. Weakness
c. Numbness and tingling
d. Uncoordinated ataxic gait

7.55 **The *most common* cause of spinal cord compression is**

a. Chronic steroid use
b. Carcinomatosis meningitis
c. Metastasis to the vertebral column
d. Primary disease of the vertebral column

7.56 **Spinal cord compression occurs by all *except* which of the following mechanisms?**

a. Vertebral collapse
b. Increased osteoblast activity
c. Displacement of bone into the epidural space
d. Direct extension of the tumor into the epidural space

7.57 **Mrs. Johnson has been treated for lung cancer, and she has complained of back pain for 2 months and now presents with weakness. Which of the following helps to explain her symptoms?**

a. Back pain is rarely a symptom of spinal cord tumors.
b. Back pain and weakness are classic symptoms of spinal cord tumors.
c. Back pain and weakness are likely caused by her chronic steroid use.
d. Back pain and weakness are likely caused by inactivity related to fatigue from her lung cancer treatment.

7.58 **Mark is being discharged from the hospital. His prostate cancer involves bone metastasis to the spine and pelvis. Which of the following developments is *not likely* to indicate a need for emergent radiation therapy?**

a. Sensory deficits
b. Worsening back pain
c. Bowel and urinary incontinence
d. Weakness of the lower extremities

7.59 **A woman with breast cancer and known bone metastasis is currently on pamidronate. Her primary complaint is weakness in both arms. She has back pain, but it is unchanged from the previous week. The *most logical* explanation for her symptoms and the correct nursing action is which of the following?**

a. Weakness in arms and legs is common with pamidronate, and she should increase her use of the arms to avoid losing muscle strength.
b. She has known bony metastasis that is no worse; the pamidronate will help the bone to heal, so it is appropriate to monitor her symptoms.
c. If she has bony disease in her spine, she should have an emergency magnetic resonance image to rule out spinal cord compression.
d. She should be encouraged not to cough, strain, or lift heavy objects because she could have osteoporosis and is at risk for disc disease.

7.60 A man with a history of lung cancer calls his doctor to report the following symptoms: dyspnea; headache; swollen face, neck, and arms; and dilated chest veins. Which of the following *best* identifies what he is describing?

a. Telangiectasia and complications of prior radiation therapy
b. Possible pneumothorax
c. Possible local recurrence with brain metastasis
d. Possible superior vena cava obstruction

7.61 Which of the following is *not* characteristic of superior vena cava syndrome (SVCS)?

a. As the superior vena cava is compressed, there is reduced venous return to the right atrium.
b. An increase in venous pressure causes venous hypertension.
c. Late symptoms include cough and dyspnea.
d. Initial symptoms include hoarseness and edema in the face, neck, and arms.

7.62 What is the *most likely* initial treatment of choice for a quickly progressing SVCS caused by non-small cell lung cancer?

a. Radiation therapy
b. Chemotherapy
c. Surgical resection
d. Administration of anticoagulants

7.63 What is the *best* surgical intervention for SVCS to provide rapid relief of symptoms prior to a tissue diagnosis?

a. The portion of the vena cava that is being compressed is repositioned surgically following resection of the tumor.
b. Percutaneous placement of an endovascular stent to bypass the obstruction.
c. A bypass graft is fashioned to redirect blood flow around the obstruction.
d. The compressed portion of the vena cava is removed.

7.64 Which of the following cancers is responsible for more than 75% of all cases of SVCS?

a. Breast cancer
b. Lung cancer
c. Hodgkin's disease
d. Kaposi sarcoma

7.65 Which of the following is the *most common* cause of SVCS?

a. Thrombus formation from intravascular devices
b. Mediastinal fibrosis
c. Thoracic aortic aneurysm
d. Malignancy in the mediastinal area causing obstruction of upper venous blood flow to the heart

7.66 In most instances of central nervous system tumors, the first, earliest, and *most sensitive* indicator of increased intracranial pressure (ICP) is a

a. Change in level of consciousness and cognitive ability
b. Change in vital signs
c. Motor and sensory function
d. Vomiting

7.67 After tumor resection, a patient suffers postoperative cerebral edema. This results from all of the following *except*

a. Surgical manipulation of the surrounding brain tissue
b. Changes in regional blood flow
c. Brain injury caused by excessive retraction
d. Seizures postoperatively

7.68 Jeffrey's intracranial pressure is acutely elevated. In acute situations like his, the drug of choice is

a. Carmustine
b. A corticosteroid
c. Vincristine
d. Dilantin

7.69 Which of the following statements regarding brain tumors is *not* accurate?

a. Metastatic brain tumors occur in 20%–40% of individuals with cancer.
b. The incidence of metastatic brain tumors is decreasing because of advances in cancer care.
c. Tumors in the lung are the most likely of all solid tumors to metastasize to the brain.
d. Radiation therapy is the primary mode of treatment and is palliative.

7.70 In balancing intracranial pressure, the mechanism that specifically maintains a normal intracranial pressure despite fluctuations in arterial pressure and venous drainage is

a. Autoregulation
b. Compensation
c. Cerebrospinal fluid displacement
d. Cerebral blood flow

7.71 Which of the following is used as sclerosing agent for the management of recurrent cardiac tamponade?

a. Rituximab
b. Gemcitabine
c. Doxorubicin
d. Bleomycin

7.72 What is the *most likely* treatment for a patient with non-Hodgkin's lymphoma and an associated SVCS?

a. Chemotherapy
b. Surgical resection
c. Radiation therapy
d. Administration of anticoagulants

7.73 Early signs of increased intracranial pressure include

a. Headache
b. Decorticate posturing
c. Widening pulse pressure
d. Increased systolic blood pressure

ANSWER RATIONALES

Please note: All page numbers referenced in the Answer Rationales sections refer to the textbook *Cancer Nursing: Principles and Practice, Seventh Edition*, by Connie Henke Yarbro, Debra Wujcik, and Barbara Holmes Gobel (Jones & Bartlett Learning, © 2011).

METABOLIC

7.1 The answer is b.
Risk of bleeding and DIC increases during periods of febrile neutropenia. This is due to the activation of the coagulation cascade by endotoxins released from bacteria. DIC is a dangerous sequelae of sepsis. This is most frequently seen in gram-negative sepsis due to the endotoxins released from the bacteria. Page 929–930.

7.2 The answer is b.
DIC always results from an underlying disease process that triggers abnormal activation of thrombin formation. Thrombin is both a powerful coagulant and an agent of fibrinolysis. Thus small clots may be formed in the microcirculation of many organs at the same time that clots and clotting factors are being consumed. The result is hemorrhage because the body is unable to respond to vascular or tissue injury. Page 929–931.

7.3 The answer is b.
Vitamin K might be administered to a patient experiencing hypocoagulability, but not the hypercoagulability caused by DIC. All the other therapies may provide short-term relief of DIC symptoms. Treatment of the underlying malignancy is vital in treating the patient with DIC as the tumor is the ultimate stimulus. Page 934–936.

7.4 The answer is d.
Qualitative abnormalities refer principally to alterations in platelet function, which may include decreased platelet adhesiveness, a decreased procoagulant activity of platelets, and decreased aggregation in response to adenosine diphosphate, thrombocytosis associated with myeloproliferative disorders, and the coating of platelets by fibrin degradation products as a result of the increased activation of coagulation factors. Page 750, 931.

7.5 The answer is c.
DIC represents the most common serious hypercoagulable state in individuals with cancer. Tests generally done to help support the diagnosis of DIC include prothrombin time (prolonged), platelet count (decreased), and the plasma fibrinogen level (decreased). Page 933.

7.6 The answer is d.
The laboratory tests that are both specific and sensitive for the presence of DIC include the D-dimer assay and the Fibrin Degradation Product titer. The other tests help to support the diagnosis of DIC, but are not specific for DIC. Page 933–934.

7.7 The answer is d.
The most common cause of acute DIC is infection and sepsis associated with cancer. It is believed that bacterial endotoxins, which are released from gram-negative bacteremia, activate factor XII of the clotting cascade. This factor can initiate coagulation as well as stimulate fibrinolysis. Page 929–930.

7.8 **The answer is b.**
Treatment of the underlying malignancy is vital in the patient with a hypercoagulability abnormality, because the tumor is the ultimate stimulus. All other therapy, although effective on a short-term basis, provides only an interval of symptomatic relief. Page 934.

7.9 **The answer is b.**
Demeclocycline (600–1200 mg daily) is an antibiotic that is most frequently used to treat chronic SIADH. It stimulates diuresis by inhibiting the effect of arginine vasopressin on the renal tubule. Page 1011.

7.10 **The answer is d.**
The criteria for the diagnosis of SIADH includes serum osmolality less than 275 mOsm/kg; serum sodium less than 135 mEq/L; urine osmolality greater than serum osmolality; urinary sodium greater than 30 mEq/L; euvolemia; decreased levels of blood urea nitrogen, uric acid, creatinine, and albumin; absence of edema; and normal renal, adrenal, and thyroid function. Page 1009–1010.

7.11 **The answer is b.**
Mr. Bradford most likely has hyponatremia secondary to SIADH. SIADH is primarily associated with small cell lung cancer. Water intoxication accounts for the signs and symptoms seen with SIADH. The early symptoms, such as nausea, weakness, anorexia, and fatigue, can be easily attributed to the cancer. However, as the hyponatremia worsens, symptoms may progress to include altered mental status, confusion, and combativeness. Page 1006–1009.

7.12 **The answer is d.**
SIADH results from ADH secretion by the tumor. The symptoms include hyponatremia, high urine sodium, high urine osmolality and low serum osmolality, characterized by mental status changes, lethargy, seizures, and confusion. Page 1009.

7.13 **The answer is a.**
Although structurally identical to normal ADH, ectopic ADH is not regulated. Atrial natriuretic peptide, a hormone arising from cardiac atrial tissue, has been identified as a cause of hyponatremia. Water intoxication accounts for the symptomatology of SIADH. Page 1006–1008.

7.14 **The answer is a.**
Serum chemistries frequently show low blood urea nitrogen, creatinine, albumin, and uric acid; this is a dilutional effect in hyponatremia associated with SIADH. SIADH occurs commonly in patients with small cell lung cancer and initially presents as nausea, weakness, confusion, and lethargy. Page 1006, 1008–1009.

7.15 **The answer is a.**
Bisphosphonates, agents to inhibit bone resorption, are used to treat hypercalcemia. Fluids are restricted to less than 500–1000 mL/day. Hypertonic saline is given intravenously with furosemide to expedite water loss. Demeclocycline is an antibiotic used to treat chronic SIADH. It stimulates diuresis by impairing the effect of arginine vasopressin on the renal tubule. Page 952, 1009–1011.

7.16 **The answer is d.**
When sepsis progresses to a state of organ dysfunction, hypoperfusion, or hypotension, severe sepsis is present. Multiple organ dysfunction syndrome, which is defined as the presence of

altered organ function in an acutely ill patient such that homeostasis cannot be maintained without intervention, is the final common pathway for the critically ill patients. The presence of multiple organ dysfunction syndrome is an important prognostic indicator for septic shock. Page 965.

7.17 **The answer is d.**
The principal feature of sepsis is arterial vasodilation, *not* vasoconstriction. Major fluid volume depletion occurs in patients with septic shock due to decreased venous tone, vascular pooling, capillary leak, and third spacing of fluid. The hallmark of septic shock is profound hypotension. Page 967.

7.18 **The answer is c.**
Although concurrent radiotherapy and chemotherapy might increase the degree of myelosuppression, the incidence of sepsis is not increased. There is a direct relationship between the number of circulating polymorphonuclear neutrophilic leukocytes (PMNs) and the incidence of infection. When the granulocyte count is less than 500/mm^3, the risk of infection is significant. As the length of therapy and the duration of granulocytopenia increase, so does the incidence of sepsis. Page 966.

7.19 **The answer is d.**
Granulocytopenia is the single most important risk factor in the development of sepsis in the patient with cancer. Age less than 1, age greater than 65, and chronic illness are risk factors in the development of sepsis. Page 966.

7.20 **The answer is c.**
The clinical picture of septic shock illustrates the cumulative effects of coagulopathy, hypotension, hypoperfusion, and, ultimately, tissue ischemia involving failure of all body systems. Page 967–969.

7.21 **The answer is c.**
The most important intervention in the management of septic shock is immediate treatment with antibiotic therapy. According to the sepsis resuscitation bundle, antibiotics should be administered within 3 hours from the time of presentation for emergency department admissions and within 1 hour from the time for nonemergency department admissions. The use of steroids for the treatment of sepsis in the absence of shock is not recommended. Oxygen therapy and intravenous fluid therapy are both indicated in the treatment of shock, but antibiotic therapy must be the immediate focus. Page 973–975.

7.22 **The answer is a.**
Acute TLS is a complication of cancer therapy that occurs most commonly in patients with tumors that have a high proliferation index and are highly sensitive to chemotherapy. Acute TLS is most commonly seen in patients with high-grade lymphoma, acute myelogenous leukemia, chronic myelogenous leukemia, and non-Hodgkin's lymphoma. Page 1015.

7.23 **The answer is a.**
Acute TLS generally occurs when the patient is initially treated. Tumor cells spill their contents into the general circulation, causing a metabolic disturbance. Renal failure and death may occur. The treatment of choice is prevention, including hydration, and intravenous or oral allopurinol and/or rasburicase to prevent hyperuricemic nephropathy. Page 1015, 1019–1021.

7.24 **The answer is d.**
Acute TLS is most often characterized by the development of acute hyperuricemia, hyperkalemia, hyperphosphatasmia, and hypocalcemia with or without acute renal failure. Page 1015, 1017.

7.25 **The answer is c.**
Uric acid crystallization in the renal tubules, causing obstruction, decreased glomerular filtration, and/or acute renal failure, is a major complication of acute TLS. Page 1018–1019.

7.26 **The answer is b.**
In TLS there is an inverse relationship between phosphorus and calcium, whereby if one mineral increases, the other decreases in the same proportion. Page 1018.

7.27 **The answer is c.**
Fluid restriction in the management of acute TLS is contraindicated. Aggressive hydration is needed, to at least 3 liters of fluid per day, with adequate urinary output and using diuretics to promote excretion of the electrolytes that have been released from lysed cells to prevent renal tubular damage. Allopurinol inhibits the enzyme xanthine oxidase and prevents the formation of uric acid, which in turn prevents uric acid nephropathy. Page 1021–1022.

7.28 **The answer is b.**
An increase in phosphate, potassium, uric acid, blood urea nitrogen, and creatinine or a 25% decrease in calcium within 4 days of chemotherapy is indicative of TLS and places the patient at risk for life-threatening arrhythmias. Page 1025–1026.

7.29 **The answer is a.**
An infusion-related symptom complex consisting of fever, chills and rigors, nausea, asthenia, and headache occur in most patients during the first infusion with rituximab. The symptoms decrease with subsequent infusions. Rituximab causes hypotension, not hypertension. Page 793, 795, 797, 800, 803.

7.30 **The answer is d.**
Anaphylactoid reactions have most commonly occurred with monoclonal antibody therapy. Most of these reactions occurred at the beginning of therapy administration to patients with lymphoma or leukemia or when administered by rapid infusion. Page 793–794, 799.

7.31 **The answer is a.**
Acute side effects that occur during infusion are most commonly fever, chills, rigors, malaise, myalgia, nausea, and vomiting. The symptoms often resolve if the rate is slowed. Page 800, 802–803.

7.32 **The answer is d.**
Vancomycin causes release of histamine from the mast cells, which causes vasodilation and the appearance of an allergic reaction. The red neck, or red man syndrome, is common with vancomycin and improves with slowing to a 90-minute infusion. Page 535.

7.33 **The answer is b.**
Hypersensitivity reactions due to cytarabine are rare and seen only within the past few years where the doses used are 10–15 times normal. Hypersensitivity reactions are frequent with paclitaxel, docetaxel, and asparaginase therapy. Page 793–794.

7.34 The answer is b.

Hypercalcemia is rare in colon cancer. Patients with lung and breast cancer account for the highest percentage of malignancy-induced hypercalcemia. However, multiple myeloma, which is relatively rare, is the underlying cause in more than 20% of malignancy-associated hypercalcemia cases. Page 940.

7.35 The answer is b.

Constipation, not diarrhea, is more likely to be observed during the early stages of hypercalcemia. Elevated extracellular calcium levels depress smooth muscle contractility, leading to delayed gastric emptying and decreased gastrointestinal motility. Page 948–949.

7.36 The answer is d.

Before excessive bone resorption can be treated, impaired renal calcium excretion must be improved, usually by correcting dehydration and removing factors that may exacerbate hypercalcemia, including thiazide diuretics. Oral or intravenous hydration with normal saline may be required. Page 951–953.

7.37 The answer is c.

Hypercalcemia is characterized by excess extracellular calcium. This condition results from bone resorption—the release of skeletal calcium into serum—and from the failure of the kidneys to clear extracellular calcium. As calcium levels rise, symptoms of hypercalcemia appear. Page 941, 944–945.

7.38 The answer is d.

Malignancy-associated hypercalcemia is a complex metabolic complication in which bone resorption exceeds both bone formation and the kidney's ability to excrete extracellular calcium. Humoral circulating factors include a parathyroid hormone-related factor and 1,25-dihydroxyvitamin D. Hypercalcemia that develops in patients with solid tumors but without bone metastases is thought to be caused by parathyroid hormone-related factor. Page 944–945.

7.39 The answer is d.

In humoral hypercalcemia of malignancy (HHM), patients secrete high levels of parathyroid hormone-related protein but have low or normal levels of 1,25-dihydroxyvitamin D and normal intestinal absorption rates. Osteoblastic and osteoclastic activities are "uncoupled" so that bone resorption exceeds bone formation. Hypercalcemia and hypercalciuria thus occur. Page 945, 950.

7.40 The answer is a.

Hypercalcemia symptoms are numerous, vague, and nonspecific, and may be difficult to distinguish from disease- or treatment-related side effects. Page 947–949.

7.41 The answer is b.

Paraneoplastic hypercalcemia often presents as confusion, disorientation, and hallucinations with bradycardia. Thiazide diuretics decrease renal excretion of calcium, which may potentiate hypercalcemia and thus should be avoided. Treatment of hypercalcemia includes vigorous hydration, pamidronate, and aggressive cancer therapy. Page 951–953.

7.42 The answer is d.

Acute promyelocytic leukemia is the cancer most commonly associated with DIC. Symptoms related to DIC correlate to where fibrin clots have lodged. Bleeding is the most obvious sign of a hemorrhagic disorder and can occur from any orifice or opening on the surface of the skin or organ. A low platelet count is a nonspecific but frequent finding in DIC. Page 929, 931.

7.43 The answer is b.

The metabolic abnormalities that are characteristic in tumor lysis syndrome include hypocalcemia, hyperuricemia, hyperphosphatemia, and hyperkalemia. These metabolic abnormalities occur when a cell is lysed as a result of chemotherapy or other precipitating event and the intracellular electrolytes are released into the vascular system. Page 1015, 1017.

7.44 The answer is c.

Jack may be experiencing an anaphylactic reaction to the paclitaxel. Whenever anaphylaxis is suspected, the initial nursing actions would include stopping the infusion, maintaining a patent intravenous line with normal saline, and preparing for CPR as necessary. Whether or not a patient is rechallenged with a chemotherapy drug after an anaphylactic reaction is dependent on the severity of the reaction. Page 802–804.

7.45 The answer is c.

A diagnosis of Burkitt's lymphoma puts Frances at high risk for tumor lysis syndrome. Based on Frances' lab values, she is already experiencing hyperuricemia. Rasburicase is indicated for the initial management of elevated plasma uric acid levels in adults with leukemia, lymphoma, and solid tumors receiving anticancer treatment expected to result in tumor lysis syndrome. Page 1022.

7.46 The answer is b.

Allopurinol blocks the conversion of xanthine and hypoxanthine to uric acid and thus is used to help prevent tumor lysis syndrome. Hydration, forced diuresis, and bisphosphonate therapy are all used to treat hypercalcemia. Page 955, 1021.

7.47 The answer is b.

Bed rest will increase bone resorption of calcium, thereby driving the calcium into the general circulation and increasing the risk of hypercalcemia. To prevent hypercalcemia in the at-risk patient it is necessary to promote ambulation and weight-bearing activities to decrease bone resorption of calcium. Page 951.

7.48 The answer is d.

The purpose of the MEWS is to facilitate prompt communication between nursing and medical staff when deterioration in a patient's condition first becomes apparent. The authors of this scoring system intended for the MEWS to result in earlier intervention in the general medical setting so that transfer to a critical care setting is either prevented or occurs without unnecessary delays. Page 970.

7.49 The answer is d.

The initial treatment for most patients with SIADH is to restrict free-water to 500 to 100 mL/day. Hypertonic saline infusions along with administration of intravenous furosemide are generally initiated for severe hyponatremia. Chemotherapy is often an offending agent that can cause SIADH and thus is not the treatment of choice for this syndrome. Page 1007, 1009–1010.

Structural

7.50 The answer is b.

A malignant pericardial effusion is the most common cardiac complication associated with cancer and indicates a poor prognosis. Malignant pericardial effusions are not easily detected by routine tests because most patients are asymptomatic. Often, clinical manifestations are vague or attributed to other causes. Page 869, 917–919.

7.51 **The answer is b.**
The signs and symptoms of cardiac tamponade are variable and depend on the rate and amount of pericardial fluid accumulation, etiology of the tamponade, and the patient's age. If fluid accumulation occurs slowly the early signs may include tachycardia, fatigue, and shortness of breath. Page 917–918.

7.52 **The answer is d.**
Gastrointestinal cancer rarely results in pericardial effusion and tamponade, probably because of its natural pattern of metastases to the liver and surrounding organs. Pericardial effusions occur most often in patients with lung and breast cancer. Page 870, 916.

7.53 **The answer is d.**
Two-dimensional echocardiogram is the most sensitive and precise method for the diagnosis of cardiac tamponade. Findings on electrocardiography are nonspecific. A chest radiograph is not a definitive diagnostic method for cardiac tamponade. Magnetic resonance imaging has limited usefulness in the diagnosis of cardiac tamponade. Page 920–922.

7.54 **The answer is a.**
Pain is the most common presenting symptom of a spinal cord tumor. Weakness is the most readily identified objective finding and may follow the appearance of sensory symptoms. Specific sensory deficits depend on where the tumor is on a cross-section of the spine. A lateral tumor affects pain and temperature, causing numbness, and tingling. Anterior tumors lead to weakness and an uncoordinated ataxic gait. Page 983–984.

7.55 **The answer is c.**
Spinal cord compression is now referred to as a skeletal-related event or a consequence of bone metastasis, reflecting the fact that almost 90% of cases are due to involvement of the vertebral column with metastatic disease. Page 980–981.

7.56 **The answer is b.**
Osteoblasts are bone-forming cells derived from normal stromal cells in the marrow. Osteoblast activity is necessary for normal bone development. Spinal cord compression occurs either by direct extension of the tumor into the epidural space or by vertebral collapse and displacement of bone into the epidural space. It can also occur by direct extension through the intervertebral foramina. Page 941, 981–982.

7.57 **The answer is b.**
Weakness is the most readily identified objective finding for spinal cord tumor. Back pain is the most common presenting symptom of spinal cord compression. Page 980, 983–984.

7.58 **The answer is c.**
All patients with bone metastasis are at risk for spinal cord compression. Urinary and bowel incontinence are signs of autonomic dysfunction and are poor prognostic signs, and will not likely respond to radiation therapy. The degree of neurological impairment prior to initiating treatment is predictive of recovery posttreatment. Worsening back pain, weakness of the lower extremities, or sensory deficits require immediate medical attention—usually radiation therapy to control tumor impingement on the spinal cord. Page 984, 987.

7.59 **The answer is c.**
Imminent spinal cord compression should be suspected in individuals who have known bone metastases, progressive back pain associated with weakness, paresthesias, bowel or bladder dysfunction, or gait disturbances. Page 983–984.

7.60 **The answer is d.**
Obstruction of the superior vena cava is a common complication of lung cancer. Dyspnea is the most common symptom. The clinical picture can include edema of both eyelids, arms, and hands; cough; and dilated collateral chest veins. Page 998.

7.61 **The answer is c.**
Initial symptoms of SVCS include dyspnea; cough and stridor; hoarseness; edema in the face, neck, and arms; and neck and chest vein distention. Page 998.

7.62 **The answer is a.**
Radiation therapy is the treatment of choice for SVCS caused by non-small cell lung cancer because non-small cell lung cancer (NSCLC) does not respond well to chemotherapy. Radiation therapy is also the choice in patients without a histologic diagnosis. Page 1002.

7.63 **The answer is b.**
Percutaneous placement of an endovascular stent to bypass the obstruction provides rapid relief of symptoms until the etiology is determined. Surgical bypass has a limited role in the management of SVCS and is used only when other management techniques have failed to relieve the symptoms of SVCS. Page 1002.

7.64 **The answer is b.**
Lung cancer is responsible for more than 75% of all cases of SVCS. Small cell carcinoma of the lung is the most common histologic type, followed by squamous cell carcinoma of the lung. Page 996.

7.65 **The answer is d.**
A malignancy in the mediastinal area causing obstruction of upper venous blood return to the heart is the most common cause of SVCS. Thrombus from intravascular devices, thoracic aortic aneurysm, and mediastinal fibrosis are nonmalignant causes of SVCS. Page 996.

7.66 **The answer is a.**
In most instances the first, earliest, and most sensitive indicator of increased intracranial pressure is a change in the level of consciousness and cognitive ability. Motor and sensory function, vomiting and vital sign changes occur, but not early on. Page 1156.

7.67 **The answer is d.**
Postoperative cerebral edema results from the surgical manipulation of the surrounding brain tissue, changes in regional blood flow, or brain injury caused by excessive retraction. Page 1169.

7.68 **The answer is b.**
In situations in which intracranial pressure is acutely elevated, corticosteroids and careful fluid management are required. Page 1169.

7.69 **The answer is b.**
The incidence of metastatic brain tumors is increasing because of advances in cancer care. Page 1165.

7.70 **The answer is a.**
In balancing intracranial pressure, autoregulation is the mechanism that specifically maintains a normal intracranial pressure, despite fluctuations in arterial pressure and venous drainage. Page 1154.

7.71 **The answer is d.**
Bleomycin, doxycycline, and cisplatin are chemotherapy drugs that are used as sclerosing agents for the management of recurrent cardiac tamponade. Interleukin-2 and OK-432 have also been used as sclerosing agents for the management of recurrent cardiac tamponade. Page 924.

7.72 **The answer is a.**
Complete relief of symptoms related to SVCS can be obtained in 80% of patients with non-Hodgkin's lymphoma with chemotherapy. Multiagent or combination chemotherapy is the standard. Page 1001.

7.73 **The answer is a.**
Headache is a common presenting symptom of increased intracranial pressure. Decorticate and decerebrate posturing, widening pulse pressure, and increased systolic blood pressure are all signs that occur late in the course of increased intracranial pressure. Page 1156.

CHAPTER 8

Sexuality

8.1 After 18 months of intensive chemotherapy, a 32-year-old woman with breast cancer reveals to you her concern regarding the effects of cancer chemotherapy on her future children. Your counsel to her would include which of the following?

a. There has been an increased incidence of birth defects in the offspring of women previously treated with chemotherapy.
b. There has been an increased risk of first pregnancy miscarriages.
c. There has been no increased risk of nonhereditary cancers among offspring.
d. There has been an increased risk of hereditary cancers among offspring.

8.2 Both chemotherapy and radiation therapy are known to have teratogenetic effects on the fetus, causing spontaneous abortion, fetal malformation, or fetal death. These complications are *most likely* to happen during which trimester?

a. First
b. Second
c. Third
d. The risk to the fetus is equal among the three trimesters.

8.3 Janie is 7 months pregnant and has recently had a lumpectomy for breast cancer. She is scheduled to begin chemotherapy followed by radiation. She is debating whether to start her chemotherapy or delay it until after she has her baby. She is concerned about the effect of the chemotherapy on her baby. Your comments and counsel are based on the following true statements regarding the effect of chemotherapy on a developing fetus *except*

a. Chemotherapy during the second and third trimesters may cause premature birth or low birth weights.
b. Chemotherapy during the second and third trimesters is not associated with a higher incidence of congenital abnormality compared with the normal pregnancy incidence.
c. Chemotherapy during the second and third trimesters is associated with a higher incidence of congenital abnormality compared with the normal pregnancy incidence.
d. Alkylating agents and antimetabolites are most often associated with fetal malformations during the first trimester.

8.4 **The fertility of which of the following patients is *most likely* to be affected by chemotherapy?**

a. Kevin, who is 7 years old
b. Dan, who is 60 years old
c. Pamela, who is 15
d. Elaine, who is over 30

8.5 **It has been suggested that women with breast cancer wait 1–5 years after the completion of adjuvant chemotherapy before attempting conception. The rationale for this recommendation includes all of the following *except***

a. Many women require tamoxifen and should avoid becoming pregnant.
b. Pregnancy shortly after completion of chemotherapy could potentially increase risk of recurrence.
c. Time is needed for recovery of ovarian function.
d. Recurrence is most likely within the first 2 years after cancer therapy.

8.6 **Which of the following statements about pregnancy and cancer is *false*?**

a. Most cancers do not adversely affect a pregnancy.
b. In general, pregnancy does not adversely affect the outcome of a cancer.
c. Therapeutic abortion has been shown to be of benefit in altering disease progression.
d. Treatment options should be evaluated as though the patient was not pregnant, and therapy should be instituted when appropriate.

8.7 **Invasion of a cervical carcinoma into underlying tissue is found in a woman during the third trimester of her pregnancy. Which of the following treatments is *most likely* to be followed?**

a. Fetal viability is awaited, and appropriate therapy is given after delivery of the baby by cesarean section.
b. Surgery or radiation therapy, without therapeutic abortion, is undertaken immediately.
c. A radical hysterectomy and pelvic node dissection are performed and combined with radiation therapy.
d. Therapeutic abortion is performed immediately and followed by standard treatment for advanced disease.

8.8 **Evaluation of the placenta for evidence of metastasis to the fetus is *most likely* to be carried out under which of the following situations?**

a. When the mother has received combination chemotherapy during the third trimester of pregnancy
b. When the mother has received low doses of radiation during the first trimester of pregnancy
c. When the mother has breast cancer or invasive cervical cancer
d. When the mother has a melanoma or lymphoma

8.9 **Which of the following is *most likely* to involve risk to the fetus whose mother is being treated for cancer?**

a. Pelvic surgery on the mother during the second trimester of pregnancy
b. Low doses of radiation associated with diagnostic x-rays
c. Chemotherapy during the first trimester of pregnancy
d. The use of anesthetic agents during surgery on the mother during the second trimester of pregnancy

8.10 In a support group you are conducting for expectant mothers with breast cancer, the following question is raised: "How likely is cancer to spread from the mother to the fetus?" You explain that only a few cancers spread from the mother to the fetus. Which among the following cancers mentioned by the group is *least likely* to spread from the mother to the fetus?

a. Melanoma
b. Non-Hodgkin's lymphoma
c. Leukemia
d. Breast cancer

8.11 Methods have been identified that may preserve fertility during cancer treatment. The *best* method to recommend is

a. Treatment of men with gonadotropin-releasing hormone (GnRH) analogs
b. Treatment of women with gonadotropin-releasing hormone (GnRH) analogs
c. Shielding of the testes or ovaries from the radiation field
d. Birth control pills for women

8.12 The American Society of Clinical Oncology developed recommendations for fertility preservation for individuals with cancer. Options considered as standard of care include all the following *except*

a. Oocyte and ovarian tissue cryopreservation
b. Semen cryopreservation
c. Embryo cryopreservation
d. Trachelectomy

8.13 The *most common* sexually transmitted disease (STD) in the United States is

a. Hepatitis A virus (HAV)
b. Hepatitis B virus (HBV)
c. Human papillomavirus (HPV)
d. Human immunodeficiency virus (HIV)

8.14 In HIV-infected women, those with the greatest risk for HPV coinfection include all *except*

a. CD4+ levels less than 200/μL
b. CD4+ levels more than 200/μL
c. RNA viral load > 20,000 copies/mL
d. Being a smoker

8.15 Most HPV infections are asymptomatic and transient, but four HPV strains are responsible for 70% of all cervical cancers. These four HPV strains are

a. 2, 11, 16, 20
b. 2, 6, 16, 18
c. 6, 11, 16, 20
d. 6, 11, 16, 18

8.16 AIDS-defining malignancies (ADM) and non-AIDS defining malignancies (NADM) are a problem in the HIV population. Of the following statements regarding the HIV population and ADMs and NADMs, which is *false?*

a. Incidence of NADMs have decreased because of HAART.
b. Incidence of ADMs have decreased because of HAART.
c. Eighty percent of the HIV populations had ADMs, and 20% had NADMs.
d. Highly active antiretroviral therapy (HAART) has had a major impact on the prognosis of HIV infection.

8.17 Of the following statements regarding HIV infection, which is *not* correct?
a. HIV infection is now pandemic.
b. HIV has a symptom-free period that may span 10 years or more.
c. HIV primarily affects natural killer (NK) cells.
d. Without treatment 9 of every 10 persons with HIV will develop AIDS after 10–15 years.

8.18 Human papillomavirus (HPV) is linked to all of the following *except*
a. Cervical, vaginal, and vulva cancer
b. Cancer of the anus and penis
c. Genital warts
d. Cancer of the oral cavity

8.19 Mrs. Smith says that she has heard of a new vaccine that prevents HPV and the chance of getting cervical cancer. Your *most appropriate* response is
a. Yes, there is a vaccine to help prevent human papillomavirus (HPV), but it is most effective prior to sexual contact.
b. Yes, there are two different types of vaccines that can help protect females from HPV-related disease such as cervical cancer.
c. Yes, there is a vaccine, but the use of condoms can also protect against HPV.
d. Yes, there is a vaccine given in three doses to protect against HPV, and it requires that you receive all three doses.

8.20 AIDS-related malignancies are a growing concern for HIV-infected individuals. The three AIDS-defining malignancies (ADMs) are
a. Cervical, anal, and urogenital cancers
b. Cervical and anal cancer and Hodgkin's lymphoma
c. Cervical cancer, Kaposi sarcoma, and non-Hodgkin's lymphoma
d. Cervical and anal cancer and Kaposi sarcoma

8.21 Your 55-year-old patient with lung cancer has completed his treatment, including three cycles of chemotherapy and radiation. He expressed some problems with erectile dysfunction and states his internist seems reluctant to address the issue. Which of the following is the *most likely* response to his concerns?
a. Erectile dysfunction is common due to the paraneoplastic component of his illness.
b. The chemotherapy and radiation are probably the cause, and it is not likely to improve.
c. Attention to his erectile dysfunction by his internist is overshadowed by his history of cancer and treatment.
d. Sexual dysfunction is to be expected in someone his age.

8.22 Advocates who claim that sexuality should be a routine part of every assessment for patients with cancer propose the following benefits *except*
a. Routine assessment decreases embarrassment on the part of the patient and practitioner if it is viewed as a normal aspect of health care.
b. It gives the patient permission to mention sexual difficulties to the practitioner.
c. It gives the practitioner permission to ask specific questions when there is reason to believe sexuality-related side effects are present.
d. It allows the practitioner to identify sexual problems and create a list of goals for the patient.

8.23 Mr. Crane is about to undergo a radical prostatectomy. He is concerned about his ability to be sexually active after his surgery. The *most important* factor that relates to sexual function after prostatectomy is
a. Age less than 50
b. Stage of disease
c. Preservation of neurovascular bundles
d. Hormone therapy postsurgery

8.24 For patients who undergo surgery for gastrointestinal cancer, possible organic sexual dysfunction is *most closely* associated with which of the following?

a. Placement of a colostomy
b. Removal of rectal tissue
c. Changes in body image
d. Responses by family and friends

8.25 Treatments for prostate cancer have the potential to alter sexual function, even though prostate cancer occurs mostly in older men. Permanent damage to erectile function with loss of emission and ejaculation is *most likely* to occur with

a. Radical prostatectomy
b. Transurethral resection
c. Bilateral orchiectomy
d. Transabdominal resection

8.26 Assessment of a patient's alteration in sexual function includes information regarding medical, psychologic, and psychosexual status. One method for assessing sexual dysfunction includes the use of the ALARM model. ALARM is an acronym for which of the following?

a. Assess, Learn, Arousal, Relearn, Medical data
b. Assess, Libido, Activity, Relearn, Meditation
c. Activity, Libido, Arousal, Resolution, Medical data
d. Arousal, Libido, Action, Resolution, Meditation

8.27 A patient is about to receive radiation for prostate cancer. He is concerned about sexual dysfunction as a result. As part of your patient education plan, you tell him that radiation therapy can cause sexual and reproductive dysfunction through all the following factors *except*

a. Primary organ failure
b. Alterations in organ function
c. Temporary or permanent effects of the therapy
d. Androgen blockade

8.28 Which of the following has been implicated in sexual dysfunction in both men and women receiving chemotherapy?

a. Depletion of the germinal epithelium
b. Treatment with estrogens
c. Combination chemotherapy, including an alkylating agent
d. Treatment with androgens

8.29 Marcia, a patient of yours, will be starting chemotherapy in 2 weeks. She asks you to explain to her the risks and side effects of chemotherapy. You tell her all of the following *except*

a. Chemotherapy can cause ovarian failure.
b. Irregular menses are a common side effect.
c. Sexual dysfunction is normal.
d. Hot flashes and night sweats are to be expected.

8.30 The traditional bilateral retroperitoneal lymph node dissection (RPLND) results in

a. Permanent erectile dysfunction
b. Impaired ability to experience a normal orgasm
c. Decreased libido and loss of testosterone
d. The loss of antegrade ejaculation and infertility

8.31 Two basic nursing interventions for alterations in sexual health encountered by cancer patients are

a. Education and counseling
b. Screening and role playing
c. Affective therapy and role modeling
d. Enhancing reality surveillance and reinforcing personal power

8.32 Sexuality in the cancer patient may be affected by the following factors *except*

a. Psychosexual changes associated with mutagenicity
b. Physiologic problems of fertility and sterility
c. Psychologic issues such as loss of self-esteem and fears of abandonment
d. Changes in body appearance resulting from therapy

8.33 Mrs. Archer has recently had a radical cystectomy with resection of nearly one-third of the anterior wall of the vagina and vaginal reconstruction. She is approaching discharge and requires teaching regarding any changes she can expect in terms of her sexuality. It would be appropriate to include all of the following in your discussion *except*

a. The diameter of the introitus and the vaginal barrel may be compromised due to the surgery.
b. Intercourse may be restricted, even painful.
c. There will be less lubrication, and she will need to practice vaginal dilation and liberal use of lubrication.
d. Orgasm will be diminished due to the clitoris being compromised

8.34 Radiation is commonly used in conjunction with surgery as treatment for vaginal cancer. Patient education before discharge would include all of the following *except*

a. Vaginal fibrosis and scarring can occur due to a loss of blood supply; therefore, vaginal intercourse is to be minimized.
b. Vaginal intercourse and the use of a vaginal dilator are encouraged to prevent narrowing of the vagina.
c. Prescribed topical estrogen cream is an effective measure to minimize functional loss.
d. Douche daily with diluted hydrogen peroxide/water mixture for 2 to 3 months.

8.35 Mr. James is scheduled for a radical cystectomy with urinary diversion. He is especially concerned about the possibility of being impotent and unable to have sex because of the urinary diversion following surgery. Your *best* response is based on which of the following?

a. Because the surgery involves removal of the bladder, attached peritoneum, the prostate, and seminal vesicles, penile sensation is altered and impotence is unavoidable in many cases.
b. He should be encouraged to talk to his surgeon because it is possible that the surgeon will do a potency-sparing cystectomy.
c. Refer him to an enterostomal therapist for information about a penile prosthesis and placement of the urinary diversion.
d. Urinary diversions today result in improved sexual adjustment due to decreased leakage and odor control.

ANSWER RATIONALES

Please note: All page numbers referenced in the Answer Rationales sections refer to the textbook *Cancer Nursing: Principles and Practice, Seventh Edition,* by Connie Henke Yarbro, Debra Wujcik, and Barbara Holmes Gobel (Jones & Bartlett Learning, © 2011).

8.1 The answer is c.
Edgar et al. (2007) identified several large international studies providing a pool of 25,000 childhood survivors and noted no increased risk of genetic abnormality in the offspring of cancer survivors. Other studies have found no increased risk of nonhereditary cancers among offspring, no increased risk of birth defects, and no increased risk of malignancies or anomalies in the offspring. Page 896.

8.2 The answer is a.
Radiation exposure during the first trimester represents the greatest risk to the fetus. In the second or third trimester, fetal death is unlikely, but growth retardation, sterility, and cataracts are common. Chemotherapy, particularly when received during the first trimester, has been related to congenital abnormalities, with approximately 10% of fetuses experiencing some type of anomaly. Page 896.

8.3 The answer is c.
Chemotherapy in the second and third trimester may cause premature birth or low birth weight, but congenital abnormalities are not increased over the normal pregnancy incidence. Page 896.

8.4 The answer is d.
Women over the age of 30 are less likely to regain ovarian function because they have fewer oocytes. Page 889.

8.5 The answer is b.
There appears to be no decrease in survival for women who become pregnant after breast cancer treatment. In fact, some researchers believe further pregnancy may actually protect against recurrence. Page 902.

8.6 The answer is c.
Therapeutic abortion has not been shown to be beneficial in altering disease progression and should not be considered unless pregnancy will compromise treatment and thus prognosis. Therapeutic abortion is most likely to be recommended when the cancer is diagnosed at an advanced stage during the first trimester of pregnancy and the effects of combination chemotherapy are likely to damage the fetus. Page 901.

8.7 The answer is a.
During the first two trimesters, surgery or radiation therapy, without therapeutic abortion, is usually undertaken. Early-stage disease may be treated with radical hysterectomy and pelvic node dissection, whereas radiation therapy is the most common treatment in advanced disease. During the third trimester, fetal viability usually can be awaited and the infant delivered by cesarean section, after which appropriate cancer therapy can be given. Page 902.

8.8 The answer is d.
Certain malignancies, notably melanoma, non-Hodgkin's lymphoma, and leukemia, are known to spread from the mother to the fetus. If the mother has any of these cancers, the

placenta should be carefully evaluated at delivery and the baby monitored for development of the disease. Page 903.

8.9 **The answer is c.**
Chemotherapy during the first trimester has been associated with fetal wastage, malformations, and low birth weight, although the incidence of fetal malformations is low and may be minimized or avoided with careful selection of agents. Maternal surgery can be safely accomplished with minimal risk to the fetus. Pelvic surgery is more easily accomplished during the second trimester. There is little risk to the fetus from short exposure to anesthetic agents after the first trimester, provided ventilation is adequate and hypotension is prevented. Low doses of radiation associated with diagnostic x-ray studies are not harmful if adequate fetal shielding is provided. Page 896.

8.10 **The answer is d.**
Only a few cancers spread from the mother to the fetus; melanoma, non-Hodgkin's lymphoma, and leukemia are the most common. Page 903.

8.11 **The answer is c.**
Appropriate shielding of the testes or ovaries or oophoropexy to position the ovaries outside the radiation field are beneficial. Studies evaluating treatment of men and women with GnRH analogs have been disappointing and inconsistent. Page 897.

8.12 **The answer is a.**
Oocyte and ovarian tissue cryopreservation remain investigational while the others are considered standards of care. Page 898.

8.13 **The answer is c.**
According to the Centers for Disease Control and Prevention, human papillomavirus (HPV) is the most common sexually transmitted disease in the US and is responsible for causing nearly all cases of cervical cancer. Page 106.

8.14 **The answer is b.**
HIV-infected women who are at greatest risk for HPV coinfection are women with CD4+ levels less than 200/μL, RNA viral load > 20,000 copies, smokers, and women of African American descent. Page 1044.

8.15 **The answer is d.**
The four HPV strains responsible for 70% of all cervical cancers are 6, 11, 16, 18. Page 1044.

8.16 **The answer is a.**
NADMs have increased because HIV-positive individuals are living longer and therefore have more time to develop cancer. Page 1035–1036.

8.17 **The answer is c.**
HIV primarily infects helper T cells, specifically CD4+ T cells. Page 1034.

8.18 **The answer is d.**
HPV is not linked to cancer of the oral cavity. Page 551.

8.19 **The answer is a.**
Vaccines against HPV are approved for prevention of cervical cancer and genital warts in females after the ages 9 to 26 and are most effective prior to sexual contact. Page 106.

8.20 **The answer is c.**
The three defining ADMs are non-Hodgkin's lymphoma, Kaposi sarcoma, and cervical cancer. The other cancers are non-AIDS-defining malignancies. Page 1035.

8.21 The answer is c.

Comorbid conditions are often ignored by physicians, and therefore survivors of cancer have significantly poorer health outcomes. Compared with matched control subjects without a cancer history, the cancer survivors were more likely not to receive recommended care for a broad range of chronic medical conditions, such as angina, congestive heart failure, erectile dysfunction, and diabetes. Investigators conclude that survivors are a vulnerable population because their history of cancer may shift attention away from important health problems unrelated to cancer. Page 882–889.

8.22 The answer is d.

All patients should be assessed because it is important to identify those who may be at high risk for sexual dysfunction. It is not the practitioner who should create a list of goals but instead help the patient discuss any problems and assist the patient to establish goals. Page 891–893.

8.23 The answer is c.

Preservation of the cavernous nerves is the most important factor related to postprostatectomy erectile function. The nerve-sparing procedure is recommended for patients with stage A or B disease who are eligible to undergo radical prostatectomy. Factors identified that promote sexual function after surgery are age less than 50, and stage of disease. In patients over 70, only 22% regain potency postoperatively, even if both neurovascular bundles are spared. Page 883.

8.24 The answer is b.

Choices a, c, and d, although all associated with sexual dysfunction resulting from gastrointestinal surgery, primarily are psychosexual and not organic issues. For all patients the removal of rectal tissue appears to be the most common denominator to organic sexual dysfunction. If the rectum remains intact, there rarely is an associated sexual dysfunction without direct tumor invasion. Page 881, 1245.

8.25 The answer is a.

Permanent damage to erectile function with loss of emission and ejaculation may occur with perineal resection or radical prostatectomy. Retrograde ejaculation is common with transurethral and transabdominal resection and erectile dysfunction with transabdominal resection. Bilateral orchiectomy causes sexual dysfunction through gradual diminution of libido, impotence, gynecomastia, and penile atrophy. Page 883.

8.26 The answer is c.

Evaluation of sexual dysfunction according to the ALARM model includes

A—Activity or sexual function
L—Libido or desire
A—Arousal and orgasm
R—Resolution or release
M—Medical data. Page 893.

8.27 The answer is d.

Radiation therapy can cause sexual and reproductive dysfunction through primary organ failure, through alterations in organ function, and through the temporary or permanent effects of therapy related to total dose, location, length of treatment, age, and prior fertility status. Androgen blockade occurs with hormonal manipulation. Page 886, 1628.

8.28 The answer is c.

Chemotherapy-induced reproductive and sexual dysfunction is related to the type of drug, dose, length of treatment, age, and sex of the individual receiving treatment and to the length of time after treatment, as well as to the use of single rather than multiple agents and drugs to combat side effects of chemotherapy. Combination chemotherapy including alkylating agents such as mechlorethamine have been shown to produce sexual dysfunction and to decrease fertility in both men and women. Androgen therapy affects sexual function in women; estrogen therapy affects sexual function in men. Chemotherapy may deplete the germinal epithelium that lines the seminiferous tubules in men. Page 887–889.

8.29 The answer is c.

Sexual dysfunction is not a normal side effect of chemotherapy. Although it is not uncommon in conjunction with breast cancer and surgery and it is more prevalent among younger women, sexual dysfunction can be treated, usually through therapy or a support group. The rest of these—ovarian failure, hot flashes, night sweats, and irregular menses—are common side effects of chemotherapy. Page 889.

8.30 The answer is d.

The traditional bilateral RPLND results in the loss of antegrade ejaculation with resultant infertility from retrograde ejaculation. The ability to experience a normal orgasm is not impaired. Page 883.

8.31 The answer is a.

Education and counseling are basic interventions for alterations in sexual health. It may be difficult for patient and family to adapt to role playing. Another problem is that patients are generally not screened for participation. Screening increases the probability of identifying patients and partners with preexisting problems that may require more intensive therapy. Page 894.

8.32 The answer is a.

Among the factors that affect a cancer patient's sexuality are those related to the biologic/physiologic process of cancer, the effects of treatment, the alterations caused by cancer and treatment, and the psychologic issues surrounding the patient and family. Physiologic problems of infertility and sterility, changes in body appearance, and the inability to have intercourse are enhanced by psychologic and psychosexual issues of alteration in body image, fears of abandonment, loss of self-esteem, alterations in sexual identity, and concerns about self. Mutagenicity and psychosexual changes are not closely related. Page 880–895.

8.33 The answer is d.

If more than the anterior third of the vaginal wall is removed, the diameter of the introitus and the vaginal barrel can be severely compromised and intercourse may be restricted. She needs instruction on vaginal dilation and to use liberal lubrication. Orgasm is not diminished. Page 882.

8.34 The answer is d.

For women receiving radiation therapy to the vagina, vaginal fibrosis and scarring with a loss of blood supply and elasticity is a major adverse effect. Frequent intercourse can minimize these effects. For patients who are not sexually active, the use of a vaginal dilator with water-soluble lubricants or prescribed estrogen cream starting 2 weeks after treatment are effective prophylactic measures to minimize functional loss. Page 1735.

8.35 The answer is d.

The new urinary diversions and neobladder have resulted in improved quality of life, decreased alterations in sexual function, and decreased odor and urine leakage. A radical cystectomy with urinary diversion, particularly if accompanied by a lymphadenectomy, can affect many aspects of sexual functioning; however, penile sensation is not altered. Erectile impotence that results after radical cystectomy may be helped by the insertion of a penile prosthesis. When the nerves crucial to the mechanisms of penile erection are spared, erectile potency has been preserved. Page 882.

CHAPTER 9

Survivorship

9.1 Demographic trends show that cancer survivors in the future will be older and more ethnically diverse. These trends include all of the following *except*

a. Older age at diagnosis
b. Increased elder population, therefore increased cancer rates
c. The US population will be 25% Hispanic by 2050.
d. African Americans, Native Americans, and Asians combined will be 25% by 2050.

9.2 Research results concerning overall survival of women with breast cancer indicate that all of the following are true *except*

a. Anastrozole is the first aromatase inhibitor to provide an overall survival benefit, compared with tamoxifen.
b. Anastrozole provides overall survival benefit for pre- and postmenopausal women.
c. Anastrozole decreases the incidence of recurrence of breast cancer by 50% in postmenopausal women treated for early breast cancer.
d. Anastrozole reduces the risk of death by nearly a third in postmenopausal women treated for early breast cancer.

9.3 Survival rates from cancer have only recently begun to improve. Which of the following *most accurately* depicts the percentage of persons surviving 10 years and beyond after diagnosis?

a. Fifty percent of adults and 60% of children survive beyond 10 years.
b. Sixty percent of adults and 77% of children survive beyond 10 years.
c. Sixty-five percent of adults and 85% of children survive beyond 10 years.
d. Sixty-five percent of adults and 75% of children survive beyond 10 years.

9.4 Your new position in a cancer clinic gives you the opportunity to counsel cancer survivors. You are aware that the adult cancer survivor's ability to achieve optimal physical, social, and psychologic function can be significantly affected by all of the following *except*

a. Socioeconomic considerations
b. Disease trajectory considerations
c. Physical function and cosmesis
d. Older age at diagnosis

9.5 The most powerful predictor of cancer survival is ____________ at diagnosis.

a. Advanced disease
b. Changes in appearance or body function
c. Comorbid physical or mental conditions
d. Access to care

9.6 Survival analysis is defined as

a. The probability that an individual will live with or without cancer for a specified period of time
b. A time interval without evidence of recurrence of disease
c. An observation of individuals with cancer and a calculation of their probability of dying over time
d. The length of time an individual with cancer survives with evidence of disease

9.7 Pruritus is a late effect that frequently accompanies jaundice in patients with obstructive biliary disease. Which of the following *best* describes the mechanism of pruritus under these circumstances?

a. Itching is primarily due to dry flaky skin.
b. Itching is caused by irritation of the cutaneous sensory nerve fibers by accumulated bile salts.
c. Itching is due to poor body hygiene and the use of deodorant soaps.
d. Itching is due to the accumulation of cholestyramine.

9.8 Sleeping disturbances can be problematic long after treatment ends. Research into the incidence of sleep disturbances indicates that sleeping difficulty is reported by approximately what percentage of patients with cancer?

a. 50%
b. 40%
c. 30%
d. 20%

9.9 Following four courses of chemotherapy, Albert shows you that his fingernails have developed transverse white lines or grooves. You explain to Albert that this symptom

a. Is a response to doxorubicin because pigmentation has been deposited at the base of the nail
b. Indicates a reduction or cessation of nail growth in response to cytotoxic therapy
c. Reflects a cytotoxic reaction to cyclophosphamide
d. Is a partial separation of the nail plate called onycholysis and is a reaction to 5-FU therapy

9.10 Because of the staging of her cancer, the size of the tumor, and a number of other factors, Marcia will undergo immediate breast reconstruction after her surgery. She is concerned about long-term effects and her body image. Her surgeon has explained that the procedure most likely to be used in her case is the TRAM flap. During your discussion of how she will look after complete healing, you explain to Marcia that this will involve removing tissue from her ____________ and tunneling it to the mastectomy site.

a. Abdominal muscle
b. Latissimus dorsi muscle
c. Lower abdomen
d. Buttocks

9.11 Depression can be a short-term or long-term effect for patients with cancer and responses to a perceived loss of self-esteem may be affective, behavioral, or cognitive. Which of the following is an example of a behavioral response associated with depression?

a. Lack of energy
b. Guilt
c. Indecisiveness
d. Suicidal ideation

9.12 The differences in incidence, mortality, and survival among various ethnic groups has been studied, and it has been determined that poverty, not race, accounts for the lower survival rate. Poverty lowers the survival rate among the many ethnic groups by

a. 5%–10%
b. 10%–15%
c. 15%–20%
d. 20%–25%

9.13 The growth of managed care and capitation have contributed to

a. A dramatic drop in coverage of prevention-oriented services
b. Driving the coverage of preventive services
c. Reduced funding for immunologic studies
d. Fewer elder care provisions

9.14 Work-related research indicates which of the following is *true*?

a. Survivors of breast, prostate, and colorectal cancer are most likely to return to work.
b. Of patients who stopped work, 78%–92% returned to work within 2 years of completion of treatment.
c. Males have more delay in returning to work than females.
d. Higher income contributes to more delay in returning to work.

9.15 Fatigue may produce anxiety or depression in some individuals with cancer. Which of the following is the *best* explanation for this effect?

a. Fatigue-induced electrolyte imbalances often trigger feelings of anxiety or depression.
b. Fatigue, anxiety, and depression have the same etiology.
c. Treatment-induced fatigue may force the individual to give up usual social roles.
d. Anxiety or depression frequently forces individuals with cancer to expend too much energy.

9.16 The primary purpose of the Health Insurance Portability and Accountability Act, or HIPAA, is to provide guidelines for which of the following?

a. Methods to provide health insurance for the uninsured
b. Measures to ensure each state honors insurance policies issued in other states within the United States
c. Methods to describe how patient documents should be written and transcribed
d. Measures to provide for electronic healthcare transactions and privacy

9.17 Which of the following does COBRA, a federal law passed in 1986, do?

a. It offers extended medical coverage to those who leave jobs.
b. It provides low-cost insurance to cancer survivors and other high-risk individuals.
c. It provides free group health insurance to individuals not otherwise covered by medical plans.
d. It prohibits employment discrimination against cancer survivors.

9.18 The National Coalition for Cancer Survivorship (NCCS) provides all of the following *except*

a. It provides referral to local support services for patients and families.
b. It addresses barriers to employment and access to health insurance.
c. It advocates for changes in healthcare delivery.
d. It offers assistance with transportation and medications.

9.19 Which of the following statements about employment among cancer survivors is *correct*?

a. Approximately 40% of cancer patients return to work after being diagnosed.
b. The work performance of cancer survivors differs little from others hired at the same age for similar assignments.
c. "Job-lock" refers to the situation in which cancer survivors are reluctant to accept new jobs that might involve increased responsibilities.
d. Most federal and state laws specifically include cancer survivors among the "handicapped or disabled."

9.20 Individuals with low annual incomes

a. Are three to seven times more likely to die of cancer than those with high annual incomes
b. Rarely experience a definable difference in survivorship or treatment outcome based solely on their economic status
c. Are twice as likely to experience recurrence, treatment failure, or death as those with higher annual incomes
d. Have the same survival rates as those with moderate incomes

9.21 Research indicates that sleep deprivation following insomnia is associated with which of the following?

a. Alterations in immune and neuroendocrine function
b. Increase in attention deficit disorder
c. Rebound hypersomnia
d. No change in cognitive function

9.22 Which of the following is *not* considered to be a predisposing factor associated with sleep disturbance in patients with cancer?

a. Female gender
b. Age
c. A diagnosis of lung cancer
d. A family history of sleep disorder

9.23 Which of the following is *least likely* to be a cause of anemia in patients with cancer?

a. Decreased red cell production
b. Iron deficiency
c. The primary disease process
d. Radiation therapy

9.24 The *most important* role of the nurse in home parenteral nutrition (HPN) is to

a. Keep records of times of infusion, intake, and output.
b. Deliver all supplies, equipment, and medicines to the patient.
c. Evaluate the patient, the home environment, and the family's ability to manage HPN.
d. Perform all infusion regimens at home.

9.25 Total parenteral nutrition for prolonged periods or at home is indicated in all *except* which of the following situations?

a. As a treatment for cancer cachexia
b. Where enteral feedings are not feasible
c. For patients with enterocutaneous fistulas
d. For patients with acute radiation enteritis

9.26 According to research, the ability to conceive or father a child after stem cell transplantation is *most likely* to be related to which of the following?

a. Initial treatment for the cancer
b. Whether or not total body irradiation is used
c. The use of colony-stimulating factors
d. The presence of graft-vs-host disease

9.27 Your patient, Melissa, is beginning her treatment for osteogenic sarcoma and is concerned that the chemotherapy and radiation therapy might cause congenital abnormalities in her future offspring. An appropriate response would include which of the following?

a. Explain that she should be thinking about her own situation instead of dwelling on what might never be.
b. Explain that this is a legitimate concern, and reassure her that research has found no higher incidence of congenital malformation in the children born of women who have had treatment for cancer than in the general population.
c. Explain that it is difficult to answer her question because there is a much higher incidence of miscarriage in women who have been treated for cancer.
d. Explain that you understand how she feels, and refer her for genetic counseling.

9.28 The late effects of cancer treatment on the endocrine system result from damage to the hypothalamus pituitary axis and/or to

a. Target organs (e.g., the thyroid, ovaries, testis)
b. The cortical areas of the brain
c. The chemical structure of key hormones (e.g., insulin)
d. Epithelial tissue (e.g., blood vessel linings)

9.29 Growth impairment as a late effect of treatment for cancer occurs as the result of

a. Overproduction of thyroxine by the thyroid gland
b. Deficient growth hormone release by the hypothalamus
c. Primary hypothyroidism
d. A disruption in pituitary control of several target organs

9.30 Research indicates that when compared to women who have no history of cancer, women who have completed their chemotherapy more than a year before participating in the study report which of the following concerning the symptom of fatigue and quality of life?

a. Worse menopausal symptoms and poorer quality of sleep
b. Excessive weight gain and lack of energy
c. Increased psychosomatic complaints and depression
d. Moderate to severe fatigue that is cumulative over time

9.31 According to a national survey, which of the following *best describes* the oncologist's view of fatigue?

a. Fatigue is a result of chronic illness.
b. Fatigue is a sensation of tiredness.
c. Fatigue is a symptom of cancer.
d. Fatigue is a result of cancer treatment.

9.32 A patient who has finished treatment 6 months ago and is considered cured returns for a follow-up appointment. His major complaint is that he is distressed because he continues to experience symptoms related to his treatment, such as fatigue and difficulty sleeping. Your response is based on which of the following concerning psychosocial late effects in cancer survivors?

a. The persistence of late and long-term physiologic symptoms often contributes to psychologic distress.
b. Fatigue is not normal, and he should be evaluated for possible recurrence of cancer.
c. Depression is common regardless of the presence of comorbid conditions.
d. Quality of life before diagnosis is unrelated to quality of life after cancer treatment.

9.33 Several years ago a patient was given concomitant radiation therapy and chemotherapy for cancer of the bladder. Recently, she developed cystitis. If this condition is a late effect of her cancer treatment, which agent is *least likely* to have been the responsible one involved?

a. Cyclophosphamide
b. Ifosfamide
c. Methotrexate
d. Cisplatin

9.34 Patients with HIV and neutropenia who have received treatment with corticosteroids or who have had prolonged immunosuppression should be monitored for which of the following?

a. Tuberculosis
b. Second malignancies
c. *Pneumocystis carinii* pneumonia
d. Elevated CD4 lymphocyte count

9.35 Late effects involving the central nervous system are *most likely* to occur in which of the following individuals?

a. A child treated for Hodgkin's disease
b. A child treated for bone sarcoma
c. An adult treated for small cell carcinoma of the lung
d. An adult treated for primary hypothyroidism

9.36 Which of the following statements about the late effects of cancer treatment is *incorrect*?

a. Late effects are believed to progress over time.
b. Late effects are believed to involve different mechanisms than those of the acute side effects of chemotherapy and radiation.
c. Late effects are severe and clinically subtle.
d. Late effects are the consequence of biologic cure.

9.37 As a nurse, you know that all of the following are part of your caregiving role *except*
a. Determining the meaning of your patient's pain
b. Deriving nursing diagnoses
c. Ensuring patient compliance
d. Assisting in selecting interventions

9.38 Adjuvant therapy with aromatase inhibitors (AIs) such as letrozole or anastrozole is known to provide a survival benefit for women with breast cancer. A troubling side effect of this therapy and one under investigation includes which of the following?
a. Increased incidence of second malignancy
b. Progressive gastrointestinal irritation
c. Significant bone loss
d. Increased risk of renal insufficiency

9.39 Which of the following agents is *least likely* to result in loss of bone mineral density?
a. Leuprolide
b. Tamoxifen
c. Anastrozole
d. Cyclophosphamide

9.40 Which of the following preventive behaviors is recommended to prevent osteonecrosis of the jaw (ONJ) associated with intravenous or oral bisphosphonate therapy?
a. Steroid therapy
b. Antibiotic flushes
c. Avoid invasive dental procedures.
d. Topical anesthetics

9.41 While teaching your 41-year-old female patient about the side effects of high-dose chemotherapy she asks you about the possibility that she may become menopausal. Your discussion is based on which of the following research findings regarding risk of menopause as it relates to high-dose chemotherapy?
a. Because the treatment is dose dense, lasting only 9 weeks, she is not likely to experience permanent menopause.
b. High-dose chemotherapy is associated with a high rate (90%) of ovarian failure.
c. She has a 55% risk of permanent menopause.
d. Data are not available to address this issue with certainty.

9.42 Your 36-year-old patient with testes cancer is completing a course of curative chemotherapy and begins to inquire about his ability to father children and whether or not they might have a higher risk of birth defects as a result of his treatment. Your *most appropriate* response would include which of the following?
a. Men with azoospermia immediately after chemotherapy will not recover a sperm count.
b. Chromosomal abnormalities have been observed in survivors and could result in miscarriages or still births, so he should not pursue fathering a child.
c. It is recommended that men wait at least 6 months after the end of cancer treatment before attempting to conceive children.
d. It is recommended that men wait at least 2 years after the end of cancer treatment before attempting to conceive children because most recurrences occur in that time period.

9.43 Your patient has prostate cancer and is undergoing leuprolide therapy. He recently began to complain of pain in his hip. He underwent a bone scan and was found to have an isolated lesion that was thought to be malignant. Biopsy was done, and a sarcoma was confirmed. This finding represents which of the following?

a. This is most likely a metastases from his prostate cancer.
b. This is histologically dissimilar from a prostate cancer and is therefore considered to be a second primary cancer and potentially curable.
c. This is most likely a benign condition because he is receiving treatment for cancer.
d. This finding represents a guarded prognosis because his immune system obviously is failing.

9.44 Mr. Svensen has had treatment for a primary kidney tumor, which was completely eradicated. Now, however, the surgeon discovers a biopsy-proven metastatic lesion in the lung. The metastatic site seems to be solitary, and Mr. Svensen is very healthy otherwise. Given these limited clues, what method of treatment will be used for his metastatic lesion?

a. Chemotherapy to provide systemic control of metastasis
b. Cytoreductive surgery to reduce the mass so combination therapy will be effective
c. Combination radiation and chemotherapy
d. Surgical resection

9.45 The *most common* second malignant neoplasms following radiation therapy are

a. Breast carcinomas and gynecologic tumors
b. Cancers of the gastrointestinal tract
c. Sarcomas of the bone and soft tissue
d. Tumors of the bladder and lung

9.46 Your patient is a 5-year survivor of Hodgkin's disease. Your annual workup is conducted with the knowledge that she is most at risk for developing which of the following second primary cancers?

a. Breast cancer
b. Leukemia
c. Lung cancer
d. Non-Hodgkin's lymphoma

9.47 Mr. Allen, a heavy smoker for 20 years, has lung cancer and has completed his radiation and chemotherapy. He is instructed to return for checkups frequently because he is also at risk for which cancer?

a. Bladder cancer
b. Melanoma
c. Sarcoma
d. Leukemia

9.48 Judith had Hodgkin's disease as a child and received mantle radiation therapy. It has been more than 20 years since her treatment. Which of the following statements is *not* correct concerning her follow-up care?

a. She needs to continue her annual physical exams and mammograms because she is most at risk for second malignancies at this time.
b. She can relax more because her risk for second malignancies decreases every year.
c. Her highest risk for second malignancies is breast cancer and lung cancer.
d. Second malignancies are most likely to occur in the field of radiation.

9.49 The risk of developing a second malignant neoplasm after treatment for a primary malignancy depends on several factors, including all of the following *except*

a. The type and dose of treatment received (e.g., radiation and alkylating agents)
b. A common underlying etiologic factor (e.g., smoking)
c. Genetic susceptibility (e.g., genetic retinoblastoma)
d. The timing of withdrawal of chemotherapeutic agents (e.g., MOPP latency)

9.50 Four years ago Ms. Smith successfully completed treatment for breast cancer. Now she is diagnosed with acute myelogenous leukemia (AML). Which is *most likely* to have contributed to Ms. Smith's AML?

a. Alkylating agents
b. Anthracyclines
c. Vinca alkaloids
d. Antimetabolites

9.51 Mantle radiation for Hodgkin's disease is associated with an increased risk of which of the following cancers?

a. Breast cancer, especially in those irradiated before the age of 30
b. Lung cancer
c. Liver cancer
d. Head and neck cancer

9.52 Mrs. Howe is undergoing adjuvant therapy for breast cancer and asks you if it is a good idea for her to exercise while she is taking chemotherapy. Which would be the *most appropriate* response?

a. Exercise can intensify her feelings of nausea, and she should avoid exercise for 3–4 days following her treatment.
b. Research shows that exercise following meals relieves heartburn and is a good idea.
c. Aerobic exercise is especially effective in relieving fatigue and is highly recommended for women undergoing adjuvant chemotherapy for breast cancer.
d. Exercise can lead to dizziness, and she should consult with her doctor before engaging in any form of exercise.

9.53 All of the following are considered an accepted means of communication for the person who has undergone a laryngectomy *except*

a. Pneumatic larynx
b. Pocket communicator
c. Esophageal speech
d. Tracheoesophageal prosthesis

9.54 Six months after his surgery Mr. Fox, after participating in extensive speech rehabilitation, learns to speak by diverting exhaled pulmonary air through a surgically constructed fistula tract directly into the esophagus. This method of speech is produced through

a. An artificial larynx made available immediately after surgery
b. Esophageal speech therapy
c. Surgical voice restoration or tracheoesophageal prosthesis
d. An oral prosthesis

9.55 After surgery, part of Ms. Eliot's rehabilitation process involves restoring the swallowing function because aspiration during swallowing is one of the major complications following supraglottic laryngectomy. Initially, ____________ will be the most difficult thing for Ms. Eliot to swallow without aspirating.

a. Soft mashed foods
b. Dry crunchy foods
c. Liquids
d. Hard bulky food boluses (especially meats)

9.56 A program that regards rehabilitation in cancer care as a dynamic rather than a passive process is *most likely* to emphasize both ongoing reassessment and

a. Customary convalescence
b. A hospital or community base
c. Redefinition of goals
d. Frequent nursing referrals

9.57 The overall goal of rehabilitation for the person with cancer is to

a. Return to baseline performance before the cancer
b. Anticipate and prepare physically for future debilitating effects of cancer
c. Achieve optimal functioning within the limits of cancer
d. Maintain an active busy life

9.58 Which of the following factors have been found to be *most closely* related to the rehabilitation needs of the patient with cancer?

a. Medical and family history
b. Type of treatment and side effects experienced
c. Cancer site and stage of disease
d. Severity or duration of disease

ANSWER RATIONALES

Please note: All page numbers referenced in the Answer Rationales sections refer to the textbook *Cancer Nursing: Principles and Practice, Seventh Edition,* by Connie Henke Yarbro, Debra Wujcik, and Barbara Holmes Gobel (Jones & Bartlett Learning, © 2011).

9.1 The answer is c.
Demographic trends of the future include a population that is older at the time of diagnosis, and because there will be more elders, the cancer rates will be increased. By 2050 the US population will be 35% Hispanic and 25% combined African American, Native American, and Asian. Page 1744.

9.2 The answer is b.
For the first time an aromatase inhibitor has shown a survival advantage over tamoxifen in early stage breast cancer for postmenopausal women. By replacing tamoxifen with anastrozole, postmenopausal women treated for early breast cancer reduce the likelihood of their disease returning by almost half and, more importantly, reduce their risk of dying by nearly a third. Page 1098, 1128.

9.3 The answer is d.
The population of cancer survivors is increasing, with 65% of adults and 75% of children surviving now beyond 10 years after their diagnosis. Fourteen percent of all survivors alive today were diagnosed more than 20 years ago. Of the 24,040 households in the 1992 National Health Interview Survey, 63% of the respondents had a cancer diagnosis more than 5 years previous and 10% had a cancer diagnosis more than 25 years previous. Page 1744.

9.4 The answer is d.
Four main considerations affect the adult cancer survivor's ability to achieve optimal physical, social, and psychological function: developmental considerations, disease trajectory considerations, physical function and cosmesis, and socioeconomic considerations. Page 1749.

9.5 The answer is a.
Advanced disease at diagnosis is the most powerful predictor of cancer survival. Page 1744.

9.6 The answer is c.
The observation over time of individuals with cancer and the calculation of their probability of dying over several time periods is called survival analysis. Page 1744.

9.7 The answer is b.
Pruritus, which frequently accompanies jaundice, is precipitated by irritation of the cutaneous sensory nerve fibers by accumulated bile salts. The use of deodorant soaps should be avoided because they tend to dry skin and intensify pruritus. Page 1330–1331.

9.8 The answer is a.
An estimated 50% of patients with cancer report significant distress related to sleep disturbances. Page 674.

9.9 The answer is b.
Beau's lines indicate a reduction in or cessation of nail growth in response to cytotoxic therapy. Page 146.

9.10 The answer is a.
The TRAM flap procedure is sometimes known as the "tummy tuck" because the muscle and fat are tunneled from the abdominal muscle to the mastectomy site. Page 237.

9.11 **The answer is a.**
Choice *b* is an affective response; other affective responses include worthlessness, hopelessness, and sadness. Choices *c* and *d* are cognitive responses; another cognitive response is a decreased ability to concentrate. Other behavioral responses include change in appetite, sleep disturbances, withdrawal, and dependency. 1945–1946.

9.12 **The answer is b.**
In the late 1970s the question of the role of poverty in the differences in incidence, mortality, and survival of different ethnic groups was first raised. The disproportionate number of African Americans in the lower socioeconomic strata accounted for the increased incidence. However, one study concluded that poverty, not race, accounted for the 10–15% lower survival rate from cancer in many ethnic groups. Page 87–88.

9.13 **The answer is b.**
Historically in the United States, cancer prevention services have not been reimbursed by payers at all levels. The growth of managed care and capitation and the increasing use of primary healthcare providers as gatekeepers are driving the coverage of preventive services. Quality control efforts by health plans carefully monitor whether patients receive necessary preventive services. However, funding for preventive services remains inadequate, even in prepaid health systems. Page 110.

9.14 **The answer is b.**
Research shows that 78%–92% of patients who stopped work during cancer treatment returned to work within 2 years of treatment completion. The most work-related research has been done with survivors of breast, prostate, and colorectal cancers, but there is no work-related research comparing patients with different cancer diagnoses. Delay in returning to work has been associated with age, low income, being female, African American, partnered, lower educational level, and receiving chemotherapy among others. Page 1751.

9.15 **The answer is c.**
Anxiety and depression can result from the disruption in lifestyle produced by fatigue. This may occur when fatigue experienced as a side effect of cancer treatment forces the individual to give up usual social roles or makes it impossible to reach desired goals. Page 772–776.

9.16 **The answer is d.**
HIPAA mandates security and privacy regulations for electronic health information. Page 1877.

9.17 **The answer is a.**
Under COBRA, group medical coverage is ensured to those whose circumstances warrant reducing or changing work hours or leaving the job. The employee is eligible for extended benefits for up to 18 months, and spouse and dependents receive these benefits for 36 months. Page 1751.

9.18 **The answer is d.**
The NCCS focuses on a wide range of issues related to quality of life for cancer survivors and their families but does not provide direct assistance with medications or transportation. Page 1751.

9.19 **The answer is b.**
Up to 80% of cancer patients return to work after being diagnosed, and their performance differs little, if any, from others hired for similar assignments. "Job-lock" refers to survivors' fear of losing medical coverage if they changed jobs. Only a few states explicitly protect those with a history of cancer. Page 1751.

9.20 The answer is a.
Individuals with low annual incomes are three to seven times more likely to die of cancer than those with high annual incomes. Page 87–88.

9.21 The answer is a.
In both laboratory and natural settings, sleep deprivation after insomnia has been associated with a decline in cognitive function, inability to engage in work or recreational activities, loss of hedonic capacity, a sharp decline in quality of life, and alterations to immune and neuroendocrine function. Page 674.

9.22 The answer is c.
Lung cancer patients are at least twice as likely to have insomnia compared to others with cancer. In the general population female gender increases the risk of insomnia twofold, and this is true in the cancer population as well. Sleep disturbance also increases with age. As with psychiatric disorders, those with a family or personal history of sleep disturbance are more vulnerable to the onset of sleep difficulties. Page 674.

9.23 The answer is b.
The causes of anemia frequently seen in patients with cancer include decreased red cell production secondary to myelosuppressive therapy (e.g., chemotherapy and radiation therapy) and the primary disease process. Page 465–466.

9.24 The answer is c.
Home care assessment for HPN begins with a visit coincidental with the arrival of equipment. The nurse should review orders for HPN with the supplying agency. The assessment should include the type and status of the venous access device, the patient's and family's knowledge of the management of HPN, and an evaluation of the home for safety factors. Adequate refrigeration should be available in the home for a 2- to 3-week supply of solutions. An electric infusion pump with a battery backup is normally part of the equipment. Choices *a* and eventually *d* are handled by the family; *b* is done by the home infusion therapy company personnel. Page 470.

9.25 The answer is a.
Total parenteral nutrition for prolonged periods or home total parenteral nutrition is indicated only in situations in which enteral feeding is not feasible because of advanced disease or severe toxicities of cancer therapies. Patients with enterocutaneous fistulas are not able to use the enteral route for nutrition because oral intake stimulates fistula output and can lead to metabolic and electrolyte disturbances. Page 838–839.

9.26 The answer is b.
The ability to conceive or father a child after stem cell transplantation is related to age and treatment with total body irradiation. Page 895.

9.27 The answer is b.
A review of the findings from 18 studies that included almost 1600 children born to 1078 mothers or fathers who had previously been treated for cancer indicated no increase in fetal wastage or in congenital defects noted in the offspring when compared to the general population. Page 895.

9.28 The answer is a.
The target organs most commonly affected are the thyroid, ovaries, and testes. Late effects can include alterations in metabolism, growth, secondary sexual characteristics, and reproduction. Page 1759.

9.29 The answer is b.

High doses of radiation to the hypothalamic pituitary axis can damage the hypothalamus and disrupt the production of growth hormone. Growth hormone deficiency with short stature is one of the most common long-term endocrine consequences of radiation to the central nervous system in children. Page 1759.

9.30 The answer is a.

Women who received chemotherapy reported low to moderate fatigue (a year posttreatment) that was significantly related to other symptoms, including poorer sleep quality and more menopausal symptoms. Page 774.

9.31 The answer is c.

The most commonly used definition of fatigue states that it is a sensation of tiredness and is a self-perceived state. The causes of fatigue are multifocal, but most studies address fatigue as a side effect of cancer treatment. This contrasts a national survey of oncologists, who reported that fatigue is a symptom of cancer rather than a side effect of treatment. If fatigue is a symptom, then cancer therapy should decrease the patient's fatigue instead of increasing it. Page 774.

9.32 The answer is a.

Fatigue is normal for many months following treatment and often occurs with other symptoms. Depression occurs most commonly when symptoms persist, lending to uncertainty in illness and fear of recurrence. The better the quality of life before diagnosis, the better the patient tolerates treatment and recovery. Page 756, 762–763.

9.33 The answer is c.

Nephritis and cystitis are the major long-term renal toxicities that result from cancer treatment. Damage to the nephrons and bladder has been documented in patients treated with cyclophosphamide, ifosfamide, and cisplatin. Page 496–498.

9.34 The answer is c.

Patients with HIV and neutropenia, who have had prolonged treatment with corticosteroids, or who have had prolonged immunosuppression should be assessed for the development of *Pneumocystis carinii*. Because symptoms are insidious, a prolonged fever that is unresponsive to antibiotics and associated with a nonproductive cough and dyspnea on exertion may indicate infection. Page 515.

9.35 The answer is c.

The late effects of central nervous system treatment, including neuropsychological, neuroanatomic, and neurophysiologic changes, have been observed most commonly in children with acute lymphoblastic leukemia and brain tumors and in small cell carcinoma of adult lung patients, all of whom received central nervous system treatment for the primary tumor or as prophylaxis against meningeal disease. Page 1768–1769.

9.36 The answer is c.

The late effects of treatment for biologic cure result from physiologic changes related to particular treatments or to the interactions among the treatment, the individual, and the disease. Unlike the acute side effects of chemotherapy and radiation, however, late effects are believed to progress over time and by different mechanisms. They can appear months to years after treatment; can be mild, severe, or life threatening; and can be clinically obvious, clinically subtle, or subclinical. Their impact appears to depend on the age and development stage of the patient. Page 1756, 1762.

9.37 The answer is c.
Choices *a*, *b*, and *d* are part of the nursing role as defined by the Oncology Nursing Society, as well as describing pain, identifying aggravating and relieving factors, determining individuals' definitions of optimal pain relief, and evaluating efficacy of interventions. Page 1852–1853.

9.38 The answer is c.
The large anastrozole, tamoxifen alone, or in combination study, known as the ATAC study, compared anastrozole, tamoxifen, and the combination of both drugs as first-line adjuvant therapy in over 9000 women. There was a significantly higher incidence of fracture with anastrozole compared with tamoxifen. Bone density in AI-treated patients was lower at 1 year relative to baseline and was further decreased after the second year. The lower bone marrow density at longer follow-up suggest that AI-associated bone loss may be progressive over time. Page 1126–1127.

9.39 The answer is b.
One of the most beneficial aspects of tamoxifen therapy is that it has bone-protective effects. This was demonstrated in the ATAC trial, where there was less evidence of fractures in the tamoxifen-only group. Page 1126–1127.

9.40 The answer is c.
Mouth rinses and antibiotics may be used to treat ONJ, but there is no evidence it helps to prevent it. Steroids are contraindicated in patients at risk for ONJ. Patients who need invasive dental work should have it done well in advance of beginning bisphosphonate therapy, and they should be well aware of the risk associated with this treatment. Page 956.

9.41 The answer is b.
Women older than 40 who develop amenorrhea have the highest risk of experiencing an abrupt permanent menopause. In contrast to standard-dose chemotherapy, high-dose chemotherapy is associated with a high rate of ovarian failure (90%), even in young women. It is the nurse's responsibility to inform patients regarding their risks associated with reproductive and hormonal sequelae of chemotherapy. Page 895–899.

9.42 The answer is c.
The effect of cancer treatment on sperm counts may be temporary or permanent. Some men with azoospermia immediately after cancer treatment eventually recover sperm counts sufficient to conceive children. Studies comparing the offspring of survivors with the offspring of survivors' siblings have demonstrated no increased risk of birth defects among the children of survivors. Because of the uncertainty about treatment-related chromosomal damage, men should wait at least 6 months after the end of cancer treatment before attempting to conceive or to harvest sperm for assisted reproduction. Page 895–899.

9.43 The answer is b.
A second primary lesion refers to an additional histologically separate malignant neoplasm in the same patient. A general rule is always to biopsy the first recurrence, because it may represent a new, curable, or treatable malignancy. Page 1770–1771.

9.44 The answer is d.
Surgery may be used to resect a metastatic lesion if the primary tumor is believed to be eradicated, if the metastatic site is solitary, and if the patient can undergo surgery without significant morbidity. Page 1441.

9.45 The answer is c.

Sarcomas of the bone and soft tissue are the most common second malignant neoplasms following radiation therapy, with the incidence peaking at 15–20 years following radiation. In a large study of survivors of childhood cancer, the risk of bone cancer was highest among children treated for retinoblastoma and Ewing's sarcoma, but also increased significantly in patients treated for rhabdomyosarcoma, Wilms' tumor, and Hodgkin's disease. In addition to sarcomas and leukemia, a variety of solid tumors have been linked to treatment with radiation, including carcinomas of the breast and tumors of the bladder, rectum, and uterus. Page 347–348.

9.46 The answer is b.

In patients with Hodgkin's disease, there is a 77-fold increased risk of the development of leukemia within 4 years of initial treatment. Page 1770.

9.47 The answer is a.

Patients with lung cancer are at greater risk for the development of bladder cancer because both tumors are associated with smoking. Page 1770.

9.48 The answer is b.

In a study of survivors of Hodgkin's disease, a 17% cumulative risk of second cancers was noted 20 years posttreatment. The most common tumors were lung and breast cancers, with 77% of the tumors occurring in or adjoining the field of radiation. Page 1770.

9.49 The answer is d.

Adults and children who have received chemotherapy or radiation therapy, or both, for a primary malignancy are at increased risk for the development of a second malignant neoplasm. Alkylating agents and ionizing radiation are the treatments most closely linked to a second malignant neoplasm. In addition to the type and dose of treatment received, the risk of the development of a secondary cancer depends on several predisposing factors, including choices *b* and *c*. Page 1767–1770.

9.50 The answer is a.

Alkylating agents have a demonstrated causative relationship to acute myelogenous leukemia (AML). AML is the most frequently reported second cancer following aggressive chemotherapy for Hodgkin's disease, non-Hodgkin's lymphoma, multiple myeloma, ovarian cancer, and breast cancer. Page 1770.

9.51 The answer is a.

The risk of breast cancer correlates with increased radiation dosage, especially if a woman is exposed to radiation in the period of young adulthood. Page 347–348.

9.52 The answer is c.

Research involving women receiving adjuvant chemotherapy for breast cancer indicates that exercise may relieve fatigue. Patients who participated in a supervised aerobic interval training exercise program showed an improvement in fatigue measured as a component of mood, nausea, and functional capacity. Page 781–782.

9.53 The answer is b.

Many patients may ultimately use all three speech methods at different times in the rehabilitation period: artificial larynx immediately after surgery; esophageal voice therapy a month or so after surgery; and, after a few months, surgical voice restoration or tracheoesophageal prosthesis. Pocket communicators are used to make intelligible speech clear. Page 1355.

9.54 The answer is c.
Tracheoesophageal prosthesis enables the patient to divert exhaled pulmonary air through a surgically constructed fistula tract directly into the esophagus. Page 1355.

9.55 The answer is c.
Liquids are the most difficult thing for the patient to swallow without aspirating. Page 1354–1355.

9.56 The answer is c.
The success of any cancer survival program depends on the commitment of the healthcare team to provide ongoing evaluation and planning for change in the lives of survivors. Under such a dynamic program, preventive and restorative goal setting become critical to a long-term survivorship trajectory that is characterized by minimal debilitation and a wellness orientation. Particular attention is also paid to the ongoing and long-range implications of financial burden imposed by cancer. Page 1770–1771.

9.57 The answer is c.
Rehabilitation refers to the process by which individuals, within their environments, are assisted to achieve optimal functioning within the limits imposed by cancer. The goals are to improve the quality of life for those experiencing cancer and to help the individual regain wholeness. Page 1770–1771.

9.58 The answer is d.
Severity or duration of disease is the factor most closely related to the cancer patient's rehabilitation needs. The physical needs frequently occurring with a variety of cancers include general weakness, limited activities of daily living, and issues related to limited morbidity. Page 1770–1771.

CHAPTER 10

End-of-Life Care

10.1 Which of the following grief reactions of an elderly woman who has lost her husband of 40 years to lung cancer would prompt the hospice nurse to suggest counseling?

a. She takes out 40 years' worth of photograph albums and wants to review her marriage and life with her deceased husband with the hospice nurse.
b. She refuses to let her sister and brother-in-law into her home anymore, blaming them for buying her husband cigarettes "all those years."
c. She plans her husband's funeral by herself, listens to all his favorite classical music pieces, and chooses passages from his Bible.
d. She delegates all the responsibility for the funeral and disposition of her husband's belongings to the children.

10.2 While describing her sadness about her husband's imminent death, the wife of your patient says, "I have never been able to accept the death of our son, and now my husband is going too." Which of the following is the *most appropriate* response?

a. "Do you feel your husband is dying soon?"
b. "What was it like for you and your husband when your son died?"
c. "Losing your son and your husband must be so difficult for you."
d. "At least your son and your husband will be together soon."

10.3 One year after the death of her husband, Mrs. Ely still cries, has difficulty concentrating, avoids activities, and rarely goes out with friends. As part of bereavement counseling, you conclude which of the following?

a. This is a normal grief reaction. She could benefit from being seen more often.
b. This is an example of a post-traumatic stress disorder.
c. Acute grief can last beyond a year, but Mrs. Ely could benefit from a support group.
d. Grieving beyond a year is often associated with unresolved guilt about the death of a loved one.

10.4 Which of the instruments below was developed specifically for eliciting information from family members about the patient's end of life?

a. McGill Quality of Life Questionnaire
b. Hospice Quality of Life Index
c. Missoula-Vitas Quality of Life Index
d. Quality of Dying and Death Questionnaire

10.5 A potential reaction of an adolescent whose parent is terminally ill is to

a. Blame the healthy parent and/or other family members for the parent's illness
b. Exhibit signs of anxiety and depression
c. Shield siblings from discussing distressing feelings
d. Openly share information and feelings with the healthy parent and other family members

10.6 As you plan your interventions for assisting a family member who is grieving because a loved one is dying, you consider all of the following approaches *except*

a. Encourage the family member to obtain support from others and shelter their feelings from the patient, which help relieve their stress.
b. Encourage the family member to be optimistic and focus on meaningful activities with the loved one.
c. Facilitate communication between the patient and family throughout the illness process.
d. Encourage the family member to obtain support from others.

10.7 Research has identified seven categories of spiritual needs of patients with cancer. The category that was *least important* was

a. Being positive
b. Finding meaning and purpose
c. Preparing for death
d. Loving others and relating to God

10.8 Research has uncovered a number of barriers to successful palliative care by healthcare professionals. These barriers include all of the following *except*

a. Lack of cultural awareness and sensitivity
b. Delays in referral to hospice services
c. Inadequate knowledge related to palliative care
d. Lack of palliative care resources

10.9 Four levels of hospice care exist based on Medicare Hospice Regulations. Which of the four levels of care below include funding by Medicare?

a. Routine home care, day care, inpatient care, and respite care
b. Continuous home care, routine home care, residential care, and extended caregiver services
c. Inpatient care, routine home care, day care, and residential care
d. Routine home care, continuous home care, respite care, and inpatient care

10.10 The establishment of a Medicare hospice benefit has placed the following regulations on hospice care *except*

a. An expected prognosis of 6 months or less
b. Primary caregiver be present in the home
c. Patient's decision to choose hospice care rather than curative care
d. Enrollment in an accredited Medicare hospice program

10.11 In some settings, inpatient palliative care is provided by consultation from a palliative care team. There are limitations to this model and include all of the following *except*

a. Absence of specially trained staff providing around-the-clock care
b. Little or no room for multiple family members to participate in care
c. A financial loss with the use of a hospital palliative care consultation service
d. Condition of roommates may prohibit flexibility in established visiting hours

10.12 Nurses may use all of the following to justify needed resources *except*

a. Feasibility studies
b. Cost-avoidance initiatives
c. Standards of quality care
d. Cost-effectiveness analyses

10.13 Along with the quantity and quality of care provided by alternative care settings, the other *important* factor that influences the selection of a care setting for the patient with cancer is

a. Its proximity to the acute care hospital
b. Its cost and the patient's financial resources
c. The professional training of its medical staff
d. Its policies relating to the multidisciplinary team approach

10.14 The Study to Understand Prognoses and Preferences for Outcomes and Risks of Treatments (SUPPORT) identified problems in end-of-life care for hospitalized patients. The shortcomings reported include all of the following *except*

a. Fifty percent of patients experienced moderate to severe pain.
b. Only 47% of physicians knew that their patients did not want cardiopulmonary resuscitation.
c. Approximately 46% of do-not-resuscitate orders were written within 2 days of death.
d. Intensive care unit stays were minimal.

10.15 Although it is true that oncology nurses hold diverse perspectives about controversial issues such as physician-assisted suicide and active euthanasia, nurses' attitudes regarding end-of-life decisions are *most significantly* influenced by which of the following?

a. Professional integrity
b. Sanctity of life
c. Personal religiosity
d. Patient autonomy

10.16 Which is preferable: the durable power of attorney or the living will, and why?

a. The living will is preferable because it prevents more suffering.
b. The durable power of attorney is preferable because it covers only terminal situations.
c. The durable power of attorney covers not only decisions in a terminal situation, but also any treatment decisions, and therefore is preferable.
d. The living will is better because healthcare providers are concerned about the ethical issues in active direct euthanasia.

10.17 The Patient Self-Determination Act provides for which of the following?

a. The patient has a right to request euthanasia, provided it is in writing.
b. The physician must by law inform patients of their right to determine the manner in which they will die.
c. On admission to the hospital, all healthcare institutions receiving Medicare or Medicaid reimbursement must ask patients whether they have an advance directive.
d. No patient admitted to a hospital that receives Medicare or Medicaid reimbursement may be denied terminal care at that institution.

10.18 According to the revised and broadened definition of palliative care from the World Health Organization the goal is to promote integration of palliative care earlier in the course of illness. As a result of this effort, which of the following *might* also occur?

a. Patients would enter hospice later rather than earlier.
b. Patients would feel less abandonment from their caregivers.
c. Reimbursement for palliative care could be captured under traditional and existing reimbursement coding.
d. Continuity of care could suffer.

10.19 Which of the following *most accurately* describes the philosophy of hospice care?

a. Patients can be made comfortable with alternative and complementary care.
b. Euthanasia is an integral aspect of care if the patient requests it.
c. Hospice care is an interdisciplinary model of caring for individuals in the final stages of an illness.
d. Hospice is specialized care for the dying that is nonphysician-based care.

10.20 Research has demonstrated that when confronted with a life-threatening illness, spirituality helps patients to accomplish which of the following before dying?

a. Define the role of religion in their lives.
b. Find a sense of meaning despite the illness.
c. Find trust in their caregivers.
d. Confirm their belief in a higher power.

10.21 Which of the following statements concerning advanced directives (AD) is *false*?

a. An AD is a legally binding contract.
b. An AD is a statement that provides very specific instructions regarding the medical care than an individual would want to receive if unable to express his or her wishes at a future date.
c. ADs may be either written or verbal and can include documents such as a living will.
d. A directive may not always be honored due to the inability of medicine to determine the terminality of the patient's condition.

10.22 When a patient at the end of life complains of dyspnea, the nurse should *most appropriately* focus on which of the following?

a. Determine degree of dyspnea by assessing arterial blood gases and pulmonary function tests.
b. Monitor pulse oximetry to determine need for oxygen.
c. Administer opioids to lessen the sensation of breathlessness.
d. Administer bronchodilators as needed.

10.23 Delirium is common in the final days of life. Which of the following nursing interventions would be counterproductive in the management of delirium?

a. Concentrate on orienting the individual to what is real and what is not.
b. Administer low-dose haloperidol to decrease anxiety.
c. Discontinue benzodiazepines because they can worsen delirium.
d. Encourage the individual to speak about a loved one that has died.

10.24 As your patient nears death, his daughter is distressed and believes he is suffering because he is unable to drink fluids. She insists you give him intravenous fluids. In an attempt to help her understand her father's condition and provide optimal end-of-life care, which of the following is the *most appropriate* response?

a. She is right; dying of thirst is painful, and you will call the doctor for intravenous hydration.
b. Assure her that he is not suffering or experiencing any discomfort from dehydration.
c. Suggest they insert a small nasogastric tube to administer fluids to prevent dehydration.
d. Suggest that she try to encourage her father to drink fluids in small amounts.

10.25 A patient has aspiration pneumonia from a tracheoesophageal fistula. He is terminal and in hospice care. The physician has ordered scopolamine (1.5 mg transdermal patch) and to increase to two patches after 24 hours. You explain to the patient and family that the purpose of the scopolamine patch is which of the following?

a. To decrease the amount of secretions
b. To manage his pain
c. To decrease anxiety
d. To help manage dyspnea

10.26 Mr. Dillon is dying from lung cancer and has had no appetite for some time. His living will asks for no life-saving measures; however, his family states they are uncomfortable with their loved one starving to death and want him to be force fed. Which of the following is *not* an appropriate rationale for intervention?

a. Artificial nutrition can lead to congestive heart failure, nausea, vomiting, and diarrhea.
b. Anorexia is an adaptive protective mechanism that leads to a gentler death.
c. Dehydration commonly accompanies other signs of impending death as the organs begin to fail.
d. If the family wants the patient to have enteral or parenteral nutrition, this is a therapeutic option.

10.27 The presence of pain during the final days of life is often difficult to assess when the patient no longer is able to report intensity or presence of pain. Which of the following would *not* be considered a pain cue in this population?

a. Changes in appearance
b. Changes in appetite
c. Changes in overt behavior
d. Changes in sounds

10.28 Your patient is in hospice care. One of his primary complaints is that he cannot get enough air. Upon examination you learn he has a normal oxygen saturation, elevated blood pressure, and minimal pain, manageable by hydrocodone. Which of the following treatment scenarios would *best* address his chief complaint?

a. Continuous pulse oximetry, low-dose oxygen therapy to treat his air hunger, and a benzodiazepine to treat anxiety
b. Chest x-ray and arterial blood gases with pulmonary function tests to rule out pneumonia along with a benzodiazepine for anxiety
c. Low-dose opioid therapy, a benzodiazepine for anxiety, position the patient upright, and provide a cool fan
d. Low-dose oxygen therapy, bronchodilators, and benzodiazepine for anxiety

10.29 As the gag reflex and reflexive clearing of the oropharynx decline, secretions accumulate in the oropharynx, and dyspnea becomes complicated. Which of the following measures is *most effective* to manage the accumulation of secretions often associated with the "death rattle"?

a. Glucocorticoids to decrease swelling and secretions
b. Benzodiazepines to sedate the patient and increase comfort
c. Oral suctioning in the posterior pharynx to clear secretions
d. Anticholinergic medications to dry secretions

10.30 Your patient has failed yet another treatment regimen and could benefit significantly from hospice care, but his wife refuses to consent to hospice care. Your *primary* intervention to facilitate acceptance of hospice care is which of the following?

a. Provide information to the husband and wife regarding response to therapy and the benefits of hospice care.
b. Suggest a "drug holiday" to allow time to pass so she begins to see that hospice is the best choice.
c. Point out that she is denying what is inevitable and that accepting hospice care is the best thing for everyone.
d. Refer the patient and family to a visiting nurse service.

10.31 Which of the following *excludes* a patient from meeting criteria for hospice care?

a. The family prefers that the nurse not talk about dying around the patient.
b. The patient explains that he wants to continue to receive the new monoclonal antibody because he is certain it will be curative.
c. The doctor orders two units of blood to be given at home along with pamidronate.
d. The patient explains they are not ready to look at funeral homes.

10.32 Palliative sedation refers to

a. The intentional taking of one's own life
b. Sedation that relieves symptoms to a level of unresponsiveness
c. Letting a a patient who is suffering die by withdrawing life-sustaining care
d. Assisted suicide

10.33 The *most frequently* addressed factors contributing to palliative sedation or euthanasia are

a. Pain and other symptom distress
b. Advanced illness and poor prognosis
c. Family history of suicide or personal suicide history
d. Hopelessness and loss of self-esteem or control

10.34 The basic medical and nursing approach toward patients in a hospice program is

a. Acute care
b. Curative care
c. Palliative care
d. Euthanasia care

10.35 The husband of a woman with end-stage breast cancer is concerned that his wife is sleeping more and is not even waking to eat or drink. The hospice nurse would explain to the husband that

a. These are signs of approaching death.
b. The pain medication has reached a high blood level and needs to be reduced.
c. There is no reason to be concerned.
d. Her oncologist should be called to obtain some direction for her care.

10.36 The hospice nurse may decide in the initial interview that patient criteria for hospice care will *not* be met because

a. The patient's spouse expresses his wish to be involved in his wife's care.
b. The patient has entered a clinical trial through the National Cancer Institute.
c. The patient has expressed that she wishes to die without the use of narcotics.
d. The patient does not wish to be resuscitated if she stops breathing at home.

10.37 In the weeks before death many patients on opioid therapy experience agitation, confusion, and difficulty sleeping, especially at night. Which of the following medications is *most therapeutic* for patients experiencing these symptoms?

a. Amitriptyline, for its anticholinergic effect
b. Lorazepam, for its sedating effect
c. Promethazine, because it potentiates the analgesic effect of opioids
d. Haloperidol, to combat confusion and agitation

10.38 Katrina has end-stage cancer with a bowel obstruction and is currently in hospice care. Which of the following would be an *appropriate* intervention to minimize her discomfort?

a. Placement of a nasogastric tube to manage nausea and vomiting
b. Enemas every other day to promote evacuation
c. Avoiding the use of opioids, because they will only make it worse
d. Octreotide acetate to minimize secretions

10.39 The elderly are at risk for under treatment of pain, especially at the end of life. To prevent under treatment of pain, all of the following strategies should be used *except*

a. Subcutaneous injections as the preferred route of administration
b. Sustained release medications when possible
c. Introduce one new agent at a time
d. Titrate slowly with sufficient intervals for assessment

10.40 Radiation is indicated for patients receiving hospice care to

a. Decrease brain metastases and prevent seizures
b. Prevent bowel obstruction
c. Decrease pain from bone metastases
d. Stop bleeding from a fungating breast mass

10.41 Your patient with metastatic ovarian cancer is very uncomfortable due to increasing ascites. All of the following may be recommended *except*

a. A bowel regimen to relieve constipation
b. To conserve energy by alternating periods of activity and rest
c. To lie on her right side to increase vascular flow
d. Small, frequent meals or snacks

10.42 During the hospice admission interview for a patient with recurrent colon cancer and metastases to the liver, a family member asks if surgery to remove the liver lesions would extend the patient's life. Your *best response* is

a. The doctor would not recommend hospice care if there was any chance for cure
b. To remove liver metastases, the surgeon must be able to completely remove all of the tumor yet have adequate liver tissue remaining
c. Liver resection is not indicated unless the colon cancer has been cured
d. There must be no other evidence of disease

ANSWER RATIONALES

Please note: *All page numbers referenced in the Answer Rationales sections refer to the textbook* *Cancer Nursing: Principles and Practice, Seventh Edition,* by Connie Henke Yarbro, Debra Wujcik, and Barbara Holmes Gobel (Jones & Bartlett Learning, © 2011).

10.1 The answer is b.
Abnormal grief may manifest itself as a post-traumatic stress disorder through dissociative flashback episodes and reactivity to cues that symbolize or resemble an aspect of the traumatic event, which is the loss of her husband. The nurse should be able to identify and recommend competent referrals for abnormal grief syndromes. It is therapeutic to review a person's life with a loved one. Listening to a family member share stories of their life with the loved one honors the meaning of their relationship and their life together. Funeral planning can be therapeutic and facilitate someone's loss as they do one last thing in a special way for their loved one. Delegating responsibilities that can be overwhelming or too painful might actually be an indicator of the grieving party being aware of their limitations and calling on their resources and support systems. Page 677.

10.2 The answer is b.
It is helpful to explore previous losses and coping mechanisms used. Page 1792.

10.3 The answer is b.
Persistent avoidance of activities and friends after the death of her husband and symptom duration more than 1 month is indication of a post-traumatic stress disorder. She should be referred to an appropriate professional. Page 677.

10.4 The answer is d.
The Quality of Dying and Death questionnaire was developed for family members to provide information. The other instruments have been developed expressly to capture the elements that are important to patients at the end of life. Page 214.

10.5 The answer is b.
Most children and adolescents whose parent is ill are well adjusted, but a significant number are at risk for moderate to high levels of emotional distress and behavioral problems. Researchers have found that children's responses vary by developmental age. Compared to younger children, adolescents report more problems with anxiety and depression. Page 1784.

10.6 The answer is a.
The family member should not deny their feelings but communicate openly with the patient. Interventions include promoting optimism and hope, providing support, and facilitating communication between the patient and family. Page 1792–1793.

10.7 The answer is c.
Preparing oneself for death was least important as compared to being positive, finding meaning and purpose, loving others, and relating to God. Page 1800–1801.

10.8 The answer is d.
Resources exist. However, professionals lack cultural awareness and sensitivity of palliative care, lack adequate knowledge, have difficulty with issues related to death and dying, and delay referral for hospice services. Page 1822.

10.9 The answer is d.

Routine home care provided by hospice staff, continuous home care with skilled nursing, respite care to give caregivers a break, and inpatient care with limitations on days are the four levels of hospice care. Funding is not provided by Medicare for residential care, day care, and extended caregiver services. Page 1819.

10.10 The answer is b.

The individual hospice program may place the requirement of having a primary caregiver present in the home but it is not a Medicare Hospice regulation. Page 1819.

10.11 The answer is c.

There is a financial benefit, not a loss, with the use of a palliative consultation team as they have demonstrated an ability to help decrease length of stay and cost savings through coordination of care. Page 1818.

10.12 The answer is c.

Increasingly, nurses are being called on to justify the resources that are needed to improve patient care. Standards of care define expectations of the professional role that nurses must practice. Feasibility studies and cost-analysis studies, including cost-avoidance initiatives and cost-effectiveness analysis, are some techniques at the nurse's disposal. Feasibility studies determine whether a new program should be developed and implemented in a healthcare agency. Cost-avoidance initiatives identify direct or indirect activities that avoid or reduce expenses while maintaining or improving clinical outcomes. Cost-effectiveness analysis is all the costs, measured in dollars, necessary to achieve a certain benefit, calculated and expressed as cost per unit of effectiveness. This technique is used to compare relative costs of several alternatives. Page 1855.

10.13 The answer is b.

The evaluation and selection of alternative care arrangements requires individual attention to the needs and goals of the patient. Two important considerations in this selection process are cost and the patient's financial resources, including insurance coverage and benefits, and the quantity and quality of care provided by alternative care settings or agencies. Page 1820–1821.

10.14 The answer is d.

The cost of palliative care services is affected by the location where that care is delivered. The SUPPORT study depicted the inadequacies of the end-of-life care being provided in the intensive care unit. Intensive care unit stays of 10 days or more were noted for 38% of patients who died. Page 1820.

10.15 The answer is c.

Hospice and oncology nurses' personal spirituality and religiousness influence their attitudes and how their care is delivered. Page 1804.

10.16 The answer is c.

The durable power of attorney is preferable. A living will gives advance directives for the final period of terminal illness, and the durable power of attorney covers any treatment situations at any stage in life. This document names an individual who will speak for the patient if the patient becomes incompetent to make decisions about health care. Page 1822.

10.17 The answer is c.

This legislation required that all healthcare institutions receiving Medicare or Medicaid reimbursement ask patients they admit to the hospital whether they have an advance directive.

If patients do not, the institution is obligated to provide written information about such directives. Page 1822.

10.18 The answer is c.
Economics is often described as a barrier to palliative care. As experts in the field address earlier palliative intervention, reimbursement for these efforts can be captured under traditional and existing reimbursement coding. However, patients making transition between treatment for curative intent to palliative intent face economic issues. Page 1816, 1821.

10.19 The answer is c.
Hospice care is a medically directed, interdisciplinary, team-managed program of services that focuses on the patient and family as the unit of service. It has been the general experience of those who provide optimal palliative care that their patients do not need or desire euthanasia. Hospice in the United States began as an antimedical establishment and antiphysician movement. This antagonistic bias has unfortunately been a major factor in preventing hospice and palliative care principles from being applied to dying patients on a broader scale. Page 1816.

10.20 The answer is b.
Spirituality greatly affects a patient's journey through a life-threatening illness and provides a sense of meaning despite the illness. Although the other selections may also be true, they are part of how one finds a sense of meaning through spirituality. Page 1798–1803.

10.21 The answer is a.
An AD is a one-person statement, not a legally binding contract. Page 1822.

10.22 The answer is c.
Although continuous pulse oximetry is used widely, patients and family members often focus on the monitor, which can increase anxiety and fear. Opioids are the first-line therapy in relieving dyspnea, without causing respiratory depression. Bronchodilators can relieve bronchospasm but can also increase anxiety. Page 1833–1834.

10.23 The answer is a.
Reality orientation is not considered beneficial in actively hallucinating patients. In fact, correcting the patient's perceptions may only increase anxiety and agitation. Be open to comments by dying patients about "going home" or seeing loved ones who have previously died. These are common behaviors seen during the dying process. Page 1835.

10.24 The answer is b.
Research demonstrates that patients do not suffer or experience discomfort due to dehydration. Tube feedings may actually contribute to decreased survival due to aspiration and abdominal distention. Family members may inadvertently try to force patients to eat or drink, leading to aspiration or simply to decrease discomfort for the patient. Page 1836.

10.25 The answer is a.
Scopolamine is used to manage excessive salivation and respiratory tract secretions. Page 1835–1836.

10.26 The answer is d.
Because the patient's living will requests no life-saving measures, the family's desire to force feed the patient is an inappropriate rationale. All the other selections are reasons why patients should not be force fed. Page 1818.

10.27 The answer is b.
Pain cues include changes in overt behaviors (aggressiveness, restlessness, and agitation), sounds (increases or decreases in verbalization or vocalization), or appearances (facial expressions or body language). Page 1830.

10.28 The answer is c.
Continuous pulse oximetry is contraindicated because it provides no useful information and serves only to exacerbate existing fear and anxiety as the family focuses on the monitor rather than on ways to provide comfort. Although antibiotics may help to treat pneumonia, extensive testing will yield information that is immaterial to the outcome. Oxygen therapy is not indicated in the absence of hypoxemia and is not effective in treating the symptom of dyspnea. What is helpful is air therapy—room air directed at the person's face. Opioids are the first-line therapy in relieving dyspnea. Opioids decrease the intensity of dyspnea regardless of the underlying pathophysiology without causing respiratory depression. Low doses of an opioid administered on an as-needed basis are generally very effective in patients with mild to moderate dyspnea who have not previously been taking opioids. Page 1834–1835.

10.29 The answer is d.
Although suctioning visible pooled secretions in the posterior oral cavity may be effective, suctioning is usually ineffective. It may be contraindicated because of the associated discomfort and because the site of the accumulated secretions is generally inaccessible. Anticholinergic medications, including scopolamine or glycopyrrolate, are effective for decreasing oral secretions once the patient is unable to mobilize them himself. Glucocorticoids are ineffective in managing fluid in the oral pharynx, and benzodiazepines only sedate the patient. Page 1835.

10.30 The answer is a.
Families often believe the information they receive from healthcare professionals regarding coping is insufficient. The family begins to prepare for the unavoidable pain of loss and the necessary adjustments that must be made (hospice care) if sufficient information is presented to them. Families desire honest communication, despite the use of denial, as well as appropriate referrals. Denial is viewed as a healthy coping mechanism that with appropriate information will help the wife gradually accept the next level of care. Page 1789–1791, 1817, 1822.

10.31 The answer is b.
The patient must desire palliative, not curative, treatment. Patients can receive treatments that are aimed at palliation, not cure. Blood is generally not given but can be, for palliative reasons, as can pamidronate. Page 1819.

10.32 The answer is b.
Suicide is the intentional taking of one's own life. Palliative sedation relieves symptoms to the patient's level of unresponsiveness in the final hours and days of life. Active euthanasia refers to direct intervention causing death, whereas passive euthanasia refers to letting a sufferer die by withholding or withdrawing life-sustaining care. Page 1837.

10.33 The answer is a.
The most frequently addressed factors contributing to palliative sedation or euthanasia are pain and other symptom distress. Page 1824, 1837.

10.34 The answer is c.
Hospice care pivots around the idea of palliative medical management. Palliative management involves a shift in treatment goals from curative toward providing relief from suffering.

Euthanasia means active interventions to hasten a person's death, and this is not the philosophy of hospice care. Page 1817–1819.

10.35 The answer is a.
The hospice team's goal is to help the family prepare for their loved one's death. Families need to be prepared for the actual time of the patient's death and what universal signs they can anticipate. Increasing sleep, a gradual decrease in need for food and drink, increased confusion or restlessness, decreasing temperature of extremities, and irregular breathing patterns may occur. Calling the oncologist would be indicating the need for intervention, when in fact the goal of care is purely palliative. The pain relief regimen should not be altered if the patient is comfortable, even if the patient is sleeping more and death is approaching. Page 1836.

10.36 The answer is b.
Clinical trials are experimental medical trials that are implemented to determine whether there is any disease response to a new antineoplastic regimen. Patients and their families often turn to an experimental procedure when there are limited, if any, options remaining that might halt their disease progress. This choice suggests that the patient has not agreed to palliative care and is still pursuing curative treatment. Further assessment is indicated to make sure this is not the case, because a patient criterion for hospice care is that the patient is agreeable to palliative and not curative care. The remaining three options are actually patient criteria for hospice care: the patient has a primary caregiver, the patient resides in the hospice program's geographic area, and some programs require that the patient have a do-not-resuscitate status before admission to the hospice program. Page 1821.

10.37 The answer is d.
Haloperidol can be used to treat opioid-induced acute confusional states (e.g., hallucinations, agitation from delirium). Page 1835.

10.38 The answer is d.
Octreotide or somatostatin is used to minimize intestinal secretions. A gastrostomy tube or a percutaneous endoscopic gastrostomy (PEG) would be chosen over a nasogastric tube, which is uncomfortable. Enemas are contraindicated and lead to cramping pain. Opioids are important, because over 90% of patients have continuous abdominal pain. Page 1235.

10.39 The answer is a.
Although the elderly metabolize medications differently than younger patients, they respond to opioids for the treatment of pain. The least invasive route of administration is recommended and sustained release medications are frequently used. Subcutaneous injections are not the preferred route of administration. Page 692.

10.40 The answer is c.
The most common indication for radiation at the end of life is to control pain from bone metastases. Page 1069.

10.41 The answer is c.
The patient should lie on her left side to increase vascular flow, facilitate lymphatic flow, and improve diuresis. Page 1567.

10.42 The answer is b.
National Comprehensive Cancer Network guidelines to remove liver metastases in patients with colon cancer indicate the surgeon must be able to completely remove all tumor yet have adequate liver tissue remaining. Page 1226.

CHAPTER 11

Professional Performance

LOCAL, STATE, AND NATIONAL RESOURCES

11.1 Which national organization issues national patient safety goals and recommendations that are updated annually and are delineated by practice setting?

a. Institute of Medicine
b. The Joint Commission
c. Occupational and Safety Health Administration
d. National Institutes of Health

11.2 Guidelines for handling antineoplastic agents have been established by all *except*

a. The US Food and Drug Administration
b. The Occupational Safety and Health Administration
c. The Oncology Nursing Society
d. The American Society of Hospital Pharmacists

11.3 Examples of useful cancer-related websites recommended for patients and families include all *except*

a. http://www.cancer.org
b. http://www.livestrong.org
c. http://www.canceranswers.org
d. http://www.cancercare.org

11.4 Which of the following does the federal government insist on before a drug can be marketed?

a. The safety of the drug only
b. The efficacy of the drug only
c. The safety and the efficacy of the drug only
d. The safety, efficacy, and long-term value of the drug

SCOPE AND STANDARDS OF ONCOLOGY NURSING PRACTICE

11.5 Which of the following *best describes* the difference between the eligibility criteria for the advanced oncology nursing certification examination for the Advanced Oncology Certified Clinical Nurse Specialist (AOCNS®) and the Advanced Oncology Certified Nurse Practitioner (AOCNP®)?

a. To qualify to be certified as an AOCNP®, the nurse must be at least master's prepared and complete an accredited nurse practitioner program, whereas the AOCNS® only requires a master's degree in nursing.
b. An AOCNS® is qualified to be certified as an AOCNP® provided he or she completes a minimum of 500 hours of supervised practice as an advanced practice nurse.
c. If a nurse is in an advanced practice role, he or she is eligible to become certified as an AOCNS® if he or she can pass the test.
d. To be eligible for the AOCNP®, the nurse must spend greater than 50% of his or her time delivering direct patient care.

11.6 Professional nurses occasionally question why it is important to be recertified on a regular basis by the Oncology Nursing Certification Corporation. Which of the following would be the *best response* to this issue?

a. Certification guarantees that the nurse is qualified to provide competent care.
b. Certification is a requirement for receiving Magnet Hospital status through the American Nurses Credentialing Center.
c. All employers recognize certification through pay differentials.
d. Certification validates that you know the most current oncology nursing practices.

11.7 Which of the following *best describes* the difference between the nurse generalist and the nurse specialist?

a. A baccalaureate degree
b. A broader scope of practice
c. Clinical experience
d. Conceptual knowledge and skills

11.8 The mission of the Oncology Nursing Certification Corporation is to advance oncology nursing through the certification process. To be eligible for the certification examination, a nurse must have accomplished all *except* which of the following?

a. Be a current registered nurse license
b. Have a minimum of 50 continuing education units in the area of oncology nursing practice
c. Have 1 year of experience as a registered nurse over the 3-year period before application
d. Have at least 1000 hours of oncology nursing practice within 2.5 years of application for a current license

APPROPRIATE SOURCES OF DATA FOR EVIDENCE-BASED PRACTICE

11.9 The Oncology Nursing Society (ONS) Putting Evidence into Practice Weight of Evidence Rules use

a. 6 levels of effectiveness for grading nursing and medical interventions
b. 4 categories from low- to high-level evidence
c. 6 levels of higher or lower strength
d. 4 grades of recommendations from very low to high

11.10 When reviewing a research survey it is important to ensure whether the survey has been validated for reliability. Which of the following is a type of research reliability measure?

a. Question and answer format
b. Test–retest format
c. External consistency reliability
d. Connect–disconnect analysis

11.11 One of the statistical methods used to determine reliability is Cronbach's coefficient alpha. Which of the following *best describes* what this statistical measure refers to?

a. It is a measure of the strength of the internal consistency of a set of survey questions.
b. It is a measure of the likeness of individuals being surveyed.
c. It is a predictive measure of the sameness of the findings as they relate to similar research findings.
d. It is a measure of whether two observers agree.

11.12 Pilot studies are useful for all *except*

a. Assessing the feasibility of a research design
b. Pretesting an instrument
c. Evaluating the risk, side effects, and compliance with a new nursing management approach
d. Determining effectiveness of an intervention

EDUCATION PROCESS

11.13 Culturally sensitive education must consider all of the following *except*

a. Addressing the person formally, such as using "Mr." or "Mrs."
b. Simple educational messages
c. Determining the preferred language and learning process
d. Determining the decision-making patterns

11.14 When providing education for patients who do not speak English, you should use all of the following *except*

a. Over the telephone interpretation service
b. Professional interpreters of the same tribe, state, region, or nation
c. Nonfamily members of the same age and gender
d. Family members

11.15 The *most important* information to include when providing education for patients receiving radiation is

a. Treatment plan and expected outcomes
b. Sensory and procedural information
c. Myths and misinformation that family members may provide
d. Side effect management

11.16 In planning a smoking cessation program, the nurse knows that the *most successful* strategy for tobacco cessation is

a. Increased taxes on tobacco products
b. The smoker's desire and readiness to quit
c. Pharmaceutical interventions
d. Nonpharmaceutical interventions

LEGAL AND ETHICAL ISSUES

11.17 In instances where the advanced practice nurse (APN) is employed by a physician, the physician is able to bill 100% of the Medicare fee schedule for the services provided by the APN as long as all of the following requirements are met *except*

a. The physician must be present in the office at the time of the patient's visit.
b. The patient is being seen for a preexisting problem.
c. The physician must countersign the patient's chart.
d. There is a medical plan of care.

11.18 The authority for the advanced practice nurse (APN) to prescribe drugs is regulated at the state level but also involves the Drug Enforcement Administration. Whether the nurse has dependent prescriptive authority or independent prescriptive authority is based *primarily* on which of the following?

a. Dependent prescriptive authority requires the APN be under the supervision of a physician when performing this task.
b. Dependent prescriptive authority permits the APN to prescribe only nonnarcotic medications independent of the physician.
c. Independent prescriptive authority is given only when the APN is certified at the doctoral level.
d. Independent prescriptive authority requires the APN to be prepared at the doctoral level, attend pharmacology courses, and to be under the direct supervision of the responsible physician.

11.19 While administering chemotherapy to your patient, she mentions she is worried she might be forced to quit her job because her boss forces her to take vacation days when she comes for therapy. She works for a small business owner but states she can always get one of the other 10 employees to cover for her. Your counsel is based on which of the following facts regarding the Americans with Disabilities Act (ADA)?

a. Provided she has coverage the employer must make reasonable efforts to accommodate her needs during therapy.
b. The patient is not required to get coverage when she is absent due to treatment.
c. She is not protected by the ADA because she works for a small business owner.
d. She should see a lawyer to learn more about her rights because she has a right to sue to keep her job.

11.20 If Ann is guilty of misappropriation in the course of conducting her research, she has *most likely*

a. Misused the research funds entrusted to her through a grant
b. Committed plagiarism
c. Tagged her study onto an existing protocol rather than initiating a new project
d. Deliberately omitted facts or fabricated data and findings

11.21 Following World War II the Nuremberg Code was established to delineate legal responsibility for patient education in the area of informed consent. Content central to this code includes all *except* which of the following?

a. The use of voluntary consent to protect human subjects in experimentation
b. The use of coercion as deemed necessary to provide quality care
c. The individual is capable of providing consent
d. An understanding of the risks and benefits

11.22 A patient with metastatic cancer is admitted to a unit with uncontrolled pain. The physician has ordered morphine as the primary pain medication. The patient frequently requests more pain medication. You suspect he is a drug abuser and has an addiction problem. The *most appropriate* nursing action would be to do which of the following?

a. Substitute other medications in the place of narcotics.
b. Refer him to a drug addiction program.
c. Call the physician to increase his pain medication.
d. Administer less potent analgesics along with the morphine to stretch the effect of the narcotic.

11.23 As safety and efficacy of gene therapy is established a number of ethical issues arise including all *except*

a. Treatment costs that make therapy available to those with insurance
b. Treatments available only in large medical centers
c. Gene therapy on healthy individuals
d. Discrimination by health insurers

11.24 One of the four ethical principles guiding clinical practice is nonmaleficence. To what does this term refer?

a. Helping the patient to balance the benefits against the risks
b. Distributing the resources in a fair and reasonable way
c. Helping the patient make decisions that are right for him or her
d. Avoiding practices that will do harm to the individual

11.25 The two *most important* ethical considerations within the realm of genetic testing and genetic information are

a. Nonmaleficence and beneficence
b. Informed consent and confidentiality
c. Informed consent and full disclosure
d. Nonmaleficence and confidentiality

PATIENT ADVOCACY

11.26 The Patient Self-Determination Act (PSDA) was passed by the US Congress in 1990. This act requires that all healthcare institutions do which of the following?

a. Ensure health care to all regardless of ability to pay
b. Provide all patients with written information regarding informed consent
c. Provide written information regarding financial obligations
d. Provide written information about advanced directives

11.27 Which of the following statements concerning advanced directives (AD) is *false*?

a. An AD is a statement made by a competent person that directs their medical care in the event that they become incompetent.
b. ADs do not address all possible medical situations, only terminal conditions due to illness or injury.
c. An AD is a legally binding contract.
d. A directive may not always be honored due to the inability of medicine to determine the terminality of the patient's condition.

11.28 The *primary* goal of the Patient Self-Determination Act is to
a. Facilitate a systematic process of eliciting and honoring patient wishes
b. Control healthcare costs in the last 6 months of life
c. Require healthcare institutions to notify patients on admission of their rights under the law to execute an advance directive
d. Facilitate a responsible use of technological intervention

11.29 A patient makes some comments about a living will that leads you to conclude the patient needs more information. You know he understands what a living will is when he says it
a. Specifies disbursement of assets
b. Addresses all possible medical situations
c. May not always be honored and implemented
d. Describes the specific types of care to be used

QUALITY ASSURANCE

11.30 Failure mode and effect analysis (FMEA) is a risk analysis technique that is used to examine which of the following?
a. Root-cause analysis
b. Pharmacy errors in drug dispensing
c. Risk analysis technique to examine the chemotherapy administration process
d. Errors in drug administration as it relates to method of administration

11.31 The *major* difference between root-cause analysis and failure mode and effect analysis (FMEA) as it relates to chemotherapy administration is which of the following?
a. They are the same process where root-cause analysis follows FMEA.
b. FMEA is designed to prevent chemotherapy errors.
c. Root-cause analysis is a prospective risk analysis.
d. Both FMEA and root-cause analysis provide a "fail-safe" process in drug administration.

11.32 Which of the following chemotherapeutic agents is lethal if injected intrathecally, and to assure patient safety it has special United States Pharmacopeia (USP) labeling and packaging that must be removed before administration?
a. Cytarabine
b. Methotrexate
c. Vincristine
d. Interferon

11.33 The Joint Commission's National Patient Safety Goals and Recommendations includes all *except* which of the following?
a. Improve safety when using oxygen.
b. Improve the effectiveness of alarm systems in patient care areas.
c. Improve safety when using infusion pumps.
d. Improve safety when stocking, ordering, and dispensing medications.

PROFESSIONAL DEVELOPMENT AND MULTIDISCIPLINARY COLLABORATION

11.34 The Balanced Budget Act of 1997 was amended in 1999 to provide Medicare Part B reimbursement to advanced practice nurses (APNs). These nurses are reimbursed at what percentage according to what physicians receive for services in the Physician Fee Schedule?

a. 90%
b. 85%
c. 75%
d. 50%

11.35 The nurse practitioner (NP) is a registered nurse who has advanced education and clinical training in a specialty area. The *primary* difference between an adult, family, pediatric, or acute care NP is which of the following?

a. Educational requirements are essentially the same.
b. A family NP is more general and not considered "advanced" compared to the other practitioner roles.
c. A family NP requires a clinical doctorate in nursing.
d. A master's degree is common but not a baseline requirement for an adult NP.

11.36 The three interacting domains of competencies of the Oncology Clinical Nurse Specialist (OCNS) practice are which of the following?

a. Patient/client, nurses and nursing practice, and organizations/systems
b. Patient/family, professional nursing practice, and institutional practice
c. Patient/client, evidence-based practice, organizational quality initiatives
d. Patient/family, nurses and nursing practice, institutional practice

11.37 According to the Oncology Nursing Society (ONS) the *primary* difference between an oncology clinical nurse specialist (CNS) and a nurse practitioner (NP) is which of the following?

a. There is no significant difference between these terms.
b. NP is a nurse who has completed an NP program at the master's or doctorate level.
c. CNSs deliver direct care to patients, whereas NPs are more like doctor's assistants.
d. All CNSs are NPs, whereas not all NPs are considered CNSs.

11.38 Specialty certification among healthcare providers has concentrated on all *except* which of the following avenues of inquiry?

a. Identification of characteristics that differentiate certified and noncertified providers
b. Describing variations in practice that are associated with certification
c. Describing the role of labor unions and demands for certification among healthcare providers
d. Linking provider certification to patient outcomes

11.39 Terrence is an oncology advanced practice nurse (OAPN) who chooses to work as a consultant rather than as a direct care provider. The OAPN in secondary care may be involved in any of the following *except*

a. Discussing the treatment plan and expected outcomes with the patients and family
b. Planning and implementing initiatives aimed at patient and family education and support
c. Pain and symptom management
d. Establishing standards for oncology practice and developing critical pathways

11.40 Which of the following is *not* required for use of the designation "oncology certified nurse"?

a. A minimum of 1 year experience as a registered nurse within the last 3 years
b. A baccalaureate degree with credits toward a master's degree
c. A minimum of 1000 hours of cancer nursing practice within the last 2.5 years
d. A passing score on the Oncology Nursing Certification Corporation certification examination

11.41 Karen is a nurse practitioner (NP) working in a collaborative practice. In general, in a collaborative practice all of the following are considered basic to success *except*

a. NPs function independently in caring for a caseload of patients in the ambulatory setting.
b. NPs function independently in caring for a caseload of patients in the acute care setting.
c. The skills of the provider are matched with the needs of the patient.
d. The physician ultimately makes the final decision regarding patient management.

11.42 The *most important* reason for multidisciplinary collaboration in determining cancer risk is

a. Individual healthcare providers always include family history in the patient assessment.
b. Individual and family risk are the same and should be shared among the care providers.
c. Although preliminary risk assessment can be done by all healthcare providers, full assessment and testing should be provided by trained genetic counselors.
d. Only physicians can refer patients and families for genetic risk assessment.

11.43 Professional barriers to successful palliative care have been identified as inadequate knowledge, lack of cultural awareness and sensitivity, difficulty with issues related to death and dying, and delays in referral for hospice services. To *best* overcome these barriers, palliative care should be

a. Provided only in dedicated inpatient palliative care units
b. Provided only in combined hospital/palliative care units with or without a community-based hospice program
c. Provided by trained providers both in inpatient and outpatient settings
d. Provided by trained providers in the setting that is most appropriate for the patient and family

11.44 Patients with head and neck cancer receive multimodality therapy. Coordination of therapy may be complicated by which of the following

a. Timing of consultations with radiation, surgery, and medical oncologists; dentists; and nutritionists
b. Timing of consultations with radiation, surgery, and medical oncologists; nutritionists; and financial counselors
c. Presence of side effects from various therapies
d. Inability to swallow oral targeted therapies and/or liquids and solids

ANSWER RATIONALES

Please note: All page numbers referenced in the Answer Rationales sections refer to the textbook *Cancer Nursing: Principles and Practice, Seventh Edition*, by Connie Henke Yarbro, Debra Wujcik, and Barbara Holmes Gobel (Jones & Bartlett Learning, © 2011).

Local, State, and National Resources

11.1 The answer is b.
The Joint Commission has National Patient Safety Goals and recommendations delineated for practice settings, for example, hospitals, ambulatory care, and home care. Page 1869–1870.

11.2 The answer is a.
Potential hazards associated with the administration of antineoplastic agents have prompted the Occupational Safety and Health Administration, Oncology Nursing Society, and American Society of Hospital Pharmacists to set guidelines for compounding, transporting, administering, and disposing of toxic chemotherapy agents. Page 394–395.

11.3 The answer is c.
The American Cancer Society (http://www.cancer.org), Lance Armstrong Foundation (http://www.livestrong.org), and Cancer Care (http://www.cancercare.org) are all reputable organizations that provide useful information for patients with cancer and their families. Page 1791.

11.4 The answer is c.
The Food and Drug Act of 1906 called for the truthful labeling of ingredients used in drugs but did not ban false therapeutic claims on drug labels. The Sherley Amendment in 1912 made it a crime to make false or fraudulent claims regarding the therapeutic efficacy of a drug, but proof of intent to defraud the customer was needed. Finally, in 1962 Congress added that drugs must demonstrate efficacy in addition to safety before they can be marketed, and a process was created by which a substance can become approved for prescription use. Page 648.

Scope and Standards of Oncology Nursing Practice

11.5 The answer is a.
To qualify to be certified as an AOCNS® the nurse must be a licensed registered nurse with a minimum of a master's degree in nursing with a minimum of 500 hours of supervised practice in an advanced practice role in oncology nursing. To be eligible for the AOCNP® the nurse must be a licensed registered nurse with at least a master's degree in nursing, but, most important, they must have successfully completed an accredited nurse practitioner program and have a minimum of 500 hours of supervised clinical practice as an oncology nurse practitioner. Page 1853.

11.6 The answer is d.
An increasing number of employers want certified nurses as employees. Although certification does not validate who we are as nurses or as people, certification does validate that nurses have met stringent requirements for knowledge and experience and are qualified to provide competent care. Nurses who are not certified may provide competent care, but earning oncology certification provides strong evidence beyond a person's claim. Page 1852.

11.7 **The answer is d.**
Cancer nursing is practiced by both nursing generalists and nursing specialists. Nursing generalists have conceptual knowledge and skills acquired through basic nursing education, clinical experience, and professional development and updated through continuing education. They meet the concerns of individuals with cancer and provide care in a variety of healthcare settings. Nursing specialists have substantial theoretical knowledge gained through preparation from a master's degree. They meet diversified concerns of cancer patients and their families and function in a broader scope of practice. Page 1846–1848.

11.8 **The answer is b.**
Nurses are not required to have continuing education units to take the exam. Page 1852.

Appropriate Sources of Data for Evidence-Based Practice

11.9 **The answer is a.**
The ONS Putting Evidence into Practice Weight of Evidence Rules use a 6-level grading system that considers effectiveness and risk-benefit ratio. Page 664.

11.10 **The answer is b.**
Surveys must be validated for reliability to ensure that the participants understand the questions in the way the researchers intended to the questions to be understood. Types of reliability measures include alternate form, internal consistency, interobserver, intraobserver, and test–retest formats. Page 40.

11.11 **The answer is a.**
Cronbach's coefficient alpha is a statistic that measures the strength of the internal consistency or homogeneity of a set of survey questions. It is an assessment that measures the extent to which items included on a questionnaire focus on a particular domain (e.g., patient satisfaction, well-being). Page 240–241.

11.12 **The answer is d.**
Pilot studies are useful to assess the feasibility of a research design; to pretest an instrument; and to evaluate the risk, side effects, and compliance with a new nursing management approach. Pilot studies do not have the power and effect size to prove the effectiveness of an intervention. Page 40–41.

Education Process

11.13 **The answer is a.**
Culturally sensitive education practices include identifying the preferred communication style such as the best way to address him or her and acceptable nonverbal communication. Page 88.

11.14 **The answer is d.**
You should avoid using family members for patient teaching and consenting purposes. Family members may not communicate the information without bias from trying to protect the patient, their own misinterpretation of the information, or a lack of comfort in discussing personal information about the patient. Whenever possible, the optimal strategy is to use professional interpreters. Page 89.

11.15 The answer is b.
While all patient education starts with what the patient already knows and includes the treatment plan, expected outcomes, and side effect management, the most important information to include for patients undergoing radiation therapy is sensory and procedural information. Page 317–318.

11.16 The answer is a.
Although some pharmaceutical and behavioral interventions have proven to be successful, the most successful approaches result from increasing excise taxes on tobacco products. Page 99.

Legal and Ethical Issues

11.17 The answer is c.
Physicians may bill for 100% of the Medicare fee schedule for the services provided by the APN as long as the following requirements for incident to services are met

1. The collaborating physician must be present in the same office suite.
2. The patient must have been seen by the physician at least once, and a plan of care must be documented by the physician.
3. The patient must not have a new problem.
4. Services must be of the type commonly provided in a physician's office.
5. The physician need not countersign the patient's chart, but the office schedule must document the physician's presence in the office at the time of the patient's visit. Page 1855.

11.18 The answer is a.
The level of prescriptive authority varies from independent prescriptive authority including controlled substances to dependent prescriptive authority excluding controlled substances. The dependent authority requires that the APN be under supervision of a physician when performing this task. The task may be prescribing controlled or noncontrolled substances. Some states may require documentation of a certain amount of pharmacology coursework, but a doctorate is not required. Page 1853.

11.19 The answer is c.
The ADA requires employers to make reasonable accommodation for employees with a disability. Cancer is considered a disability under the ADA. Scheduling changes would be considered reasonable, for example, but turning a full-time job into a part-time job is not required. The ADA applies to employers with 15 or more employees, so patients with disabilities who are employed by small businesses are not protected. Page 1750.

11.20 The answer is b.
Misappropriation refers to an intentional or reckless act of plagiarism or a violation of the confidentiality associated with the review of scientific manuscripts or grants. Page 226.

11.21 The answer is b.
Central to this code is the use of voluntary consent to protect human subjects in experimentation. Such consent assumes not only the ability to consent and freedom from coercion, but also that there is an understanding of the risks and benefits and that the subject is giving an informed consent. Page 225.

11.22 The answer is c.
Failure of the nurse and her employer to fulfill their obligations and responsibilities could result in increased pain and suffering, leading to emotional and mental anguish. Ethically,

regardless of whether the patient is "addicted," the nurse has a responsibility to first do no harm and call the doctor for more pain medication. Page 700.

11.23 The answer is d.
The Genetic Information Discrimination Act prohibits health insurers from discriminating against an individual based on his or her genetic information to determine health insurance eligibility or premiums. Page 595.

11.24 The answer is d.
The four ethical principles guiding clinical practice are autonomy, nonmaleficence, beneficence, and justice.

- Autonomy is the process of helping patients make the decisions that are right for them.
- Nonmaleficence means to do no harm.
- Beneficence is shown by helping the patient balance the benefits against the risk of harm.
- Justice is the distribution of resources in a fair and reasonable way. Page 225.

11.25 The answer is b.
While nonmaleficence (first do no harm) and beneficence (opportunity for benefit) are important ethical principles in genetic counseling, providing informed consent and maintaining confidentiality are considered to be the most important principles to ensure. Page 141–143.

Patient Advocacy

11.26 The answer is d.
The PSDA requires that all healthcare institutions receiving Medicare or Medicaid reimbursement ask the patients they admit if they have an advance directive. If patients do not, the institution is obligated to provide written information about such directives. Page 1822.

11.27 The answer is c.
An AD is a one-person statement, not a legally binding contract. Page 1822.

11.28 The answer is c.
The Patient Self-Determination Act may also serve to control healthcare costs in the last 6 months of life and to facilitate a responsible use of technological intervention. However, these are not the primary goals of the act. The act does not necessarily facilitate a systematic process of eliciting and honoring patient wishes. Page 1822.

11.29 The answer is d.
Patients can become confused about what a living will is. It does not specify disbursement of assets. It does not address all possible medical situations. The words *artificial* and *extraordinary* are often used in an advanced directive (AD); however, these words can be interpreted differently. A directive may not always be honored and implemented. An AD is a one-person statement, not a legally binding contract. Page 1822.

Quality Assurance

11.30 The answer is c.
Promoting a culture of safety involves a philosophical shift from error measurement to proactive assessment of potential harm. Failure mode and effect analysis is a prospective risk analysis technique that can be used to examine the chemotherapy administration process. It is a systematic, multidisciplinary, team-based approach to error prevention, which is why the other choices are not correct. Page 1874.

11.31 The answer is b.
FMEA is a prospective risk management approach that allows cancer centers to potentially prevent chemotherapy errors rather than react to them, as is done in root-cause analysis, which is a retrospective process conducted after chemotherapy errors have occurred. The fundamental purpose of FMEA is to recommend and take actions to reduce the likelihood of process errors (failures). Page 1874.

11.32 The answer is c.
Errors in the route of administration for vincristine prompted United States Pharmacopeia labeling requirements and standards for vincristine packaging, which include cautionary labeling that states "FATAL IF GIVEN INTRATHECALLY. FOR IV USE ONLY. DO NOT REMOVE COVERING UNTIL MOMENT OF INJECTION." Cytarabine, methotrexate, interferon, and thiotepa have all been given safely intrathecally. Page 416–417.

11.33 The answer is a.
Additional safety goals include improve patient identification procedures, improve communication, perform the correct surgical procedure on the correct patient and correct site, and reduce the risk of healthcare-acquired infection. Page 1870.

Professional Development and Multidisciplinary Collaboration

11.34 The answer is b.
The Balanced Budget Act of 1997 was amended in 1999 to provide Medicare Part B reimbursement to APNs at 85% of what physicians receive for services in the Physician Fee Schedule. State-specific practice acts determine the extent to which APNs can receive Medicaid reimbursement, if at all. It is important to realize that Medicare is the federal mandate for reimbursement fee structures for APNs regardless of state-specific practice acts. Page 1854.

11.35 The answer is c.
Except for family NPs, a master's degree is now considered the minimum education required for entry: family NP requires a clinical doctorate in nursing. Page 1848.

11.36 The answer is a.
The three interacting domains of competencies of OCNS practice are patient/client, nurses and nursing practice, and organizations/systems. Page 1848.

11.37 The answer is b.
The ONS recognizes nurses who have become experts in coordinating and providing direct and indirect care to people with cancer through study and precepted clinical practice in oncology at the graduate level as oncology CNSs. The term *NP* describes the nurse whose educational preparation includes completion of an NP program at the master's or doctorate level. The role of the NP is to provide comprehensive clinical care to individuals, with an emphasis on health promotion, disease prevention, diagnosis, and management of acute and chronic diseases. The ONS recognizes NPs who have expertise in the specialty of oncology as oncology NPs. Page 1846–1848.

11.38 The answer is c.
Few studies have evaluated specialty certification in the healthcare professions or described links between provider certification and patient outcomes. Three avenues of inquiry have been typical of the research on specialty certification among healthcare providers. These include identifying characteristics that differentiate certified and noncertified providers, describing variations in practice, and linking provider certification to patient outcomes. Labor unions do not have a role. Page 1852–1853.

11.39 The answer is a.
As a consultant, the OAPN in secondary care is involved in planning and implementing initiatives aimed at patient and family education and support. The OAPN's expertise is also used in symptom management, and OAPNs are often important members of multidisciplinary pain and symptom management teams. They also may act as consultants to an institution in establishing standards for oncology practice and developing critical pathways. Page 1846–1847.

11.40 The answer is b.
The Oncology Nursing Certification Corporation administers a certification program for cancer nurses. A certification examination is offered twice yearly. Nurses with a registered nurse license, 1 year experience as a registered nurse within the last 3 years, and a minimum of 1000 hours of cancer nursing practice within the last 2.5 years are eligible to take this examination. Page 1852–1853.

11.41 The answer is d.
In a collaborative practice NPs function independently in caring for a caseload of patients, whether in the ambulatory or the acute care setting. Care is provided based on competence: The skills of the provider are matched with the needs of the patient. Page 1849.

11.42 The answer is c.
All healthcare providers can do a preliminary cancer risk assessment. Patients and families can then be referred to trained genetic counselors for a full risk assessment and testing. Page 147–148.

11.43 The answer is d.
Palliative care should be provided by professionals who have knowledge related to palliative care, cultural issues, issues of death and dying, and appropriate timing of referrals. Providers working together can ensure successful palliative care in hospital, outpatient and home settings. Page 1822–1823.

11.44 The answer is a.
Patients with head and neck cancer are evaluated for all treatment modalities. Prior to beginning therapy, a dental assessment is done to address dental caries and oral infections. The nutritionist is consulted at diagnosis since many patients are malnourished at the time of diagnosis, and further compromise is expected due to the side effects of treatment. Page 1347–1350.